CW01064235

Fish's
SCHIZOPHRENIA

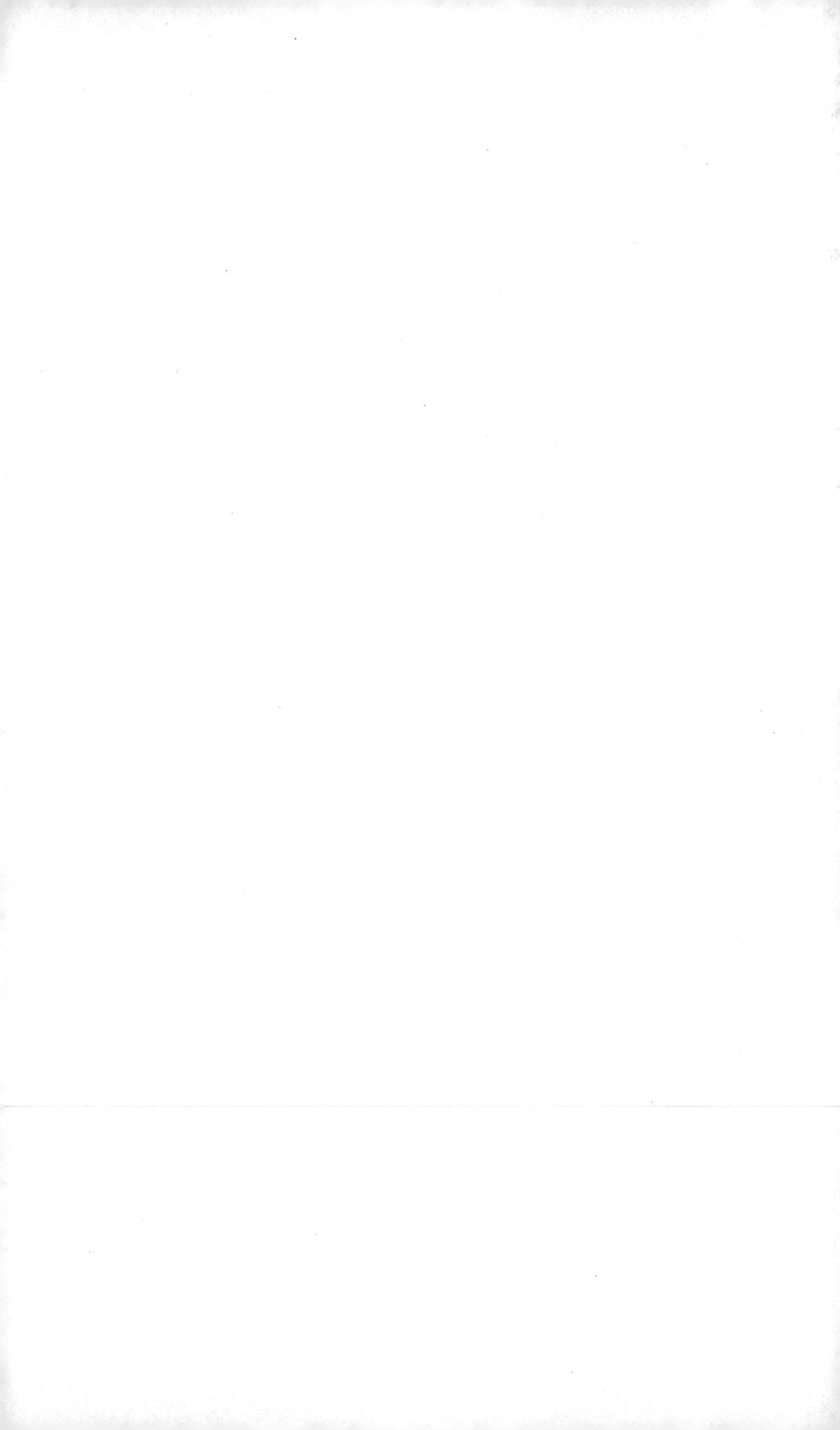

Fish's Schizophrenia

Edited by

MAX HAMILTON

MD, FRCP, FRCPsych, FBPsS

Emeritus Professor of Psychiatry, University of Leeds
Formerly Honorary Consultant to General Infirmary at Leeds
St James's University Hospital, Leeds
Stanley Royd Hospital, Wakefield

THIRD EDITION

WRIGHT · PSG
Bristol · London · Boston
1984

Published by
John Wright & Sons Ltd, 823–825 Bath Road, Bristol BS4 5NU, England.
John Wright PSG Inc., 545 Great Road, Littleton, Massachusetts 01460, USA.

First Edition 1962
Second Edition 1976
Third Edition 1984

British Library Cataloguing in Publication Data
Fish, Frank
Fish's Schizophrenia.—3rd ed.
1. Schizophrenia
I. Title II. Hamilton, Max
616.89'82 RC514

ISBN 0 7236 0751 6

Library of Congress Catalog Card Number: 83–40044

Typeset and printed in Great Britain by
John Wright & Sons (Printing) Ltd
at The Stonebridge Press,
Bristol BS4 5NU

PREFACE TO THE THIRD EDITION

Frank Fish wrote this book with the intention of providing a clinically orientated text and to give English-speaking psychiatrists an account of the developments in German post-Kraepelinian work. The continued demand for this book has shown that he satisfied a real need and it has been my endeavour to continue along the lines he laid down.

Updating this edition has been a considerable task. In the past decade there has been a tremendous increase in research on the schizophrenias with the result that some of the bits of the jigsaw puzzle are fitting together and we might even hope that we shall soon have some notion of what the picture will be.

For this edition the chapter on aetiology has again been considerably revised as well as updated. In addition to the revisions in the previous edition to the chapters on paranoid states, prognosis, and treatment, the chapters on special varieties of schizophrenia and differential diagnosis have also been considerably revised. Throughout the text references to recent work have been included and some out-of-date work deleted. In consequence, only the chapters on the concept, symptomatology and varieties of schizophrenia still closely resemble the version of the first edition. The last chapter on Theories of Schizophrenia (which might better be described as Philosophical Interpretations) might be considered unnecessary but has been retained because I think it is unique among textbooks on schizophrenia.

I wish to express my thanks to Mrs J. M. Brierly, my personal assistant, for her help with the search for references, the preparation of the manuscript and the checking of proofs.

M. H.

PREFACE TO THE FIRST EDITION

This book is an expansion of a series of lectures on schizophrenia which were given to the first group of postgraduate students to take the new course for the second part of the Diploma in Psychiatry of the University of Edinburgh. The aim of these lectures was to present those aspects of the subject which had been neglected in English-speaking countries and to relate them to the well-known current views. This book has, therefore, a different bias from that of most other books on this topic that have been published in Britain and the United States in recent years. Although there is nothing new in this book, it is hoped that this presentation of the ideas of the classical German-speaking psychiatrists will be useful to those who find the vague concepts of 'psychodynamic' psychiatry of little value in clinical practice and research.

Wherever possible the author has acknowledged the major source of the topic under discussion, since it would have been too cumbersome to include all references in the text. However, the subject and author indexes refer to the bibliography as well as to the text, so that the reader can find any additional references that he may require.

The influence of many different workers is apparent throughout the book. In the clinical sections the author has depended to a large extent on the clear descriptions of Karl Kleist and Karl Leonhard. In the more theoretical sections the author has been influenced by the ideas of Karl Jaspers, Kurt Schneider, and Klaus Conrad. Although it is not directly quoted in this book, there is no doubt that the famous Volume 9 ('Schizophrenie') of Bumke's *Handbuch der Geisteskrankheiten* has had a marked effect on the whole book. Finally the author would like to express his thanks to Professor T. Langan's clear and penetrating book, *The Meaning of Heidegger*, without which he would have been lost for ever in the Heideggerian undergrowth.

F. J. F.
1962

ACKNOWLEDGEMENTS

I am indebted to the Pergamon Press for permission to reproduce Table 2 which appeared in *Transmission of Schizophrenia*, edited by D. Rosenthal and S. S. Kety in the article by E. Slater.

I am also indebted to the editor of the *British Journal of Psychiatry* for permission to use Figure 3 in the paper by Luc Ciompi (1980, **136**, 413–420).

I should like to express my thanks to F. K. Schattauer Verlagsgesellschaft mbH, Stuttgart and New York, for permission to use Figures 3 and 5 in the paper by J. Angst et al., 'Statistische Aspekte des Beginns und Verlaufs schizophrener Psychosen' G. Huber (ed.) *Verlauf und Ausgang Schizophrener Erkrankungen*.

CONTENTS

Chapter		Page
1	The Concept of Schizophrenia	1
2	Aetiology	5
3	Symptomatology	38
4	The Classification of Schizophrenia	78
5	Paranoid States	98
6	Special Varieties of Schizophrenia	111
7	Course and Prognosis	127
8	Treatment	140
9	Diagnosis and Differential Diagnosis	160
10	Theories of Schizophrenia	172
	References	202
	Further Reading	216
	Index	223

'In writing the history of a disease, every philosophical hypothesis whatsoever, that has previously occupied the mind of the author, should lie in abeyance. This being done, the clear and natural phenomena of the disease should be noted—these, and these only. They should be noted accurately, and in all their minuteness; in imitation of the exquisite industry of those painters who represent in their portraits the smallest moles and the faintest spots. No man can state the errors that have been occasioned by these physiological hypotheses. Writers, whose minds have taken a false colour under their influence, have saddled diseases with phenomena which existed in their own brains only; but which would have been clear and visible to the whole world had the assumed hypothesis been true. Add to this, that if by chance some symptom really coincide accurately with their hypothesis, and occur in the disease whereof they would describe the character, they magnify it beyond all measure and moderation; they make it all and in all; the molehill becomes a mountain; whilst, if it fail to tally with the said hypothesis, they pass it over either in perfect silence or with only an incidental mention, unless, by means of some philosophical subtlety, they can enlist it in their service, or else, by fair means or foul, accommodate it in some way or other to their doctrines.'—*Thomas Sydenham.*

Chapter 1

The concept of schizophrenia

Schizophrenia was originally delimited as a mental illness in which severe irreversible personality changes occurred. The historical development of the concept is well known. Morel, in 1852, reported a series of cases of severe intellectual deterioration starting in adolescence and he called this illness *démence précoce*. In 1871 Hecker described hebephrenia, an illness which occurred in puberty and led to a 'silly' deterioration. In 1874 Kahlbaum drew attention to a mental illness in which stupor occurred in the absence of disease of the nervous system; he called this illness 'tension insanity' or catatonia. In 1891, Pick described a 'simplex' syndrome which remained after the two groups described by Hecker and Kahlbaum had been separated from the broad category of Morel. He emphasized the 'simple deterioration' accompanied by a minimum of other symptoms in his residual group. Three years later these groupings were incorporated into Sommer's textbook. In 1893, in the 4th edition of his textbook, Kraepelin brought together the syndromes of *démence précoce*, hebephrenia, catatonia, and dementia paranoides and called this group of illnesses 'psychological degeneration processes'. In 1899 he used the term 'dementia praecox' to designate this group of illnesses because intellectual deterioration was a common feature and the illness usually occurred in young people. However, he later admitted that some patients did recover from dementia praecox, about 2·5 per cent, and that the illness could occur in the middle-aged. In the 8th edition (1913) of his textbook, he defined dementia praecox as follows: 'Dementia praecox consists of a series of clinical states which have as their common characteristic a peculiar destruction of the internal connections of the psychic personality with the most marked damage of the emotional life and of volition.' Contrary to what is commonly believed, he did not consider course and outcome as the only criteria for recognizing the disorder; indeed, he developed a very subtle nosography which allowed for a diagnosis to be made at a very early stage.

As Kraepelin regarded disorders of emotion and of volition as important features of schizophrenia, he set apart a group of paranoid mental deteriorations in which the disorders of emotion and volition were not very marked. This group of illnesses he called 'paraphrenia'.

In 1911 Eugen Bleuler introduced the term 'schizophrenia' in an attempt to get away from the confusion caused by the words 'dementia praecox'. He defined schizophrenia on the basis of symptomatology and course when he wrote as follows: 'By the term dementia praecox or schizophrenia we designate a group of psychoses whose course is at times chronic, at times marked by intermittent attacks and which can stop or retrograde at any stage, but does not permit a full *restitutio ad integrum*. The disease is characterized by a specific type of alteration of thinking, feeling, and relation to the external world which appears nowhere else in this particular fashion.'

Although Bleuler held that schizophrenia always left behind a defect of the personality, he believed that in some cases the defect was so slight as to be undetectable. He occupied a middle position between Kraepelin and Freud inasmuch as he went beyond pure psychological description and considered psychological processes as relevant both to the general understanding of the illness and to the genesis of the whole gamut of 'accessory symptoms'. He and his pupils used the term 'schizophrenia' for a large number of mild illnesses which many other psychiatrists did not consider to be schizophrenic. Thus schizophrenia became a very fashionable diagnosis in Switzerland and has remained so to the present day. Other workers, especially Kleist, have adopted the viewpoint that schizophrenia is an illness which always leads to a defect state. *Table 1* shows the difference in schizophrenia admission rates in four different continental psychiatric clinics. The different concepts of the disorder are clearly reflected in these figures.

Table 1. ADMISSIONS TO UNIVERSITY NEUROPSYCHIATRIC CLINICS
(After Kleist and Kolle)

Cases	*Munich* 1925	*Zürich* 1925	*Frankfurt* 1925	*Kiel* 1929
Total admissions	2524	743	1625	
Manic depressives	284	27	104	
Schizophrenia and paraphrenia	496	321	152	276
Percentage of schizophrenics and paraphrenics	19·6	43·2	9·4	12

The immediate problem facing anyone who claims that schizophrenia is a recoverable illness is to define what is meant by a schizophrenic symptom. The only useful criterion is that of understandability which was introduced into psychiatry by Jaspers (1910).* The examiner determines whether a given symptom can be understood or not by feeling himself into the situation of the patient and assessing whether the symptom can be understood logically or emotionally as

* *See* the discussion of 'Understanding Psychology', in Chapter 10.

arising from the patient's affective state, his previous personality, and the current situation. This approach is somewhat vague and subjective, since some examiners are prepared to understand much more than others. Nevertheless, there are some symptoms which, when clearly expressed, cannot be understood at all and are therefore schizophrenic. It must be stressed that the understandability of a symptom means that the symptom can be understood by a naïve observer, since many different schools of psychopathology claim to understand any symptom on the basis of their special theories. A non-understandable symptom in the Jasperian sense is one in which the form of the symptom cannot be understood or empathized with, although frequently the content can be understood to some degree. Of course, schizophrenic symptoms in this sense can occur in psychoses due to coarse brain disease, so that they are therefore only diagnostic of schizophrenia in the absence of evidence of organic disease.

Given these two criteria, we have a disorder, or group of disorders, which can have an acute or slow (chronic) onset. The acute condition may show a more or less complete recovery, or may become chronic. The chronic type may progress to deterioration or remain static; its course may also show acute episodes.

The opposing view which regards schizophrenia as an incurable disease is faced with a problem of a different kind, namely, the classification of those phasic psychoses which are completely dissimilar from manic-depressive illness and which are not followed by any permanent defect. If these illnesses are not schizophrenic, it is necessary to classify them into a separate group. Schröder (1920a, b) isolated a group of degeneration psychoses which were phasic in character and which did not fit into any of the typical manic depressive illnesses. Kleist (1923) also called this type of illness 'degeneration psychoses', by which he inferred that it was a genetically determined psychosis indicative of familial degeneration. Later, however, he called these illnesses 'cycloid marginal psychoses', and since then Leonhard (1959) has given an exhaustive account of these illnesses, which he calls 'cycloid psychoses'. The nature of these disorders will be discussed in a later chapter.

Much work has been carried out in recent years on attempts to distinguish these syndromes from schizophrenia on the one hand, and manic-depressive disorder on the other, using symptomatic, genetic, and prognostic criteria. This work will be considered in a later chapter.

Both these conflicting concepts of schizophrenia can be justified by appealing to the concepts of disease entities used in physical medicine. The question has been asked, for example, 'Can a disease entity be established on the basis of the course of the illness?' There is no doubt that leukaemia and Addisonian anaemia were originally isolated on the basis of their incurability. Nevertheless, one could not deny that a patient had suffered from acute nephritis if his condition improved and there was no evidence of residual kidney disorder. In fact, it may be argued that the kidney disease and the vicious circle due to hypertension might be a good model for schizophrenia. Thus, acute schizophrenia which becomes chronic might be due to a vicious circle produced by some neural mechanism which comes into action if the schizophrenic process is severe enough or lasts long enough. It does not seem legitimate to assume that schizophrenia must always lead to deterioration and to exclude acute schizophrenic syndromes with complete recovery from the group of schizophrenias. Certainly such syndromes must be isolated for purposes of study and further research. We should, therefore, be grateful to the Frankfurt School for emphasizing the importance of these illnesses.

Schizophrenia has always been defined as a 'functional' disorder, i.e. one which is not caused by coarse brain disease. The recognition that schizophrenic-like symptoms, and even the complete syndrome, may occur in those suffering from some kinds of epilepsy, in toxic conditions, e.g. chronic amphetamine intoxication and treatment with corticosteroids, has aroused new interest in the physical factors which may underlie or contribute to the development of the disorder. Technological advances have produced non-invasive techniques for examining the brain and its activities, starting with the EEG and going on to air-encephalography, regional blood-flow studies, computer-assisted tomography, and, the most recent, nuclear magnetic resonance. Biochemical research and the clarification of the mode of action of neuroleptic drugs have further advanced our understanding of the nature of the disturbance in the brain which underlies schizophrenia. The mystery of 'functional' is becoming less mysterious.

In the present work schizophrenia will be considered to be a group of mental disorders not primarily produced by coarse brain disease and in which many different clinical pictures can occur. The form and content of the symptoms in these disorders cannot be understood as arising emotionally or rationally from the affective state, the previous personality, or the current situation.

Chapter 2

Aetiology

General Principles

It is unfortunate that personal prejudices play such a part in psychiatry. The distorting effect of such preconceived ideas is seen in all discussions of the aetiology of schizophrenia. Most psycho-analytically orientated psychiatrists and psychologists seem to need to believe that all psychological illness is curable and that the only legitimate method of treatment is some form of psycho-analytic therapy. This is, of course, out of keeping with the ideas of Freud. This emotionally determined attitude leads most present-day psycho-analytic authors to avoid all discussion of the genetic basis of schizophrenia, despite the fact that Freud believed that fixation points in libidinal development might be determined genetically. However, the desire for omnipotence on the part of the neopsycho-analysts is not the only factor in their rejection of the genetic basis of schizophrenia. Perhaps just as important is the incorrect idea that if a disease is genetically determined, it must of necessity be incurable or untreatable and is certainly not amenable to psychotherapy. There is, of course, no justification for this belief as far as physical illness is concerned. Genetically determined metabolic disorders such as diabetes mellitus, galactosaemia, and phenylketonuria can be treated by substitution therapy or diet.

Apart from these prejudices, inaccurate concepts of the causation of physical illness have been introduced into discussions of the aetiology of schizophrenia. Thus the simple idea that a bacterium or virus is the sole cause of an infectious disease has led many people to look for a single cause of schizophrenia. It is, of course, true that the bacterium is the *sine qua non* of the infectious disease, but many other factors such as the number of organisms, the endocrine balance, the immunological constitution, and so on, may determine the onset of an infectious illness. So that, given the infecting organism, cultural, social, climatic, and genetic factors may determine the occurrence of the illness. As it is impossible to understand the symptomatology of schizophrenia as a simple exaggeration of normal psychological reactions, one is forced to the conclusion that the essential factor in the disease is some inborn constitutional predisposition. However, this does not exclude the possibility that the onset of schizophrenia may be determined by psychological and social stresses of many kinds.

A further difficulty in determining the aetiology of schizophrenia comes from the different concepts of the nature of the illness. For example, Adolf Meyer (1906) believed that schizophrenia depended upon a special personality and constitution which developed a habit-disorganization due to lack of adaptation. So that for Meyer and his pupils, schizophrenia was not a sharp break in the personality, but it was an understandable development of an abnormal personality. Of course, schizophrenia may develop so insidiously that the exact point at which the abnormal personality became ill is uncertain, and for a time the illness appears to be merely an accentuation of the previous personality. In this the view is held that schizophrenia is an illness which begins at a definite point of time, which distorts the whole personality, and which cannot be understood as arising out of the previous personality as a simple psychological development. The Meyerians tend to regard the childhood behaviour disorders and adolescent difficulties as essential parts of the schizophrenic illness. Since these disorders are very common it seems better to consider them as contributory causes of schizophrenia, but not as manifestations of the illness itself.

Aetiology can best be considered in terms of constitutional and environmental factors. These correspond closely to the division into inner and outer, or predisposing and precipitating factors. The distinction is not absolute, because of considerable overlap between the two groups. For example, cerebral injury at birth is environmental or external but at the time when the illness develops, it is a constitutional or predisposing factor.

CONSTITUTIONAL FACTORS

Inheritance

Family Incidence

The expectation of schizophrenia for the European population is about 0·85 per cent, ranging from 0·51 to 1·23 per cent. The latter figure is for Switzerland and probably reflects the influence of Bleuler's ideas.

There is no doubt that the incidence of schizophrenia among the relatives of schizophrenics is much higher than in the general population. *Table 3* gives the generally accepted figures.

Karlsson (1973, 1982) stated that the risk of schizophrenia in first-degree relatives was raised four-fold over that of the general population, as was also the risk of other forms of 'functional psychoses'. The higher figures previously accepted were based on the inclusion of these other conditions as schizophrenia. He added that the risk in

Table 2. EXPECTATION OF SCHIZOPHRENIA FOR THE GENERAL POPULATION
(After Slater, 1968)

Date	*Country*	*N (Age corrected)*	*Expectation (%)*	*S.E.*
1931	Switzerland	899	1·23	0·368
1936	Germany	7956	0·51	0·088
1942	Denmark	23 251	0·69	0·054
1942	Finland	194 000	0·91	0·021
1946	Sweden	10 705	0·81	0·087
1959	Japan	10 545	0·82	0·088
1964	Iceland	4913	0·73	0·121

Table 3. EXPECTATION OF SCHIZOPHRENIA FOR RELATIVES OF SCHIZOPHRENICS
(After Zerbin-Rüdin, 1967)

Relationship	*Expectation*	*S.E.*
Parents (uncorrected)	4·4	0·23
Sibs (parents free of schizophrenia)	8·2	0·32
Sibs (parents not free of schizophrenia)	13·8	1·33
Children	12·3	0·94
Uncles and aunts	2·0	0·24
Half-sibs	3·2	1·00
Nephews and nieces	2·2	0·30
Grandchildren	2·8	0·62
First cousins	2·9	0·34

more distant relatives was somewhat higher than in previous reports. More recent figures were given by Gottesman and Shields (1976), who stated that the age-corrected risk of schizophrenia in siblings of probands was about 10 per cent. With one schizophrenic parent, the risk to the children was approximately 14 per cent and with both parents schizophrenic it was appoximately 46 per cent.

These figures indicate that schizophrenia can be regarded as a familial disorder, but by themselves prove nothing about the mode of transmission. As they stand, they can be interpreted either in genetic terms or as indicating familial influence.

Studies of Twins

Monozygotic twins have the same genetic constitution, whereas dizygotic twins, even of the same sex, have a genetic relationship which is the same as that of ordinary siblings. All studies have shown that the concordance rate is much higher in monozygotic twins than dizygotic twins, and this despite different methods of assessment and whether there has been a correction for age or not. The earlier results are shown in *Table 4* in which any schizophrenic-like illness occurring in the co-twin counted as a concordant pair and there was no age connexion.

More recent studies, which permit use of the proband method as described by Allen et al. (1967) are shown in *Table 5*. These give lower concordance rates for monozygotic twins since they are based on population studies, but the difference still remains. An extreme example is that of Pollin et al. (1969) who found, among nearly 16 000 twins who were veterans of the US armed forces (a highly selected healthy group), 11 pairs of monozygotic twins who were concordant for schizophrenia and 69 pairs who were discordant. The corresponding figures for dizygotic twins were 6 and 140. It could be argued that

Table 4. CONCORDANCE FOR SCHIZOPHRENIA IN TWINS (*After Gottesman and Shields, 1966*)

		MZ pairs			*Same sex DZ pairs*		
Investigator	*Date*	*N*	*C*	%	*N*	*C*	%
Luxenburger	1928	19	11	58	13	0	0
Rosanoff et al.	1934	41	25	61	53	7	13
Essen-Möller	1941	11	7	64	27	4	15
Kellmann	1946	174	120	69	296	34	11
Slater	1953	37	24	65	58	8	14
Inouye	1961	55	33	60	11	2	18
Total		337	220	65	458	55	12

Table 5. CONCORDANCE (PROBAND METHOD) FOR SCHIZOPHRENIA IN TWINS

		MZ pairs			*DZ pairs*		
Investigator	*Date*	*N*	*C*	%	*N*	*C*	%
Kringlen, Norway	1967	69	31	45	96	14	15
Fischer et al., Denmark	1969	25	14	56	45	12	26
Tienari, Finland	1971	20	7	35	23	3	13
Allen et al., USA	1972	121	52	43	131	12	9
Gottesman and Shields, UK	1972	26	15	58	34	4	12
Total		261	119	46	329	45	14

this difference could be accounted for by special environmental factors related to monozygotic twins and not dizygotic. For example, the former might be more liable in the course of psychological development to confusion of identity and weak ego formation. If that were so, it would be expected that there would be more monozygotic twins among samples of schizophrenics than in the population as a whole, but this has not been found. The strongest argument against such specific environmental factors comes from studies of monozygotic twins reared apart. Sixteen of such pairs have been reported and the concordance rate in them is 62·5 per cent, a figure which is of the same order as that of monozygotic twins brought up together (Shields and Slater, 1967).

It is obvious that all such studies tend to under-estimate concordance rates because the co-twin may show symptoms at a much later age (though many studies correct for this). For example, a follow-up 7·8 years after the first report on 16 discordant monozygotic twins (Belmaker et al., 1974) found that 1 co-twin had become schizophrenic, 3 had developed psychopathology of a possibly schizophrenic nature, the remaining 12 remaining stably discordant. Even in the absence of obvious symptoms, the twins discordant for schizophrenia often have significant character abnormalities (among the men) and neurotic symptoms (in the women), particularly when the sick twin suffers from the more 'nuclear' symptoms (Cadoret, 1973). Incidentally, Rosenthal (1962) has pointed out that concordance is about twice as high in male as in female twins.

Abe (1969) examined the probability that the co-twin of a proband would remain well over the course of time. He showed that a negative exponential curve would fit the data and that extension of the curve to 25 years gave an ultimate concordance rate of 75·7 per cent. This is close to the figure of 76·3 per cent given by Slater (1953).

A particularly interesting and very important 'twin study' was carried out by Fischer (1971). She identified, from the Danish twin register, 21 pairs of monozygotic twins born between 1870 and 1920, in which one or both had become schizophrenic or had developed a 'schizophreniform psychosis'. Among the 47 children born to the schizophrenic twins were 3 who had become schizophrenic and 1 who had committed suicide. Among the 25 children born to the normal co-twins, 3 had become schizophrenic. After age-correction, the risk in the former group was 9·4 per cent and in the latter group 12·3 per cent. Although the latter risk is higher, the difference is not statistically significant. Since it is reasonable to assume that the upbringing of the children born to the normal co-twin is likely to be less deleterious than that of the schizophrenic twin, whereas the genetic influences are the same, the evidence favours the latter theory.

Twin studies provide clear evidence of the importance of genetic factors, but the incomplete concordance of monozygotic twins indicates just as clearly that other factors are involved in the appearance of the illness. What these might be will be considered below, but it is appropriate to consider here a paper which makes an astonishing and significant contribution to this fundamental problem.

Boklage (1977) pointed out that although monozygotic twins had the same genetic constitution, they were often discordant for certain deviations of brain development to which they were specially prone. These showed other evidence of having genetic aetiologies and involved symmetry of embryonic development. He found that among 15 concordant pairs of monozygotic schizophrenic twins 4 pairs included one non-right hander, which is about the same as that found in pooled normal monozygotic twins, but among 13 discordant pairs 12 pairs included one or more non-right handers ($\chi^2 = 26{\cdot}5$, $P = 0{\cdot}0001$). The right-handed schizophrenics were of the 'nuclear' type and more severe than the left-handed. These differences were not found in dizygotic twins. In effect, discordance appears to be related to abnormalities of cerebral development.

Adoption Studies

A neat way of separating genetic factors from familial influence (mode of upbringing, inter-familial relationships) is to determine the incidence of schizophrenia in children of schizophrenics adopted away early in life and brought up in foster families, and compare it with that found in appropriate control groups. When the comparison is with other adopted children, it must be remembered that the mothers of such children are not necessarily representative of the population as a whole. Horn et al. (1975) found that two groups of unmarried mothers compared with pregnant married women and 18-year-old women, when tested with the Minnesota Multiphasic Personality Inventory (MMPI), had significantly higher scores on 9 clinical scales and especially on psychopathic deviancy and schizophrenia. Unfortunately, the unmarried mothers were not tested before they were pregnant, so we shall never know what was the basis of the high scores.

Heston (1966) compared 47 children of schizophrenics with 50 controls. All these were adopted children who had been separated from their mother within a few days of birth. He found that 5 of the 47 children in the index group became schizophrenic but none of the controls. Fisher's exact test gives a P of $0{\cdot}024$, which is statistically significant. Sociopathic personality disorders were also more frequent in the former group. In a similar study by Rosenthal et al. (1968), 39 adopted children of schizophrenics were compared with a control series of adopted children from normal parents. In the former group,

3 were schizophrenic, 6 were borderline schizophrenic, and 4 were schizoid or paranoid, whereas in the latter group 3 were borderline schizophrenic, 3 were schizoid, and 2 had a paranoid personality. For the total figures, chi-squared (corrected) equals 3·09 and $P = 0{\cdot}08$, which is just not significant. An extension of this investigation was reported by Rosenthal et al. (1971): the adopted children of 52 parents with schizophrenia spectrum disorder and 24 suffering from other mental disturbances developed schizophrenia spectrum disorder in 14, various other conditions in 10, leaving 52 who were mentally normal. Among the 67 control children from normal parents, 12 received a diagnosis of mental illness. The test of significance gives $P = 0{\cdot}09$.

The problem was examined from the opposite side by Kety et al. (1968). These investigators looked at the prevalence of mental illness in the biological and adoptive families of adopted schizophrenics. They found 33 index cases, 19 of whom had been adopted before the age of 1 month and the rest before 1 year, and compared them with 33 controls, 20 of whom had been adopted before 1 month and the rest before 1 year of age. They were able to trace 463 relatives of these 66 cases. The index cases had 150 biological relatives and 74 adopted ones, and the controls had 156 and 83, respectively. Case records of these relatives were examined and given a diagnosis as appropriate. Using the term 'schizophrenia spectrum disorder' to cover the diagnostic categories of schizophrenia, uncertain schizophrenia, and inadequate personality, it was found that in the 150 biological relatives of the index cases, 13 (8·7 per cent) had this general diagnosis whereas in the 156 biological relatives of the controls, only 3 (1·9 per cent) had this diagnosis. Fisher's exact test gives a probability (one tail) of 0·007, which is highly significant. In the case of the adoptive relatives, the diagnosis of schizophrenia spectrum disorder was given to only 2 out of 74 relatives of the index cases (2·7 per cent) and 3 out of 83 (3·6 per cent) of the controls. The difference is not statistically significant.

These investigators (Kety et al., 1975) continued with their work and finally located 512 relatives, of whom 119 had died. They obtained full interviews or adequate information on 341 and found that the incidence of schizophrenia spectrum disorder had now risen from 8·7 to 21·4 per cent in the biological relatives of the index cases, and from 2·7 to 5·4 per cent in the adoptive relatives. For the control cases, the corresponding figures had gone from 1·9 per cent to 10·9 per cent and from 3·6 to 7·7 per cent. To make it clear, we may note that 10·9 per cent of the biological parents of the controls had this diagnosis, whereas the corresponding figure for the adoptive parents of the schizophrenic index cases was only 5·4 per cent. To avoid obscuring the point with too many figures, it can be said that even if the diagnosis was confined to 'definite' or 'definite plus uncertain' schizophrenia, the biological parents of the index cases still showed a much greater incidence of illness than either the adoptive parents or the biological and adoptive parents of the controls.

In order to test the hypothesis of genetic as against environmental factors even more rigorously, the investigators examined the data on the sub-sample of children who had been adopted before the age of 1 month. The diagnosis of schizophrenia spectrum disorder was given to 9 out of 93 (9·7 per cent) of the biological relatives of the index cases and to none of the 92 biological relatives of the controls. The exact test gives a probability of 0·002. In the cases of the adopted relatives, the index cases had 2 out of 45 (4·4 per cent) as against the controls with 1 out of 51 (2 per cent) receiving the diagnosis. The difference is not statistically significant. Of particular interest is the fact that, as the authors point out, 'more than half of the schizophrenia spectrum disorders were found in their paternally related half-siblings with whom the index cases should have had in common not even an *in utero* environment but only some genetic overlap'. The evidence is clear: in the case of adopted children who became schizophrenic it is the biological relatives (with whom the children have had minimal contact) who have an increased risk of developing schizophrenia as compared with the general population, and not the adoptive relatives.

Among the 33 index cases, 7 were diagnosed as acute schizophrenic reaction and none of their biological relatives was found to suffer from schizophrenia-related disorders. The other 26 cases were diagnosed as chronic schizophrenia for 16 and borderline schizophrenia for 10. The biological families of these two groups showed the same pattern of schizophrenia-related disorders. This raises the question of the relationship between acute schizophrenia and the other forms of this disorder.

Alanen (1966) compared the extent of mental illness and symptoms among the parents of schizophrenics with the parents of neurotics and found that the former group was significantly worse. On the basis of these findings, it could be argued that if schizophrenia is psychologically and sociologically transmitted, then adoptive parents of schizophrenics would show a large amount of mental abnormality, but if it were genetically transmitted they would not. Furthermore, if child-rearing practices are important in the development of schizophrenia, then the characteristics of the biological parents of schizophrenics would be found in the adopted parents of schizophrenics. Wender et al. (1968, 1971) investigated 10 couples whose adopted children had become schizophrenic, 10 couples whose (biological) child had become schizophrenic, and as a further control group 10 couples whose adopted child was normal. They rated these parents on a scale (based on that of Alanen) which ranged from Grade 1 normal, Grade 3 mild character neurosis, Grade 6 borderline schizophrenia to Grade 7 schizophrenia. They found that the mean grade for the parents in the first group was 3·3 for the fathers and 3·5 for the mothers; for the second group it was 4·2 and 4·9 and for the third group 2·6 and 3·0, respectively. Thus the biological parents of children who became schizophrenic had the largest score for abnormality, the adoptive parents of schizophrenics had less and the adoptive parents of normals had least. In general, the statistical tests show that the difference between the biological and adoptive parents of schizophrenics is significant, but the difference between the adoptive parents of schizophrenics and those of normal children is not. These data are obviously very important but the authors were careful to point out that there were methodological difficulties in their investigation: the sampling of cases was not systematic, the interviewers knew to which group the parents belonged, and the parents of schizophrenics were frank and outspoken but the others were guarded during their interviews. Nonetheless, Rimmer et al. (1979) confirmed that the personal and social characteristics of adoptive parents of schizophrenics do not differ from those of controls.

A further method of examining the influence of upbringing is to study cross-fostered groups. Wender et al. (1974) compared three groups of adopted children: an index group with 'schizophrenic spectrum' parents, a control group with no recorded family diagnosis, and a cross-fostered group whose adoptive parents suffered from schizophrenic spectrum disorder but whose biological parents were free from that diagnosis. Among 38 cross-fostered subjects, interviewing and examination of case records gave a diagnosis of chronic schizophrenia in 9, acute schizophrenia or schizo-affective disorder (certain and doubtful) in 9, borderline schizophrenia in 4, doubtful schizophrenia or schizoid in 6, and 10 refused to provide information. They found a greater prevalence of psychopathology among the index group, but no such increase in the cross-fostered group. Although the authors warned that the numbers were small and the sample an unusual one, making extrapolation unwise, this investigation points in the same direction as the others: genetic factors are much more important for the development of schizophrenia, than the mode of upbringing.

High-risk Groups

In 1962, Schulsinger and Mednick investigated 207 children of chronic and severely schizophrenic mothers and compared them with 104 matched controls who had no history of schizophrenia in either parents or grandparents. The 'high-risk' children had a mean age of

15·1 years. Eight years later (Mednick, 1970), 20 of these children had developed schizophrenia.

A further follow-up (Schulsinger, 1976) carried out during 1972–74 traced 173 index cases (among the missing were 3 who had died, 4 who had committed suicide, and 1 probable suicide) and 93 controls. Three methods of assessment were used: the Present State Examination (and CATEGO diagnosis), DIAGNO II, and interviewers' judgement. Comparing the high-risk with the low-risk groups, the ratio of diagnosis of schizophrenia by these methods was 10 : 1, 30 : 6, and 13 : 1 respectively. Including cases with 'schizoid' and 'paranoid' personality, the ratios became 35 : 3, 20 : 1, and 71 : 5. For alcoholism the ratio was 10 : 1 and for drug abuse 12 : 3. Based on 15 cases out of a total of 173, the morbidity risk was 17·2 per cent or 23·8 per cent according to the method of calculation. For 9 cases admitted to hospital, it was 10·3 per cent or 14·3 per cent.

Useful short reviews of work on high-risk groups are those of Shields (1977) and Garmezy (1977).

The point of high-risk research is to find predictors of the development of schizophrenia, leading to the possibility of prevention. The work is still in its earliest stages and inferences must be regarded as tentative. Mednick et al. (1978) examined their data by a method of 'path analysis' and suggested that predictive variables differ between males and females. In the former, a schizophrenic outcome is directly related to early childhood separation (a consequence of early onset of schizophrenia in the mother) and abnormal autonomic responses; in the latter to the mother's early onset of schizophrenia, but only slightly to abnormal autonomic responses. Hanson et al. (1976) have suggested that possible predictors in high-risk children are: (1) Poor motor skills in childhood, (2) Large intra-individual inconsistencies in performance on a diverse set of cognitive tasks, and (3) Schizoid-like behaviour, including apathy, withdrawal, and emotional flatness mixed with emotional instability, irritability, and negativism.

Psycho-physiological Researches

Zahn (1964) investigated the level of skin conductance of schizophrenics at rest and also the spontaneous fluctuations. He found that the resting level was raised, indicating a high level of activation, and the fluctuations were greater than in normal controls. The rate of habituation of orientation responses was also slower.

Gruzelier and Venables (1974) confirmed these results, but found that many patients had no orientation response. They found also that resting conductance was asymmetrical in schizophrenics (and also in personality disorders), being higher on the left when conductance was low and on the right when it was high. Horvath and Meares (1979) found that it was in non-paranoid schizophrenics that habituation to repeated stimuli was slow or absent; in paranoid cases the responses were normal. They showed a different impairment, responding to a novel disinhibiting stimulus as if it were familar.

It is appropriate to mention here the work of Saletu et al. (1975) who examined EEG auditory-evoked potentials in 62 high-risk children and compared them with 63 matched controls. The former group showed significantly shorter latencies but no difference in amplitude. They also had greater intra-individual variability of latency in the early part of the recording and less in the later part, than the controls. The authors pointed out that these differences were similar to those between adult schizophrenics and normal subjects.

The most important findings in high-risk groups are those which have shown resemblances in electrodermal reactions between children who subsequently become schizophrenic and adult schizophrenics. In the high-risk study mentioned above, Mednick (1970) compared the 20 subjects who had become schizophrenic (the 'sick group') with 20 subjects from the controls (the 'control group') and 20 others from the high-risk group (the 'well group'). When tested on the galvanic skin response (GSR) to a loud noise, the sick group showed a much shorter latency time than the other two groups. With repeated stimuli, 69 per cent of the well group showed slowing of latency, i.e. habituation, but the sick group showed no signs of this and the latency time even decreased. The recovery of the GSR to the base rate was also very much faster in the sick group than in the other two groups. The GSR response to an irritating noise of 96 decibels was then conditioned to a stimulus tone of only 54 decibels. The period of conditioning was then followed by a series of extinction trials. Whereas the conditioned GSR showed rapid extinction in the two control groups the sick group continued to show response. Thus, on all these tests, the sick group was clearly different from the well group and the control group.

The previous history of these groups provides an explanation of the findings. One or more serious pregnancy or birth complications had occurred in 70 per cent of the sick group as compared with 15 per cent of the well group and 33 per cent of the control group. There was a marked correspondence between these birth complications and the anomalous electrodermal reactions. All the differences between the galvanic skin responses in the sick and well group could be explained by these complications which had occurred in the sick group, i.e. pregnancy and birth complications were associated with onset of rapid response, poor habituation of response, very rapid recovery of response, and poor extinction of the conditioned response. The complications recorded included anoxia, prematurity, prolonged labour, placental difficulty, umbilical cord complications, mother's illness during pregnancy, multiple births, and breech presentations. The schizophrenics were found to have had the most complicated births, and the borderlines the least complicated births (Parnas et al., 1982). These findings were interpreted in terms of a 'diathesis-stress' model, i.e. that birth complications could decompensate borderline individuals towards schizophrenic breakdown.

The author pointed out that the hippocampus in the temporal lobe is particularly sensitive to anoxia. It can therefore be inferred that the birth injuries had caused some damage to the hippocampus in the temporal lobe. The hippocampus is part of the limbic system, which is concerned with the organization and integration of emotional behaviour. Changes in autonomic function are an important part of emotional responses, e.g. to unpleasant stimuli. The abnormal psycho-physiological results in the tests, found in the sick group, can therefore be ascribed to damage to the hippocampus. Mednick then went on to compare his findings with those found in rats that had undergone experimental hippocampal lesions. These animals show relatively fast response latency and poor habituation in the galvanic skin response and they also show great resistance to experimental extinction of conditioned behaviour. The animals are also hyperactive and the author compared this with the teachers' report on the sick group who 'were disciplinary problems, domineering, aggressive, created conflicts, and disrupted the class with their talking'.

The diminished activity of the limbic system is accompanied by a relatively high state of arousal arising from the reticular system. Experimental direct stimulation of the reticular system has been shown to produce a lowering of the threshold for critical flicker fusion, in other words, a high state of arousal facilitates the recognition of a fast flicker. Skin conductance and skin potential are also increased during states of arousal. Venables and Wing (1962) found a high correlation between these two measures of arousal in non-paranoid schizophrenics. They also found a high correlation between arousal, as measured by these two indices, and withdrawal. It would therefore appear that this most prominent symptom of schizophrenia is related to an imbalance between the activity of the limbic and reticular systems, due to a deficiency in the former.

In high-risk studies, interim findings are all that is possible (until all the subjects have died), but at least one report is worth mentioning for its intrinsic interest. Venables et al. (1978) described the first results from a controlled trial. They tested 1800 children aged 3 years on skin conductance, skin potential, and electrocardiogram and found four types of response: (1) Hyper-responders who showed a large amplitude and quick recovery of skin conductance response to a stimulus, (2) Those who showed a medium amplitude with very long recovery, (3) A control group with medium amplitude and medium recovery time, and (4) Non-responders. A sample was taken, of which half went to nursery schools and the other half were left in the community.

Three years later, when the subjects were 6 years old, their behaviour was tested in a standard play situation. In group 3 the schoolchildren spent more time in constructive play and less in watching the others than the community children. Among group 1, the hyper-responders, all the children engaged in a high level of constructive play and interaction; correspondingly, the amount of time spent in watching was decreased. In group 2, the schoolchildren engaged in much interaction with correspondingly low constructive play and watching. In group 4 (non-responders) all the children showed the same high level of watching and the same low level of constructive play and about the same low level of positive interaction (the nursery group being slightly better).

The authors pointed out that in other high-risk studies, hyper-responders were liable to develop schizophrenia with first-rank symptoms, non-responders were similar to adult schizophrenics who showed defect states, and medium responders with long recovery times suggested psychopathic or criminal tendencies. The authors concluded that electrodermal tests at 3 years of age differentiated between groups who at 6 years showed differences in behaviour and different responses to nursery schooling, and that the types of behaviour shown were 'not in discord' with the results of work on high-risk groups and adult schizophrenics.

Genetic Models

The value of a definite theory of the mode of inheritance of schizophrenia is that it may eventually form the basis of a rational treatment or detection of pre-morbid cases and also provide a guide for practical methods of prevention, e.g. genetic counselling. There are three possible types of inheritance: monogenic, polygenic, and genetic heterogeneity. The last implies many different genes, some dominant and some recessive, which independently give rise to schizophrenia, presumably through distinct metabolic pathways. These different genes would be maintained in the population by spontaneous mutation. A similar theory accounts for the specific types of severe subnormality.

Monogenic theories require supplementary hypotheses to modify them, since segregation according to Mendelian laws does not occur. For example, if the children of two schizophrenics were always schizophrenic this could be accounted for by a single recessive gene. This does not occur. Even with modifiers, the siblings of schizophrenics would be more often affected than the children. The data show (*Table 3*) that the expectation in children is 13·9 per cent; in siblings 9·7 per cent if the parents of the index case are free from schizophrenia and 17·2 per cent if they are not.

If there were a number of different recessive genes giving rise to schizophrenia, then the incidence of schizophrenia among the children of two schizophrenics would be low. In fact, it is high, different investigations giving figures which range from 38 to 68 per cent. Among the data which favour a monogenic theory, the family trees constructed by Karlsson (1966) are extremely convincing. These show clearly a major gene which is either inherited or not. Before this, Leonhard (1934) had described a family in which a schizophrenic illness occurred as a simple Mendelian dominant. Böök (1953) was the first to propose the theory of a dominant gene not fully penetrating. This theory was put into quantitative form by Slater (1958) and further developed to deal with more recent data (Slater and Cowie, 1971). Taking the base-line risk of schizophrenia in the general population as 0·85 per cent and the risk in sibs as 8·5 per cent, he demonstrated that a population frequency of the gene of 3 per cent with a manifestation rate of 13 per cent in the heterozygotes would give theoretical expected risks for all relatives which best matched the observed data. The expected figures give a good fit to the observed ones, except that the observed risks of 13·9 per cent in children of schizophrenics is 40 per cent higher than the theoretical figure of 8·5 per cent. In second-degree relatives the theoretical figure is 4·7 per cent as compared with the observed of 2·6 per cent which is about 25 per cent lower. It may be added that a polygenic theory would also give a low expectation rate for the children of schizophrenics but it would be about right for second-degree relatives. An additional point in favour of a monogenic theory is that the risk to sibs when one parent is schizophrenic is 1·6 times the risk when neither parent suffers from the disorder. Support for a polygenic theory are the facts that schizophrenia can appear in the children of normal parents and that the close relatives of such patients have higher risks of schizophrenia or schizophrenia spectrum disorder than the general population. The risk decreases from monozygotic twins to first-degree relatives and again to second-degree relatives. Further support is given by the data which show that the more cases there are in the family the greater is the risk, and also that the greater the severity in the proband, the greater the risk to the relatives. For example, in monozygotic twins, if the proband is severely ill the concordance rate is 77 per cent, but only 27 per cent if the proband is mildly ill. The figures for dizygotic twins are similar but lower (Gottesman and Shields, 1966). Ødegaard (1970) showed that the risk to siblings is 2·5 times greater in families where two or more of the parental generations have suffered from schizophrenia than in those families which had none. Although it would appear that schizophrenics are not less fertile than normal, their marriage rate is below that for the general population and therefore they are effectively less fertile (Stevens, 1969). In such circumstances, the persistence and stability of the risk in the general population are more easily explained by a polygenic theory than a monogenic one.

The distinction between these two theories is not absolute. Monogenic theories require additional factors which become equivalent to polygenic effects, and polygenic theories require some contribution by dominant or non-additive genetic factors. It is therefore not possible at present to make a choice between these two theories.

The survival in the population of the genes for schizophrenia presents a difficult problem, but it is always possible that they give some biological advantage. Carter and Watts (1971) compared the relatives of schizophrenics with the relatives of matched controls in two general practices and found that there was a significantly low incidence of virus infection in the former and, in one practice, they appeared markedly protected against accidents. The possibility of increased fertility has been discounted by Buck et al. (1975). The advantages may be not so much biological as social. Heston (1966), in his study of adopted children from schizophrenic mothers, found that although half of them showed a significant excess of psychosocial disability, as well as schizophrenia and sociopathic personality disorders, the other half 'were notably successful adults. They possessed artistic talents and demonstrated imaginative adaptations to life which were uncommon in the control group.' A careful study by Karlsson (1970) of Icelanders born between 1881 and 1910 came to similar conclusions. He found that the close relatives of psychotic individuals had a significantly increased probability of being considered persons of eminence. Their rate of listing in *Who's Who* was double that expected, both for general listing and that based on artistic or scholastic achievement. The social advantages of heterozygotes is also taken into account by the two-gene model of Maricq (1975).

To summarize this section, the epidemiological study of schizophrenia shows that it is frequently a familial disorder. The transmission of schizophrenia appears to be chiefly genetic as shown by the adoption studies. The evidence from these indicates that the probability of the children of schizophrenics themselves developing schizophrenia is much about the same whether they are brought up by their parents or are adopted. The important influence of genetic loading is demonstrated by the studies of concordance in monozygotic and dizygotic twins. The nature of the genetic transmission cannot yet be decided. There is good evidence in favour of a dominant gene and equally good evidence in favour of a polygenic theory. Both theories require supplementary modifications which makes their consequences very similar, e.g. absence of full penetration. In view of the social and biological disabilities arising from schizophrenia, an explanation is required for the persistence of the genes in the general population. Some evidence is beginning to appear that when the genes of schizophrenia are insufficient to give rise to mental illness, their possessors may have social gifts and even biological advantages.

Central Nervous System

Epilepsy

The relationship between schizophrenia and epilepsy has given rise to much controversy. The notion that they were mutually inhibitory led to the introduction of convulsive therapy. This may be true in some circumstances, but the weight of evidence is now in favour of some association between these two disorders. Slater et al. (1963) found that in mental disturbances associated with epilepsy the clinical picture closely resembled schizophrenia, although there were minor differences. In epileptics, mystical delusional experiences were very common and visual hallucinations were much more frequent than in schizophrenia. In these patients, the paranoid type of disorder predominated, the warmth of personality was better preserved, and the mental symptoms were episodic and fluctuating. As a matter of interest, Slater (1969) reported that on follow-up about one-third of the patients had remitted, a third had improved, and in the last third symptoms had become more 'organic' in type.

The possibility that the concurrence of schizophrenia and epilepsy is merely fortuitous was considered carefully by these writers, in the same paper. Assuming the incidence of schizophrenia and epilepsy in the population to be 0·8 and 0·5 per cent respectively, and taking other factors into account, they calculated that 3·5 new cases per year could be expected in London's population of 10 million. Having found 69 cases over an 11-year period in two hospitals alone, they concluded that this was greater than chance expectation. Furthermore, the incidence of schizophrenia in the first-degree relatives of the patient was no greater than would be expected in a sample of the general population. This provides some evidence against the theory that the epilepsy makes manifest a latent tendency towards schizophrenia. Concerning the type of epilepsy in these patients, the authors reported that EEG studies showed a large preponderance of temporal lobe lesions.

The nature of the lesion appears to be of some significance. Taylor (1975) examined the resected tissue from patients who had had temporal lobectomy for intractable psycho-motor epilepsy and compared 41 cases of mesial temporal sclerosis with 47 patients in whom he found 'alien tissue' (small tumours, hamartomas, and focal dysplasia). He found that 2 patients in the former group were psychotic as against 11 in the latter group. Alternatively, 11 out of 13 psychotic patients had 'alien tissue', while it was found in only 36 out of the 75 non-psychotics. He added that schizophrenia-like psychoses in the 'alien tissue' group tended to be females and especially left-handed females. The significance of this interesting work is not yet clear.

Flor-Henry (1969) compared two groups of temporal lobe epileptics, 50 in each group, one of which had experienced psychotic episodes and the other had not. He found that psycho-motor seizures and frequent temporal fits were inversely correlated with psychosis and that temporal lobe epilepsy in the 'dominant' hemisphere was associated with schizophrenic symptoms, but with manic-depressive disorder in the 'non-dominant' hemisphere. He concluded that epileptic psychoses were fundamentally related to the epileptic process and not to non-specific damage.

Disorders of the Nervous System

For long it has been believed by many psychiatrists that schizophrenia is due to a disorder of the brain, but the evidence for this has been a long time coming. Coarse brain disease is commonly associated with non-specific organic psychiatric syndromes, but all of the symptoms which appear in schizophrenia have been found on occasion to occur in damage to the brain in specific localities, as has been pointed out by, for example, Kleist (1960). The association that is found between cerebral disease and schizophrenia-like symptoms immediately raises two questions: whether the association arises from coincidence, and whether the disease merely makes manifest a latent tendency to schizophrenia. Davison and Bagley (1969), in their exhaustive review, came to the conclusion that the association between schizophrenia and cerebral tumour and injury was significantly greater than chance. Furthermore, there was no evidence for predisposition to schizophrenia in these cases. Even more important is their conclusion that the association is with lesions in the temporal lobe. Excluding epilepsy, the association with other diseases of the brain is less clear.

The relationship can be approached from the opposite direction. Malamud (1967) reported his autopsy findings on 18 cases of cerebral tumour who had first been diagnosed as suffering from mental disorder. Of 9 cases of tumours of the temporal lobe, 4 had received the diagnosis of schizophrenia, 4 of depression, and 1 of anxiety state;

2 cases of tumour of the cingulate region had received a diagnosis of schizophrenia, and of 7 tumours of the third ventricle 4 had received such a diagnosis, 2 had been diagnosed as psychoneurosis, and 1 as mania. He drew attention to 'the possibility of the existence of a direct causal relationship between the anatomic location of the lesion and the psychiatric symptomatology', and made a cautious inference that the limbic system must play a significant role in the overall picture. Falconer et al. (1964) found mesial temporal sclerosis in 47 cases out of 100 temporal lobes resected for the treatment of temporal lobe epilepsy, and mesial focal lesions in many of the other cases. They considered that hypoxic episodes in infancy and early childhood played a more important role in the development of these lesions than birth trauma. These papers, and many others, make clear that it is damage to the limbic structures in the temporal lobe which links temporal lobe epilepsy with schizophrenia.

Studies of monozygotic twins discordant for schizophrenia provide confirmatory evidence. Stabenau and Pollin (1967) reported on 14 such pairs which they had studied, together with data from 84 other pairs reported in the literature. They found that the schizophrenic member of the pair showed the following features twice as often as the co-twin: CNS illness as a child, birth complications, neonatal asphyxia, lighter at birth, weaker and shorter. In comparison with the co-twin the index case as a child was neurotic, submissive, serious, quiet and shy, stubborn, dependent, and was obedient and sensitive. In a subsequent paper the authors (Mosher et al., 1971) reported that in 11 out of 15 such discordant pairs, the index case showed significantly more abnormal neurological signs than the normal co-twin. Nevertheless, the authors were careful to point out that the sample was small, that not all the index cases were clearly schizophrenic, and that the 'clearly' schizophrenic cases did not show more signs than the 'probably' schizophrenic.

Birth complications and neonatal asphyxia which are known to damage the mesial temporal lobe therefore potentiate the development of schizophrenia in the presence of an hereditary disposition. Lesions in the same region are associated with schizophrenia-like symptoms, and temporal lobe epileptics are liable to develop schizophrenia. Three different approaches to the problem lead to the same conclusion. Finally, Flor-Henry (1972), in his critical review, demonstrated that schizophrenic and paranoid symptoms (and also psychopathy) were related to limbic dysfunction in the dominant temporal lobe, whereas affective psychoses and depressive neuroses were related to dysfunction in the non-dominant temporal lobe.

The development of further non-invasive methods of investigating the brain, especially computer-assisted tomography (CAT scans), has led to a great amount of work on the organic background of schizophrenia, encouraged by earlier findings of neuro-psychological deficits in these patients. For example, Rochford et al. (1970) found 'soft sign' deficits (gait, balance, co-ordination, graphesthesia, and stereognosis) in 23 out of 26 schizophrenics and in 25 out of 27 personality disorders but in only 1 of a mixed group of 12 depressives. Similar results have been found by others. Quitkin et al. (1976) found evidence of soft signs in schizophrenics with pre-morbid asociality (and patients with emotionally unstable character disorders) but not in other types. Cox and Ludwig (1979) found significantly more soft signs in schizophrenics than in four other groups of psychiatric patients and controls. Torrey (1980) used graphesthesia and face–hand tests on 84 schizophrenics and found abnormalities in 80 per cent of acute–sub-acute cases, which was significantly more than the 49 per cent he found in sub-chronic–chronic cases. They were associated with longer history and earlier onset, but not with any of the background factors he examined, including CAT scans.

Crow and Mitchell (1975) pointed out that 25 per cent of 237 chronic in-patient schizophrenics believed that they were 5 or more years younger than their real age. Among them were 12 per cent who believed themselves to be within 5 years of their age at admission (although they were 28 years older) and 5 per cent who believed themselves to be of an age within 1 year of admission. Subsequently, Crow and Stevens (1978), comparing 77 chronic schizophrenics with 'age disorientation' with 222 patients who did not show this sign, found that the probands were less likely to give correct answers on their date of birth, present year, and duration of stay in hospital. The errors tended to be consistent with their concept of their own age. Despite their deficit, some of them were aware of the current year. There was thus a continuum of time disorientation, which was similar to the deficits found in organic dementia. The authors interpreted these findings as arising from a failure of learning mechanisms.

Early damage to the right hemisphere, or any interference with its function, is likely to diminish the tendency to right-handedness. For example, Andreasen et al. (1982) found that there was more evidence of ventricular enlargement in left-handed than in right-handed patients. Torrey (1980) had noted that abnormalities with his tests were more pronounced on the right hand, implicating the 'dominant' hemisphere. Chagule and Master (1981) used a strict test of right-handedness on 93 schizophrenics and found that only 30 passed compared with 74 in a group of 150 controls. Affective psychotics and neurotics did not differ significantly from the controls. These results must be considered in relation to the extensive work which has shown that left-handedness is less common among schizophrenics than in the general population.

Work with the EEGs of schizophrenics had shown that there were disturbances of function in the left hemisphere. These have been confirmed by Serafetinides et al. (1981), who reported that out of 30 male patients, the 8 who had predominant 'left-hemisphere symptoms' (conceptual disorganization, grandiosity, hostility, suspiciousness, unco-operativeness, and unusual thought content) showed a higher amplitude in the beta II band on the left than on the right. For the 6 patients with predominant 'right-hemisphere symptoms' (somatic concern, anxiety, tension, mannerisms, posturing, and depressed mood) these changes were on the right side.

Measurement of the regional cerebral blood-flow, by the xenon isotope method, has shown that although the mean blood-flow is normal in schizophrenics, compared with controls, a high flow in frontal structures is less common and in post-central structures it is more common (Ingvar and Franzén, 1974). In chronic older schizophrenics the flow is low frontally and relatively high in the occipito-temporal areas (Ingvar, 1974). The 'static' differences are accompanied by 'functional' differences. These researchers (1975) measured the regional blood-flow in 27 chronic schizophrenics and 15 non-schizophrenic controls during the administration of psychological tests. In the controls there was an increased blood-flow in the frontal regions but little or no change in the patients. There was no difference between the two groups for changes in post-central structures.

Work which has demonstrated that enlargement of the lateral cerebral ventricles is common in chronic schizophrenics goes back a long way. One of the most important earlier studies is that of Haug (1962). He found that of 137 chronic schizophrenic patients, 84 (61 per cent) showed enlargement of the lateral ventricles in the pneumoencephalogram, being present chiefly in the older patients and those with a long history of illness. In a follow-up repeat examination of 24 patients, he found further enlargement in 4 of the 8 patients whose clinical condition had become aggravated, a most important observation.

These results have been confirmed with the technique of computer-assisted tomography. For example, Weinberger et al. (1979a), comparing 58 chronic schizophrenic patients with 56 volunteer controls, found that the patients had larger ventricles than the controls; 53 per cent were more than 2 standard deviations above the control mean and 40 per cent were outside the range of the controls. The enlargement was present in 44 patients who had never had electroconvulsive therapy. Enlarged ventricles were found also in 7 non-chronic schizophrenics. Cortical atrophy, using defined criteria, was found in 19 (32 per cent) of the 56 patients (1979b).

An earlier paper by Johnstone et al. (1976) had indicated some of the implications of these findings. They were the first to find that chronic schizophrenics had larger ventricles (in CAT scans) than controls. In all the patients there was a highly significant correlation of −0·70 between cognitive function and ventricular size. When they compared 9 age-disorientated patients with 9 matched patients, they found a tendency in the former group to have larger ventricles, poorer cognitive function, fewer positive symptoms, and more negative symptoms. In contrast, Nasrallah et al. (1982), although confirming the ventricular enlargement, were unable to find any differences between schizophrenic sub-types.

Several reports have been unable to demonstrate such enlargement. For example, in the study by Benes et al. (1982), who compared 11 schizophrenics with 26 controls, their patients had a mean age of 21·2 years (S.D. 5·5), a length of illness of 4·5 years (S.D. 4·3 years), and a stay in hospital of 1·1 years (S.D. 1·0). In contrast, the figures for the patients of Weinberger et al. (1980a, b) were 30·4 (S.D. 7·5), 12·2 (S.D. 6·4), and 7·5 (S.D. 4·0) respectively. It would therefore appear that enlargement of the ventricles is a slow process, and this is the implication of the results of Tanaka et al. (1981), who found ventricular enlargement in older schizophrenics but not in younger ones.

The large proportion of chronic schizophrenics who suffer from 'negative' symptoms (apathy, withdrawal, mannerisms, mutism) have CAT scans which indicate the presence of cerebral atrophy, and often show age disorientation and cognitive defects, are also likely to have a poor response to medication (Weinberger et al., 1980a) and a history of inadequate adjustment in childhood (Weinberger et al., 1980b). Abnormal CAT scans are much less common in acute schizophrenia. It would appear that the presence of cerebral damage leading to atrophy is an important factor in producing a chronic outcome and deterioration. Alternatively, we may consider that there are two kinds of schizophrenia; that which has an acute onset with more or less complete recovery, and that (often accompanied by cerebral damage and atrophy) which tends, with or without an acute onset, to chronicity and deterioration.

Biochemistry and Drug Action

Dopamine Hypothesis

Although the symptoms of schizophrenia can be alleviated by drugs, this does not logically imply that the disorder has a biochemical basis. However, the fact that drugs can produce a condition closely resembling schizophrenia does provide evidence for such a theory. Chronic intoxication with amphetamine produces a condition which is indistinguishable from paranoid schizophrenia (Connell, 1958). Similar effects have been reported arising from abuse of phenmetrazine and diethylpropion. In volunteers, increasing doses of amphetamine have led to paranoid changes. Intravenous injection of methylphenidate has produced an exacerbation of symptoms in patients recovering from acute schizophrenia.

Amphetamine and its related compounds are potent releasers of the neuro-transmitter dopamine. L-Dopa, which is a dopamine precursor, is used for the treatment of Parkinson's disease and has been reported to produce psychotic symptoms as side-effects. When it has been given to schizophrenics who are suffering from drug-induced Parkinsonism, it has sometimes produced an exacerbation of the symptoms.

It has been shown that neuroleptic drugs block the action of dopamine and this has been demonstrated in several ways. The effect of dopamine on dopaminergic receptors is to stimulate adenylate cyclase and produce a release of cyclic AMP, and this response is prevented by neuroleptics. In this way the blocking effect of neuroleptics can be measured accurately (Iverson et al., 1975). The effect can be shown even on individual neurons. Dopamine terminals are found in the cingulate gyrus and limbic areas of the cerebral cortex, but the major dopamine pathways in the brain rise from neurons in the substantia nigra and terminate in the caudate nucleus. This is the pathway which is degenerate in Parkinson's disease. The extrapyramidal signs and symptoms of Parkinson's disease therefore appear when there is a deficiency of the dopaminergic system (and are treatable with the dopamine precursor L-dopa), and the commonest side-effect of neuroleptic drugs is the appearance of Parkinsonism.

When measured in this way, dopamine-blocking effects of neuroleptics are directly related to the clinical potency, but with some important exceptions, e.g. butyrophenones and pimozide. However, Creese et al. (1976) showed that the ability of neuroleptics to inhibit the binding of haloperidol and dopamine on post-synaptic dopamine receptors was closely correlated with their clinical potencies, and this included the exceptions. In fact, Seeman et al. (1976) found that this was true of all the clinically effective drugs which they had tested.

It would appear that these two methods of measurement are related to two kinds of receptors D_1 and D_2, and it is the latter which is most closely related to the neuroleptic-blocking effect and the symptoms of schizophrenia. This work suggests that there is an excessive activity of dopaminergic neurons in schizophrenia. However, it has long been known that true Parkinson's disease (with its dopamine deficiency) can occur in schizophrenics. This is confirmed by post-mortem studies of schizophrenic brains, which do not show an increase in concentration of dopamine or its metabolites (homovanillic acid and dihydroxyphenylacetic acid). What has been found is an increase in the number of dopamine receptors, as shown by spiroperidol binding. This increase is almost certainly not the result of treatment with neuroleptics, as it can be found where there has not been any treatment with these drugs, and has not been found in the brains of cases of Huntington's chorea who have received them. The increase is greatest in the nucleus accumbens, putamen, and caudate nucleus (Owen et al., 1978). It can be inferred that the essential change is not an increase in dopamine activity but a hypersensitivity of the dopaminergic systems. Crow et al. (1977) were even more specific. They showed, in work on rat brains, that the clinical potency of chlorpromazine, thioridazine, and fluphenazine corresponded to the effect of these drugs on the nucleus accumbens, but that on the neostratum corresponded to the extra-pyramidal side-effects of these drugs.

The molecular structure of the phenothiazines and thioxanthenes consists of a three-ringed nucleus, with a side-chain attached to the middle ring. (*See Fig.* 5, p. 147.) This structure is often depicted with the side-chain at right angles to the nucleus, but in fact the chlorine, or other substituent, at the R_2 position, pulls the side-chain over to that side. Phenothiazines which have no substitution at the R_2 position, e.g. promethazine, do not possess any neuroleptic action.

In the thioxanthenes, the side-chain is connected to the heterocyclic nucleus by a double bond, which fixes the position of the side-chain so that it points to one end or the other of the nucleus (*cis–trans* isomerism). The thioxanthenes have two forms, alpha- and beta-isomers. The former is a considerably greater dopamine blocker than the latter and X-ray analysis shows that the alpha-isomer has the *cis* configuration, with the amine side-chain on the same side as the R_2 substitution. In a clinical trial on acute schizophrenics comparing the two isomers of flupenthixol with a placebo (Johnstone et al., 1978), it was found that the patients receiving the beta-isomer and the placebo improved about the same amount, but those on the alpha-isomer had a significantly greater improvement at the third and fourth weeks of treatment.

This suggests that the neuroleptic action arises from the shape of the molecule. Horn and Snyder (1971) pointed out that the *trans* form of dopamine (the active form) could be superimposed on the X-ray crystallographic structure of chlorpromazine. The neuroleptic butaclamol exists in two stereo-isomeric forms, only one of which is a dopamine blocker, thus confirming the hypothesis. Furthermore, it does not have a substituent at the R_2 position and resembles the tricyclic anti-depressants more than the conventional neuroleptics. A neuroleptic and dopamine-blocking effect therefore depends more on the shape than on the precise composition of the molecule.

The corpus striatum and caudate nucleus contain large amounts of acetylcholine as well as dopamine. When the latter is blocked, as with neuroleptics, the symptoms of Parkinsonism appear and this can be counteracted by anti-cholinergic (muscarinic) drugs such as benztropine and procyclidine. Neuroleptics also have an anti-cholinergic (muscarinic) effect, sometimes very powerful. The most potent in this respect are thioridazine and clozapine, and the weakest are flupenthixol, trifluoperazine, and spiroperidol. The ratio of anti-cholinergic to anti-dopaminergic effect varies widely, thioridazine and clozapine having the highest ratio and flupenthixol and spiroperidol the lowest. Thus some neuroleptics have a built-in anti-cholinergic effect which prevents the appearance of side-effects from the anti-dopaminergic action.

Differences in response to treatment run parallel with differences in dopaminergic function. Rotrosen et al. (1976) investigated the effects of injection of apomorphine (a direct-acting dopamine agonist) on the secretion of growth hormone, in schizophrenic patients (chronic patients during an acute exacerbation) and control subjects. The patients responded very differently from the controls. There was a high secretion of growth hormone in those who later failed to respond to neuroleptic treatment, and a low secretion in those who did respond. The controls were intermediate. No such differences were seen in response to L-dopa (which is an indirect agonist) given orally. There was an inverse relationship in individuals to these two drugs.

The clinical significance of this becomes clear when the drug trial mentioned above (Johnstone et al., 1978) is considered in detail. It was found that the symptoms which responded to alpha-flupenthixol were thought disorder, delusions, and hallucinations ('positive' symptoms), and this applied equally to those patients who were deteriorated and to those who were not. Angrist et al. (1980) administered D-amphetamine (0·5 mg/kg) to 21 schizophrenics and followed this by treatment with haloperidol. The symptoms which were exacerbated by amphetamine and subsequently responded to the neuroleptic drug were the 'positive' symptoms of thought disorder, hallucinations, delusions, tension, excitement, mannerisms, hostility, suspiciousness, and unco-operativeness, and the 'negative' symptom of emotional withdrawal. Motor retardation and blunted affect remained static.

The lack of response to amphetamine of 'negative' symptoms corresponds to a general resistiveness to the drug by chronic schizophrenics. Kornetsky (1976) gave 20 mg of D-amphetamine in the evening to 9 such patients (under double-blind conditions) without affecting their sleep. A dose of 40 mg did not affect their performance on a digit symbol test and a continuous performance test for brain damage, though it decreased their scores on symbol copying and increased it in tapping speed.

The dopamine theory of schizophrenia has many lacunae, as its protagonists freely acknowledge, but it has so much to back it that it is impossible to see how it could be completely replaced. One serious deficiency is that it does not account for the delay, lasting more than 2 weeks, in the response to neuroleptic medication. Its relation to the mode of action of the neuroleptic drugs should be limited to the acute symptoms of schizophrenia. Its relevance to the effect of neuroleptics in chronic schizophrenia is not clear. Such improvement in symptoms as occurs does not appear to help these patients to respond better to social influences (Hamilton et al., 1960).

An excellent account of the current status of the theory, and one which also mentions the possibility of a viral factor in the aetiology, is to be found in the two papers by Crow (1980, 1981).

Other Neuro-transmitters

Neuroleptics, including the butyrophenones and pimozide, also diminish the uptake of gamma-aminobutyric acid (GABA) which is an inhibitory neuro-transmitter. Baclofen (a GABA homologue) has a weak affinity for GABA-binding sites. It has been reported that administration of this drug led to an exacerbation of symptoms in schizophrenics. Sodium valproate (dipropylacetic sodium) blocks the breakdown of GABA and increases its level in the brain. It has been said that sodium valproate can produce an amelioration of schizophrenic symptoms, but this has not been confirmed by Lautin et al. (1980), even with doses running up to 3000 mg daily.

Noradrenaline is more prominent in the human forebrain than either dopamine or 5-hydroxytryptamine (Farley and Hornykiewicz, 1977) and evidence is accumulating that there is increased noradrenergic activity in the brains of schizophrenics (Gomes et al., 1980). Yorkston et al. (1977) found that propanolol (a beta-adrenergic blocker) was an effective treatment for schizophrenics who had not improved on neuroleptics. It is relevant to mention here that chlorpromazine, which was the first of the neuroleptics to be introduced and is probably still the one most commonly prescribed, blocks noradrenergic receptors as effectively as it does dopaminergic ones.

Endocrine and Metabolic Disorders

That schizophrenia is inherited genetically provides the one unequivocal fact for a biochemical basis for this disorder. Nevertheless, it must be remembered that although schizophrenia can have devastating effects on the patient's social life, from a crude biological point of view it is a remarkably trivial disorder. A patient can become schizophrenic in the early twenties, or even as a teenager, and yet live to a ripe old age. Whatever biochemical 'lesions' may be present will therefore not be related to fundamental vital processes. It is therefore not surprising that biochemical investigations of urine, blood and cerebrospinal fluid have not until recently yielded findings which can be regarded as steps in understanding the constitutional basis of schizophrenia. The one exception is Gjessing's findings (1932–53) in periodic catatonia.

Although schizophrenic symptoms can occur in various endocrine disorders, no specific endocrine disturbances have been shown to have any aetiological significance. Much interest has been shown in the endocrine changes, especially prolactin and growth hormone, following treatment with neuroleptics, and it is possible that these may be of value in monitoring and selection of treatments.

Intoxications

Hallucinogens

It is now accepted that the hallucinogens, e.g. mescaline, lysergic acid diethylamide (LSD), have no bearing on schizophrenia. Their most prominent effect is visual sense deceptions and they also produce a mild clouding of consciousness. Auditory hallucinations, which are so prominent in schizophrenia, are not prominent.

Organic hallucinosis, which is sometimes caused by sub-acute coarse brain disease, resembles schizophrenia more than any other psychosis. In this condition the patient hears continuous auditory hallucinations in a state of clear consciousness and has delusions of persecution which are a logical result of the hallucinations. These symptoms most commonly occur in alcoholism, but may occur in sub-acute infections of the lung, brain trauma, cerebral anoxia, and carbon monoxide and carbon disulphide poisoning. They may also occur in general paresis which has been treated with malaria. If the damage to the brain is reversible, then organic hallucinosis disappears in a few weeks. Some epileptic psychoses resemble paranoid schizophrenia and in the absence of a history of epilepsy may lead to difficulties of diagnosis.

Amphetamine Psychosis

A paranoid psychosis with bodily and auditory hallucinations may occur in amphetamine addicts. In this condition, clouding of consciousness is often absent and the clinical picture may be indistinguishable from paranoid schizophrenia. (*See above*, p. 25 and p. 28.)

Personality and Physique

The role of the personality in the causation of schizophrenia has been the subject of discussion for a long time but less so in recent years. It has been claimed that the pre-morbid personality of schizophrenics is usually abnormal and schizoid in type. The schizoid personality is a quiet, shut-in person who shows little emotion, is usually unsociable, and indulges in excessive private fantasy. The incidence of abnormal pre-morbid personalities in schizophrenia has been investigated by many workers. Arnold (1955) found that in a series of 500 schizophrenics, 32·2 per cent had normal pre-morbid personalities, in 26·2 per cent the nature of the pre-morbid personality was uncertain and not ascertainable, 26·2 per cent had schizoid personalities, and 15·4 per cent had abnormal personalities of a non-schizoid variety. M. Bleuler (1972) found that only 64 per cent of a series of schizophrenics had pre-morbid schizoid personalities. The findings of Holmboe and Astrup (1957) are shown in *Table* 6.

Table 6. OUTCOME AND PRE-PSYCHOTIC PERSONALITY IN ACUTE SCHIZOPHRENIA
(*After Holmboe and Astrup*)

	Outcome			
Pre-psychotic personality	*Recovered*	*Improved*	*Deteriorated*	*Total*
Schizoid	13	11	36	60
Sensitive	32	18	33	83
Self-assertive	19	9	11	39
Cycloid	7	5	6	18
Hysterical	6	2	3	11
Neurotic	13	5	8	26
Harmonious	22	8	17	47
Incomplete information	1	0	4	5
Total	113	58	118	289

This table is also relevant to the discussion of prognosis in Chapter 7.

Apart from semantic troubles, there are several difficulties in the way of accurate assessment of pre-morbid personality. The amount of information about the previous personality may be slight or the reliability of such information doubtful, and the doctor and the relatives often tend to be wise after the event. At times it is difficult to determine the exact point of onset of the illness so that personality change due to illness is mistaken for the pre-morbid personality. Since many adolescents have difficulty in growing up, and behave badly, it is often difficult to decide whether the unusual behaviour before the appearance of obvious symptoms has been due to an adolescent disturbance or to early undiagnosable schizophrenia. It seems likely that in some cases the schizophrenic illness has been provoked by severe adolescent difficulties, so that the schizophrenia emerges against the background of an adolescent crisis. The more one deals with human beings in adolescence and early adult life, the more one is forced to the conclusion that it is unwise to assume that personality is firmly fixed before the age of 25 years, so that assessments of the pre-morbid personality in young schizophrenics are not very reliable.

In English-speaking countries a considerable number of psychiatrists believe that the abnormal pre-morbid personality is an essential feature of schizophrenia and that the illness is a morbid psychological development of the personality. It is difficult to understand how such symptoms as hearing one's own thoughts spoken aloud and formal thought disorder can be understood as due to a development of a personality. If this idea is rejected, then there must be some other explanation of the excess of abnormal pre-morbid personalities in schizophrenics. One explanation is that abnormal personalities are extremely common in the general population and are in fact no more common in schizophrenia. The incidence of psychopathy in the general population is difficult to estimate. Ekblad (1948), in a series of recruits to the Swedish Navy, found an incidence of psychopathy (using the definition of K. Schneider) of 15 per cent. In a survey of a rural population, Essen-Möller and his associates found an incidence of psychopathy of 7·5 per cent in males. Johanson (1958), in a series of 71 male schizophrenics, found an incidence of abnormal and schizoid personalities which was considerably higher than that found by Ekblad in a normal population, but the difference was not statistically significant. Even here, the study of twins provides some information although, as usual, the data can be interpreted in two ways. Cadoret (1973) reported on monozygotic twins discordant for schizophrenia. A high proportion of the co-twins were found to have character disorder (higher among the males) or neurotic symptoms (higher among the females).

Granting that there is an excess of abnormal pre-morbid personalities among schizophrenics, it is not necessary to suppose that there is a direct connexion between the abnormal personality and the illness. An abnormal personality is more liable to place himself in a stressful situation than a normal person and, having done so, will, because of his abnormal personality, be more likely to become very disturbed than a normal person. Since it is legitimate to assume that psychological stress may precipitate schizophrenia in a predisposed person, it is therefore to be expected that there will be many more abnormal pre-morbid personalities among any group of schizophrenics than there are in the general population.

Interest in the body types associated with mental disorders has faded. In general, it can be said that in a representative sample of schizophrenics there will be more thin, ill-thriven, gawky subjects than in the general population. The impression given by the studies on body build and psychosis is that the change in body build with age may account for a good deal of the difference in incidence of pyknic body build among schizophrenics and manic depressives. There is a further criticism, namely, that the patient's body build may influence the psychiatrist's diagnosis.

ENVIRONMENTAL FACTORS

Childhood Development and Family Relationships

Environmental theories on the aetiology of schizophrenia are not alternatives to genetic theories but supplementary to them, for the actual rates of concordance in monozygotic twins leave plenty of room for environmental factors. Adoption studies show that modes of upbringing are not all that important, but there is some evidence that inter-familial relationships play a part. It has become clear that maternal deprivation, unhappy, disorganized, and broken homes can give rise to an increase in delinquency but there is no evidence that the same is true for the incidence of neurosis in the children. It is even less likely, therefore, that they will give rise to schizophrenia.

Alanen (1958) studied the mother–child relationship in 100 schizophrenics in whom the illness began under the age of 30 years, and compared them with the mothers of 20 neurotic patients and 20 normal persons as controls. More than half of the mothers of the schizophrenics were affected by disorders exceeding the psychoneurotic level and some of the mothers were manifestly psychotic, others being schizoid or borderline psychotics. Several of them showed very accentuated blockage or constriction of affective life, poor self-control, and inability to feel themselves into the inner life of other people. They showed a schizoid pattern of inter-personal relationships, they were dominating, lacked understanding, and did not respect the child as an independent person. However, the investigation also showed that the disorders in the fathers were not less marked. Further work (Alanen, 1968) emphasized the importance of the entire interactional dynamics of the family network rather than the mother–child relationship alone. The parents of the patients had greatly disturbed marriages. The atmosphere of the family showed two predominant patterns, being either chaotic or rigid. In the former there was faulty identification and the atmosphere was incoherent and irrational, often disproportionately dominated by one parent's psychotic or borderline level of thought and behaviour disorders. The latter group showed pathogenetic emotional relationships, rigidity of roles, and emotional impoverishment, together with unbending attitudes and expectations that one or both parents directed to the children. The future schizophrenic patient could not achieve sufficient independence but remained in heightened dependence upon his parents.

Singer and Wynne (1965) studied samples of conjoint family therapy sessions and also the protocols of projective tests. On this basis they concluded that the parents of schizophrenics were unable to focus attention selectively on shared percepts or feelings, or keep internal and external states discreet. They tended to communicate in such a way that the listener tries to understand, but ends up distrusting his own understanding. In consequence, meaningful communication within the family becomes almost impossible. Their special method of evaluating the Rorschach test made extensive use of the concept of sharing foci of attention and of sharing 'sets' and role relationships (Singer, 1967; Wynne, 1967). They found that peculiarities of speech and language usage, mostly not of the kind found among schizophrenics, differentiated most significantly between the parents of schizophrenics and controls. This work was to some extent confirmed by Hirsch and Leff (1975) who found that the speech of the parents of schizophrenics did show abnormalities, e.g. vagueness and odd associations, but the differences from controls were very much less than those of Wynne. Much of the differences between the schizophrenic and control groups was related to the talkativeness of the fathers of the more severe schizophrenics. None of the forms of behaviour observed in the families of schizophrenics was unique to them. Rather, the differences were a matter of frequency of behaviour. The characteristics of the parents of childhood psychotic patients were quite markedly different from those of the parents of schizophrenics who became ill in adolescence or young adulthood (Singer and Wynne, 1963).

In a prospective study by Doane et al. (1981) on disturbed adolescents followed up after 5 years, it was found that those subjects, whose parents had both a pathological style and a high level of deviance in communicaton, developed schizophrenia-like disorders, at a statistically significant level. This confirms the Wynne and Singer findings, but the authors point out cautiously that parents living with a more disturbed child may develop disturbed ways of interaction.

Lidz (1968) and his colleagues (Lidz et al., 1957a, b) came to similar conclusions. In some of the families there was a marked marital schism in that the parents were hostile to each other and attempted to undermine the affection of the children for the opposite partner. In other families there was a marital skew, i.e. one partner was grossly abnormal and the other partner accepted the grossly abnormal ideas and attitudes. They obtained objective confirmation of their findings by means of a special method of scoring the object sorting tests which discriminated between the parents of schizophrenics and the parents of normal controls at a high level of statistical significance (Wild et al., 1965). According to Lidz, schizophrenia is a way of life adopted by the patient to escape from insoluble conflicts induced by a family environment that encouraged irrationality.

Bateson et al. (1956) investigated the parent–child relationship in schizophrenics and claimed that the parents used a 'double-bind' technique in order to control the child. This consists of the parents giving the child a negative injunction and threatening punishment if he does not obey; at the same time he is given a second injunction which conflicts with the first and which is usually not expressed in words. Thus the child is trained to think illogically and finally becomes schizophrenic because of the intolerable stress produced by the 'double-bind' relationship. The emphasis here is on the importance of the content of the communication, which is the exact opposite of the theories of Wynne and Singer who emphasize the importance of the style rather than the content. It may be added that Hall and Levin (1980), using audio tapes and transcripts of family interactions, were unable to confirm the 'double-bind' hypothesis.

Much of this work has been severely criticized in a review by Mednick and McNeil (1968) who pointed out the great methodological difficulties which had not been overcome in this kind of research. Since the patients were already schizophrenic, the consequents of schizophrenia could not be separated out from the aetiological aspect. Even the examination of childhood records is liable to bias in selection.

In addition, the investigations of the parents of schizophrenics are open to the objection that only the parents of young schizophrenics can be investigated. However, in over 40 per cent of cases schizophrenia begins after the age of 30 years. One would expect to find a high incidence of unusual parents and families among young schizophrenics, because such factors are liable to produce a disturbed adolescence, and therefore to bring to light a genetically predisposed schizophrenic illness which in more favourable circumstances might not appear until much later in life, if at all.

Social Isolation

In 1939 Faris and Dunham showed that the incidence of schizophrenia was highest in the central areas of Chicago where social isolation was greatest, whereas the incidence was lowest in the wealthy residential areas on the periphery of the city. These results were confirmed by several other investigations in different American cities. Hare (1956) investigated the incidence of schizophrenia in the city of Bristol and suggested that a pre-psychotic drift to areas of social isolation probably accounted for some of the increased incidence of schizophrenia in the central areas. The importance of 'downward social drift' was made clear by the work of Goldberg and Morrison (1963). They found the usual excess of patients from social class 5 among young male schizophrenics (first admissions) but showed that social class of the fathers of the patients was similar to that of the whole population. This was confirmed in the USA by further work in Detroit (Dunham, 1965). A high concentration of schizophrenic patients was again found in the socially isolated areas, but this was largely due to migration of these patients into those areas. It would appear that since then further changes have occurred and even the specific concentration has now disappeared (Levy and Rowitz, 1973).

Sundby (1955) investigated the incidence of schizophrenia in Norwegian merchant seamen and found that it was higher than in the general population, but the incidence of schizophrenia in the families of the seamen was lower than in a control group of schizophrenics. There was also a high incidence of psychopathic traits in the premorbid personalities of the seamen and Sundby felt that this had determined their choice of the Merchant Navy as a career. This seems to show that predisposed unstable persons tend to choose a career which leads to social isolation and difficult inter-personal relationships, and this in its turn may lead to the development of schizophrenia.

Roth (1957) has pointed out that the statistics of the Registrar-General for England and Wales (1950–51) show that 45 per cent of the total number of schizophrenics come from social class 5 which is only 18·4 per cent of the total population. He has also shown that isolation due to social or physical factors is commonly found in association with 'late paraphrenia'.

One of the most important of these is deafness, as had been pointed out by Kraepelin, which gives a paranoid colouring to the symptoms. Thus, Kay and Roth (1961) found hearing impairment in 40 per cent of their late paraphrenics and pointed out that ageing, social isolation, and deafness were of aetiological importance. Houston (1954) found a higher prevalence of paranoid schizophrenia among deaf patients than among those who were not deaf. Cooper and Curry (1976) found more frequent bilateral conductive deafness among late paranoid schizophrenics than among control groups.

Psychological Stress

It is extremely difficult to assess the role of psychological stress in the precipitation of schizophrenic illnesses. Brown et al. (1973) have described a method for deciding whether a life-event can be regarded as precipitating mental illness or playing a causative part. With this method, they were able to demonstrate that life-stresses merely precipitated the onset of schizophrenia, but were formative in the depressions. Clancy et al. (1973) found that precipitating events could be found in 10 per cent of schizophrenics as compared with 35 per cent in primary affective disorders. These events bore little relationship to the personal or social characteristics of the patients or to the clinical picture of the resulting disorder. Holmboe and Astrup (1957) have evaluated the precipitating factors in their series of 255 schizophrenic and schizophreniform psychoses. In 19 there was acute mental trauma, in 149 prolonged psychological conflicts, in 22 social misery or isolation, in 37 physical illnesses, including childbirth, in 19 intoxications, mainly alcoholic, and in 51 no specific causative factors were mentioned in the case notes.

Indirect evidence is found in the work of Wallis (1972) who found, among 512 Naval personnel discharged for schizophrenia, that a greater severity of psychological stresses preceding the onset of illness was associated with a better prognosis. The implication is that constitutional and precipitating factors are inversely related and indicates that psychological stresses can precipitate the development of schizophrenia.

Physical Illness

There is no doubt that physical illness, and also childbirth, may precipitate a schizophrenic illness. Sometimes it is not easy to be sure of the diagnosis of schizophrenia because an affective disorder may be provoked by a physical illness and the clinical picture may be made atypical by the continuing physical illness. Affective disorders in the puerperium are often somewhat atypical owing perhaps to the concomitant endocrine changes.

Chapter 3

Symptomatology

The main symptoms of schizophrenia can be grouped as disorders of thought, perception, emotion, and motor behaviour. Disorders of consciousness and memory may occur but are not pathognomonic. Since symptoms never occur on their own, but in connexion with other symptoms in symptom complexes, it is somewhat artificial to deal with the individual schizophrenic symptoms in isolation. Nevertheless, it is necessary to present the facts in an orderly way.

Thought Disorder

The term 'thought disorder' is often used somewhat loosely. However, for the purposes of description and discussion, it can be divided into the following four groups:

1. Disorders of the form of thought.
2. Disorders of the stream of thought.
3. Disorders of the possession of thought.
4. Disorders of the content of thought.

This is a purely artificial scheme, but is a useful way of organizing knowledge.

Formal Thought Disorder

This is diagnostic of schizophrenia if coarse brain disease can be excluded, since a rather similar disorder occasionally occurs in subacute organic states. Schizophrenic formal thought disorder can be defined as a gross disorder of conceptual thinking in the absence of coarse brain disease and in the presence of direct or indirect evidence that the patient had an adequate intellectual performance in the past. The direct evidence is the presence of a vocabulary that is much greater than could be expected from the low level of conceptual thinking, whereas the indirect evidence is the information from outside sources that the patient was of average intelligence at some time in the past.

Formal thought disorder is one of the unifying features of schizophrenia. All schizophrenics show some formal thought disorder if their illness lasts long enough. The subject is of such importance that the views and descriptions of certain authors will now be presented briefly. The description of the phenomena and the terms used depend largely on the investigator's psychological approach, so that apparent differences between different investigators are often merely differences in terminology.

E. Bleuler (1924) described formal thought disorder in terms of 'association psychology'. He considered that the basic disorder was a disorder of association which in its turn led to an increase in autistic thinking. The absence of a central determining idea leads to the sequence of thought being determined by incidental associations such as sound, alliteration, or non-essential details, so that the association between one idea and the next is not obvious. This disorder of association leads to a changeableness and lack of clarity of the concepts which are falsely constructed by condensation, displacement, and symbolism. In condensation, ideas which have something in common are lumped together regardless of logic, whereas in displacement an associated idea is used in place of the correct one. By symbolism, Bleuler meant the misuse of symbols, usually the use of symbols in a concrete way, as, for example, when a patient said, 'I hear a stork clapping in my body', by which she meant she believed that she was pregnant. Apart from this false elaboration of concepts there is also a decay of concepts, in that the boundaries between different concepts are not maintained so that parts of one concept may be incorporated in another. The weakness in association allows the affects to dominate the train of thought and this leads to an increase in autistic (dereistic) thinking, by which is meant fantasy thinking which is not goal-directed. It is of particular significance that disturbance of association improves under the influence of neuroleptics (Namyslowska, 1975).

Since the outstanding feature of schizophrenic formal thought disorder is the lack of genuine causal links, Cameron (1944) has called it 'asyndetic thinking'. He considers that the patient uses clusters of more or less related sequences of thought instead of well-knit sequences so that there is a general vagueness or woolliness of thought. The patient is unable to restrict his thinking to the task in hand, to eliminate all unnecessary material, and to focus his thoughts upon any given topic. There is a tendency to use imprecise approximations and to substitute terms or phrases instead of the more exact expressions. Cameron calls these imprecise approximations 'metonyms' and points out that, apart from the metonyms, the patient tends to have an idiosyncratic speech in that he uses an asocial dialect which is full of personal idioms. Cameron has also called attention to two other psychological disorders in asyndetic thinking, namely, interpenetration of themes and over-inclusion. When the protocols of schizophrenic speech are studied, two different streams of thought can be isolated. There is one which deals with the current task or situation and the other which is due to a preoccupation with personal matters, so that the goal-directed stream of thought is interfered with by a stream of preoccupation which is mainly based on fantasy. In over-inclusion, the patient cannot maintain the boundaries of the problem and restrict his operations within the limits of the problem. Thus the patient is unable to narrow down the operations of his thought and bring into play organized attitudes or specific responses which are readily available in the normal subject. This disorder of thought does not prevent the schizophrenic from making generalizations and he can often set up many different hypotheses and shift from one hypothesis to another. However, his generalizations are not very useful since they include too much, are too involved, and are inexplicably entangled with private fantasy.

Goldstein (1944) has attempted to explain schizophrenic thought disorder by means of his modified *Gestalt* theories and his concepts of concrete and abstract attitudes. When the subject has the concrete attitude, he is unable to escape from a given object or situation and he therefore experiences things in their uniqueness, so that his behaviour is determined by the immediate claim which some particular aspect of the object or situation makes upon him. The subject with an abstract attitude deals with his experiences from a conceptual point of view so that he perceives objects as representatives of a class or as accidental examples of a category, because the individual unique qualities of the object are neglected. This abstract attitude allows the patient to assume a mental set voluntarily, to shift at will from one aspect of a situation to another, to keep in mind different aspects of the situation, to grasp the essentials of a given whole, and to see the relations of the parts to the whole. It also allows a subject to plan ahead intentionally, to assume an attitude to the mere possible, to think and perform symbolically, and to detach the ego from the external world.*

Goldstein considers that an impairment of the abstract attitude is partly responsible for the schizophrenic formal thought disorder, since the concrete attitude causes the schizophrenic to be unduly influenced by external stimuli which arise at any given moment. The patient is abnormally bound to external stimuli as long as these stimuli are connected with the reality which the patient is experiencing. As a result of the concrete attitude, words cease to have a generic meaning and tend to have an individual character, so that words which indicate categories or classes are used in a way which does not correspond to the generalizations which they normally signify. The patient chooses words according to the peculiar way in which he is experiencing a certain object or situation. Physiognomic concreteness

* Goldstein claims that the abstract attitude is not the same as intelligence, but it is difficult to see how it differs from intelligence. Thus, one textbook defines intelligence as 'the capacity to discern relevant qualities and relations and to deduce relevant correlates'.

occurs, that is, the striking superficial aspect of objects plays an undue part in determining the significance of the object for the patient because he is bound to immediate experience. Cutting and Ryan (1982) attempted to test experimentally Goldstein's theory of 'concrete thinking' but were unable to confirm it.

Goldstein considers that symptoms in coarse brain disease are due to 'isolation', that is, parts of the nervous system are isolated from the whole of the nervous system. This isolation produces a change in the threshold of excitability and forces the patient to respond to every stimulus, so that reactions are more easily evoked and tend to be carried out in a rigid way. Disorganization of the figure–ground relationships is also produced by isolation. Goldstein considers that such schizophrenic symptoms as lack of ability to concentrate, increased rigidity and distractibility of intellectual performance, forced responsiveness to stimuli, and pathological fixation to stimuli are due to isolation. Disorganization of the figure–ground relationships in schizophrenia is also due to this disorder. In normal conceptual thinking, the essential aspects of the situation act as the 'figure' which stands out against the 'ground' composed of non-essential aspects. This figure–ground relationship demands ability to extract essentials from the situation and to introduce the relevant relationships which are not phenomenally present. Both these abilities depend on the abstract attitude. Adequate figure–ground relationships are not possible in schizophrenia because the patient cannot distinguish between the essential and non-essential. Stable figure–ground relationships may never be set up, since the patient is unable to maintain adequate boundaries. In particular, the boundaries between the ego and the external world disappear, so that the self is no longer experienced as standing out against a background of the environment.

Impairment of the abstract attitude and 'isolation' occur in organic psychiatric syndromes as well as in schizophrenia. However, Goldstein claims that the disorders take a simple inane form in organic defect and the patient's behaviour in such conditions is based upon simple 'means–end' relationships which can easily be understood by the observer. In the organic state thought is non-conceptual and behaviour is based on a simple stimulus response mechanism. Concreteness of perception occurs in schizophrenia, but the perception is not based on a simple 'means–end' relationship but on personal idiosyncratic ideas. The world of the schizophrenic is animated by personalized ideas and is very much richer in material than that of the organic. The physiognomic aspects of perception play a much greater role in thought and behaviour in schizophrenics than in patients with severe brain damage.

Carl Schneider (1930) investigated schizophrenic speech and

thought in great detail. A brief account of his views will be given here since they are essential for an understanding of his interesting classification of schizophrenia. He described four characteristics of schizophrenic speech: fusion, derailment, omission, and drivelling. Fusion consists of a blending together of heterogeneous elements of speech into a senseless unity, for example, 'As soon as the skull has gone smash and one still has flowers with difficulty.' In derailment, speech proceeds along a given path but then suddenly slips into a new direction, for example, 'Councillor, that lies on the parquet floor, if one watches correctly, since there is putty in there.' The content of the new thought in derailment can be seen to consist of ideas which lie close to the original train of thought. Omission occurs when a part of a thought in the main stream drops out so that the stream of thought is interrupted, for example, 'I and what is also so comic, consequently the nun has not known me any more.' In the drivelling expression of thought there are sequences of thought which are fairly well formed and organized, but which are mixed up together in confusion, for example, 'And once the ladies' tailoring trade for men and the men's tailoring trade for women causes a jacket to be applied, which is buttoned on the side which is put opposite.' Thus the grammar and syntax of the sentences are quite good but the content is utter drivel.*

Kleist (1914) has discussed the problem from the neurological point of view and has compared schizophrenic speech disorder with aphasia. He considers that disorders such as literal paraphasia, verbal paraphasia, agrammatism, and paragrammatism can be found in the speech of schizophrenics. Literal paraphasia, which is a common aphasic symptom, consists of a disorder of production of a sound or sequence of sounds in a given word. This symptom is occasionally seen in catatonic schizophrenics. Verbal paraphasia, in which the correct word cannot be found or a word is used incorrectly, can be regarded as a disorder of word storage or word usage. In schizophrenia the patient is usually able to find a word which he wants, but often he uses the same word to designate many different things. Kleist considers this to be a disorder of word storage and uses the term 'stock word' to designate these words which are used repeatedly with different meanings. In some cases the impoverished word store leads the patient to use concrete words instead of abstract ones. When this occurs in acute schizophrenia it may lead to an apparent increase in the richness of the vocabulary and thus give the impression of a true increase in verbal ability.

Verbal paraphasia may affect secondary word formations, that is, derivations or combinations of words. In schizophrenia word forma-

*All the examples have been taken from *Die Psychologie der Schizophrenen*, by C. Schneider, 1930, Thieme, Leipzig.

tions may be incorrectly constructed or there may be an impoverishment of the word store which leads to the use of stock word formations. In some cases patients make combinations or derivations of words in a uniformly correct way. Thus one patient used the word 'vessel' for nearly all objects and called a watch a 'time vessel'. Occasionally, the disorder of the co-ordination of secondary word formations may occur, so that the secondary word formations are used in a disordered and exaggerated way. For example, a patient called a candle 'a night illumination object'. Agrammatism and paragrammatism, which are disorders of word sequence, are frequently found in schizophrenia. In agrammatism there is a simplification and coarsening of the word sequences so that all the less necessary words are omitted and the meaning is conveyed in agrammatical speech. On the other hand, the word sequence in paragrammatism is quite well formed, but the phrases and sentences are often incorrectly selected, mixed up, and contaminated with one another. The following quotation from Kleist illustrates these two speech disorders:

> Here is an example of agrammatism in a description which an old catatonic has given of two pictures. I compare this with the description of the first of these two pictures by a patient with paragrammatism. (In the first picture there is a mother with three children at a table. The two girls are writing, the boy turns up the lamp and holds a paper with writing on it over the top of the lamp in order to dry it. The mother is raising her finger in warning. In the second picture the lamp has fallen over and burst, the oldest girl runs away with her dress on fire, the boy is screaming and mother has seized the youngest girl's arm and turns to run away.)
>
> The catatonic describes the first picture as '. . . that is a rich table with woman (Q. the girl who is writing?) the woman is written (Q. the boy?) is rich to light . . . correctly on (Q. the other girl?) is correctly to writing woman.' The second picture: (Q. mother with the child on her arm?) 'Woman and son (Q. the girl running away? slanting body posture!) woman is rich lying (Q. screaming boy?) son is also a lamentation.' In this patient the word 'rich' penetrated all his verbal utterances, like a kind of associated movement.
>
> The description of the first picture by a paranoid with paragrammatism now follows: 'The impression of the picture makes it possible for one at present to bring into connection a living-room in which the apparent family members by the lady of the house with her three children at a table covered by a green table cloth outside the lit lamplight observed the employment of her loved little ones and she proves herself the housewife apparently to be working efficiently at crochet work. The observations of the children leads or led—according to the picture established here—shows a change of the body position of the person on the picture is represented . . . the mother shows at the same time a threat to the one lad, holds possibly on to the lamp already burning a piece of writing to dry on the warmth which rises up from out of the lamp glass, and certainly from the side of the mother an instruction about the consequences on the remaining fire small things had come to utterance because the oldest of them both the girls, according to her dress or according to her apparel as such made discernible, attention of the mother listening her employment with writing work have . . . has taken up.'

Apart from the speech disorders, Kleist has described three kinds of thought disorder, i.e. incoherence, paralogia, and alogia. In incoherence there is no understandable connexion between one thought and the next. However, in paralogia concepts either do not emerge or only emerge in an incomplete way, so that derailment into neighbouring concepts takes place and displacement and mixing up of different memory images (presentations) occur. Since the patient appears to have difficulty in organizing the raw material of his thought, Kleist considers paralogia to be a sensory thought disorder. In the third variety of thought disorder, alogia, the patient is unable to form relationships and to use acts of thought which have previously been accomplished, so that no new thoughts emerge. Kleist regards this inability to produce thought as a motor thought disorder. Unfortunately, it is not easy to distinguish this type of thought disorder from the poverty of speech and thought due to defective motivation, delusional aversion, catatonia, lack of attention, or mental deficiency.

Neologisms, or new word formations, are very common in the speech of schizophrenics. Since this symptom has been analysed in great detail by Kleist, it is convenient to discuss it at this point. A neologism may be a completely new word whose derivation cannot be understood, or it may be a word which has been incorrectly built up but its origins are clearly understandable, logically and grammatically, as due to a misuse of the accepted methods of word formation. Sometimes a neologism is an accepted word which is being used in an unusual way so that an old word acquires a new meaning. Kleist considers that some neologisms are due to speech disorder, so that literal paraphasia may produce neologisms due to sound distortions, and verbal paraphasia may lead to the production of new words or the use of known words in a special way. This means that some neologisms are in fact stock words. When verbal paraphasia takes place in connexion with secondary word formation, neologisms occur which are stock secondary word formations. The same disorder gives rise to unusual word derivations or to the construction of unusual word combinations which appear as neologisms. In severe agrammatism all particles and adverbs are omitted and a long string of inadequately related words is produced. This gives rise to the type of neologism which has been called a 'word monstrosity'. In other patients, the neologisms appear to be related entirely to some delusional experience and the patient uses a neologism to describe or designate a delusional experience or idea which is outside his normal experience. This type of neologism can be called a 'technical neologism' and can be regarded as a personal jargon invented to describe the peculiar schizophrenic experiences. In other patients the neologisms seem to be due to auditory hallucinations and the patient reproduces them or may feel himself obliged to use certain words to placate the hallucinatory voices or to protect himself from them.

Mannerisms and stereotypies may lead to the repeated use of distorted words so that in some cases neologisms are really catatonic symptoms.

It has been repeatedly shown that the mental speed of schizophrenics is slower than in normal subjects and that reaction times of schizophrenics are slower and more variable. The mental slowness can be explained on the basis of over-inclusion, since if a schizophrenic includes too much in his conceptual thinking it will take him much longer to produce the correct result. It has been shown that the score of schizophrenics for concreteness in the Goldstein–Sheerer Object Sorting Test correlates highly with their score on the Epstein Test of Over-inclusion (Payne and Hirst, 1957). Thus it is probable that Goldstein's concept of concreteness can be reconciled with Cameron's concept of over-inclusion. Some of the results of tests of schizophrenic thought disorder and behaviour suggest that schizophrenic subjects are more susceptible to reactive inhibition, as defined by Hull, and this could be a contributory cause of schizophrenic mental slowness.

There appear to be two major varieties of schizophrenic thought disorder. In one, the patient is unable to produce any thoughts, while in the other, the patient produces a wealth of unusual thoughts. Kleist has designated this inability to think as 'alogia', but this term is unsatisfactory. It might be better to designate this disorder as 'negative formal thought disorder'. The opposite variety of formal thought disorder has been called 'paralogia' by Kleist, but this term is open to the objection that it has already been used by English-speaking authors to designate *Vorbeireden* (talking past the point). In order to avoid any misunderstanding it is better to refer to this type of thought disorder as 'positive formal thought disorder'. Over-inclusion, that is, the inclusion of irrelevant material in the train of thought, is the outstanding feature of positive thought disorder and may take one of two forms, fusion or derailment. The blending of heterogeneous elements into a forced unity which occurs in fusion is probably the same as the phenomenon which Freud called 'condensation'. As mentioned previously, Bleuler considered that condensation was one method of construction of false concepts in schizophrenia. Derailment, which is the slipping of the train of thought into another direction, is probably the same as displacement in which a neighbouring concept is substituted for a relevant concept. Bleuler's symbolism and the physiognomic concreteness of Goldstein and other authors can be understood as special cases of derailment. The irregularity of the train of thought in schizophrenia, which ranges from incoherence to omission, can also be explained by over-inclusion, since fusion and derailment produce an irregular progression of thought and a loss of direction.

It is interesting that the concepts which Freud introduced to describe thinking in dreams are applicable to schizophrenic thinking. Apart from Freud, a large number of other investigators have drawn attention to the similarities between thinking in tired sleepy subjects and schizophrenics. Fusion and derailment are quite often found in hypnagogic and hypnopompic states. However, the absence of any gross change in the level of awareness in schizophrenia must make us cautious in drawing any conclusion about two apparently similar thought disorders in such basically different conditions.

It is possible to erect a theory of schizophrenic thought disorder on the basis of Cameron's other concept of the interpenetration of themes. Thus it could be supposed that the thought disorder is due to some process which is continually distracting the patient's thinking. Hassol et al. (1952) have carried out an interesting experiment using the concept of the interpenetration of themes. The subject was asked to tell a story about a TAT card* and this was recorded. A little later he was asked to tell another story about the same TAT card while the original story was being played back into earphones. These investigators rated the second story for scatter,† and claimed that scatter in these subjects was much greater than in those who produced a second story to the same TAT card without being subjected to any interference. This experiment supports the theory that mental activity in schizophrenia is continuously being interfered with by some interrupting process which is not of constant intensity but varies in severity. Since auditory hallucinations are extremely common in schizophrenia, and in many cases their severity is roughly proportional to the severity of the formal thought disorder, it is possible that auditory hallucinations are also produced by this interrupting process. It has been shown that when white noise‡ is played into the ears of schizophrenics while they are performing intellectual tests an improvement occurs in their test scores. The idea behind this experiment was that schizophrenics have defective motivation and will therefore perform better if adequately motivated by being placed in an unpleasant situation and being told that they would be released from it when they had finished the test. Results of this experiment could also be explained as being due to the successful blocking of a variable interrupting process by a constant white noise.

---

* A card from the thematic apperception test: Murray, H. A. (1943), *The Thematic Apperception Test.* Cambridge, Mass.: Harvard University Press.

† This is defined by Cameron as follows: 'We call a verbal statement "scattered" when it lacks a reasonable degree of organized sequence, when it includes imprecise, substitute, or approximate words or phrases (in place of more precise definitive ones), or when it is broken by pauses which are not followed by material that continues the trend in operation before the pause.'

‡ Noise in which all audible frequencies are equally represented.

Before passing on to consider other schizophrenic abnormalities of thinking it is convenient to consider here three symptoms—*Vorbeireden*, perseveration of theme, and self-reference of thinking—which are frequently encountered in association with formal thought disorder, although they cannot be considered to be due to this disorder. The term *Vorbeireden* has been taken over from the German to designate talking past the point, since no adequate English word exists, and the term 'paralogia' which has been used by some authors for this symptom has many different meanings. Patients showing this symptom talk somewhat irrelevantly, but there is internal evidence that the task set by the examiner has been understood by the patient who is deliberately talking about some allied subject. This symptom classically occurs in hysterical pseudodementia, but is by no means uncommon in acute and chronic schizophrenics. Sometimes it seems to be due to a childish playful attitude, while in other cases it seems to be an attempt to avoid contact and escape from the interview situation. Finally, it may be a catatonic phenomenon of the nature of forced responsiveness. As the patient is obliged to respond to the question immediately, he says the first thing that comes into his head. Thus, in these patients, *Vorbeireden* is the result of a catatonic disorder and of formal thought disorder. In most cases it is not possible to determine how much of the *Vorbeireden* is due to mental sets not directly connected with conceptual thinking as such, and how much is due to positive formal thought disorder. Perseveration of theme can be considered as a special variety of over-inclusion and it occurs when the patient is unable to divert the train of thought from a given direction. This occurs in some paranoid schizophrenics and the patient tends to carry over material from one task into the next. Finally, there is the symptom of persistent self-reference of all problem-solving thinking. The patient is unable to think about any problem without referring it to himself in some way, so that a disorder of conceptual thinking occurs which is based on a paranoid attitude.

Disorders of the Stream of Thought

Thought blocking is the most important disorder of the stream of thought and occurs when the train of thought stops and a new one begins which is not connected with the previous train of thought. In the early stages of the disorder, before deterioration sets in, this can be a terrifying experience. When this symptom is well marked or is complained of spontaneously, then it is diagnostic of schizophrenia. However, it must be remembered that tired or anxious patients have difficulty in maintaining the stream of thought and so may give the impression that they have thought blocking. Blocking must be distinguished from inhibition of thinking which may occur in the depressive states, including schizophrenia. In inhibition the stream of thought is slowed down in a uniform way, while in blocking it is slowed down and stopped in an irregular manner. Some schizophrenics have pressure of thought so that their thoughts come crowding into their minds and seem to be partly out of their control. However, this symptom is not characteristically schizophrenic unless it is attributed to some outside agency. Bleuler (1924) drew attention to the fact that some patients have an abnormal brevity of associations. Thus a problem or topic occupies their thoughts for a brief period and only a few associations occur instead of the wealth of associations which such a topic would normally arouse; nevertheless, there is no increase in the speed of thinking. This is really a disorder of the form rather than of the stream of thought and serves to remind us of the artificial nature of our classification of the thought disorder.

Disorders of the Control of Thought

These disorders are probably the subjective experiences associated with the disorders of thinking which have previously been discussed. Thinking, like all conscious activities, is experienced as an activity which is being carried out by the subject or, to use a clumsy German expression, there is a quality of 'my-ness' connected with thought. In schizophrenia this sense of possession of one's own thoughts may be impaired and the patient may suffer from alienation of thought, which can be experienced as thought deprivation, thought insertion, or thought broadcasting. In thought deprivation the train of thought ceases and the patient experiences a loss of thought. This may be a subjective experience associated with thought blocking or omission. Precisely the opposite experience occurs in thought insertion when the patient is certain that alien thoughts have been inserted into his mind. It is possible that this is a subjective experience associated with the sudden experience of a new train of thought following blocking. Thought broadcasting is a strange experience, which is neither delusional nor hallucinatory, in which the patient has the certain knowledge that everyone else is participating in his thoughts. This may form the basis of the delusion that his thoughts are being read. Schneider regards all these disorders of the control of thought as schizophrenic symptoms.

The other important disorder of the control of thought is obsessional thinking, and although it is not diagnostic of schizophrenia it does occur in a small proportion of schizophrenics. Thus, in a series of English schizophrenics admitted to a university psychiatric clinic, 3·5 per cent were found to have had obsessional symptoms at some time in their lives. The obsession is distinguished from the schizophrenic disorders of the control of thought in that the patient feels compelled to think his *own* thoughts against his will, but his thoughts never lose that quality of 'my-ness'. It appears that the extent and severity of the obsessional symptoms in schizophrenia are inversely related to the severity of the illness. This has led to the suggestion that the obsessions are a defence against the schizophrenic illness and prevent the progress of the disease. Since two concurrent events are not necessarily related as cause and effect, it is just as feasible to suggest that the mildness of the schizophrenic illness and the presence of obsessional symptoms are both due to some common pathoplastic factor. Sometimes obsessions appearing at the onset of a schizophrenic illness develop into delusions later on. The incidence of schizophrenia in obsessional states depends very much on the observer's criteria for the diagnosis of schizophrenia. Since it has been shown that schizophrenic psychoses associated with obsessional symptoms have a good prognosis, it is probable that these illnesses are really atypical psychoses.

Disorders of Thought Content. Delusions

Delusions are, of course, a characteristic feature of schizophrenia. However, the textbook definition of a delusion, that is, 'a false unshakeable belief which is out of keeping with the patient's cultural and educational background', is not very helpful. The application of *verstehende* psychology to this problem has produced some interesting concepts, but the lack of any experimental investigation of these concepts has meant that very little progress in our knowledge of delusional phenomena has taken place in the past 30 years. Jaspers (1953) has differentiated between delusions which arise on an understandable basis and those which can be traced back to some experience which cannot be understood. He calls the first variety 'delusion-like ideas', and the second 'true delusions'. The delusion-like idea can be understood as secondary to some other psychological change, such as an endogenous or reactive emotional state, unpleasant experiences, illusions, hallucinations, and changes in consciousness. Delusions of this kind occur in many different psychiatric illnesses, including schizophrenia. However, the true delusion which is based on a primary delusional experience is a characteristic schizophrenic symptom. Gruhle (Berze and Gruhle, 1929) expressed this idea of the primary nature of the schizophrenic delusion when he defined it as the establishment of a reference without cause. The basic weakness of this approach is the lack of definition of understandibility, since some investigators are more tolerant of minor discrepancies than others.

In a primary delusional experience an abnormal consciousness of significance occurs in connexion with a given experience. Delusional mood, delusional states of consciousness, sudden delusional ideas, and delusional perceptions are phenomena of this kind. Since it appears that something is becoming manifest in connexion with a given psychological event, Conrad (1958b) has suggested that the word 'apophany'* should be used to designate these delusional experiences.

Delusional (apophanous) mood is usually a strange, uncanny mood in which the environment appears to be changed in a threatening way but the significance of the change cannot be understood by the patient who is tense, anxious, and bewildered. Occasionally, the patient has a feeling of joy and gladness, and, although puzzled, he is not unhappy. Finally, a delusion may crystallize out of this mood and with its appearance there is often a sense of relief. The delusional idea or delusional perception which occurs in delusional mood cannot be understood psychologically as arising from the mood. Since it is difficult to differentiate delusional mood from unpleasant bewildered states due to anxiety this symptom cannot be used in diagnosis. Usually delusional moods can only be described retrospectively because during their occurrence the examiner is experienced by the patient as a part of the threatening environment. The intravenous administration of sodium amylobarbitone to a patient in a delusional mood may interrupt the condition and allow the patient to describe his experiences.

In delusional perception an abnormal significance, usually in the sense of self-reference, despite the absence of any emotional or logical reason, is attributed to a normal perception. For example, Schneider (1959) had a patient who saw a dog lift its front paw and he knew immediately that this signified that he was being persecuted. It is necessary to be perfectly clear about the nature of the delusional perception and to distinguish it from misinterpretations of the environment based on delusional attitudes. Thus, for example, when a patient with delusions of persecution says that certain noises are due to spies, this is not a delusional perception but a delusional misinterpretation. Schneider believes that delusional perception is diagnostic of schizophrenia, whereas the sudden delusional idea is not. In his attempt to differentiate sharply between these two phenomena he has stressed the two-membered nature of delusional perception in contrast to the one-membered nature of the sudden delusional idea. In delusional perception he considers that there is a link from the patient to the perception and a second link from the normal perception to the unusual significance. This is an artificial concept, because many

---

* This word is derived from the Greek and means 'to become manifest'. Conrad uses it for all delusional experiences in which a new experience becomes manifest to the patient. This term has the advantage over the clumsy German expressions which have been used for these phenomena in that it can be turned into an adjective, so that one can talk of 'apophanous ideas', 'apophanous perceptions', and so on.

experimenters have shown that the establishment of the significance or meaning of a perceived object is the final step in perception, and because the abnormal significance and the accurate perception of the object in delusional perception often occur simultaneously. A further objection to this concept of two-memberedness of the delusional perception is that it has allowed Schneider to extend the term 'delusional perception' to include the attribution of an abnormal significance to a memory image.

The sudden delusional (apophanous) idea or autochthonous delusion appears abruptly in the patient's mind, is fully elaborated, and unheralded by any related thoughts. Since the manic depressive and psychopathic personalities may have sudden delusional ideas, the form of this symptom is not a diagnostic of schizophrenia, but if the content of the delusional idea is very bizarre then it is highly likely to be schizophrenic in origin. Consequently, patients who suddenly get the idea that they are God, Christ, the King of England, and so on, are very likely to be suffering from schizophrenia. It is unfortunate that some writers in the English language have not distinguished between the different delusional phenomena and have suggested that all 'primary delusions' including sudden delusional (apophanous) delusions, are diagnostic of schizophrenia.

It seems that most of the earlier investigators of delusional experiences have allowed themselves to be mesmerized by the 'non-understandable' nature of these phenomena. There is, of course, no reason why apophanous experiences should not be subjected to psychological and physiological experimental investigations. So far research of this kind has not been carried out, but Matussek (1952) has attempted to explain one variety of delusional perception by means of *Gestalt* theory. All the older authors, such as Jaspers, Gruhle, and Schneider, were quite certain that there was no perceptual change in delusional perception, but that the phenomenon was due to thought disorder. However, Matussek has pointed out that there are really two varieties of delusional perception: one in which the abnormal significance arises out of verbal relationships, and the other in which the abnormal significance arises from the perception itself. The first variety resembles the verbal tricks of the obsessional ruminator who is able to discover unpleasant reminders of his obsessional ruminations in any environment. An example of this verbal type of delusional perception is the patient who heard a floorboard squeak when one of his colleagues came into his office, and looked down to see the linoleum on the floor. He then said to himself: 'Lino, that means don't lie.' Thus the abnormal significance was based on a play upon words brought about by an experience. In the other variety of delusional perception the unusual significance seems to occur during the act of perception itself, and this had led Matussek to suggest that there is a loosening of perceptual integration which causes the essential properties of the perceived object to come into prominence and acquire a special significance.

The primary delusional experiences form the basis of paranoid delusions, and are woven together with feelings of bodily change, experiences of passivity, hallucinations of all kinds, products of formal thought disorder, and misinterpretations based on mood and delusional attitudes. The final result is a group of secondary delusions in which the basic primary delusional experiences are embedded. Apophanous experiences do not occur in chronic patients and it is usually impossible in these patients to isolate the earlier apophanous experiences from the current delusions. The commonest delusions in schizophrenia are paranoid* in content. The paranoid patient may believe that he is being persecuted by one or more persons or by organizations such as the Freemasons, the Jews, the Catholics, or the Communists. Since violent dislikes of well-organized groups of believers are well within the range of normal behaviour, it may be some time before the abnormality of a patient's persecutory delusions is fully realized. Hallucinations, especially auditory hallucinations, often play a great part in the formation of persecutory delusions and the voices may directly or indirectly indicate the nature of the persecutors. Bodily hallucinations and feelings of passivity may confirm the patient's belief that he is being interfered with. In fact, persecutory delusions cannot be considered in isolation but are best understood as an attempt by the patient to rationalize his extraordinary experiences, which are completely outside his normal experience. Although paranoid phenomena, such as auditory and bodily hallucinations, are very common in defect states, chronic schizophrenics with well-held persecutory delusions with a good deal of affect behind them are not frequently found in mental hospitals. Even in acute shifts the drive behind the delusions is very variable. Thus some patients protest vigorously against their alleged persecutors and may attack or abuse them, while others accept their persecution in a more or less resigned way. Sometimes the patient is extremely cautious about expressing his persecutory delusions and will not talk about them except to his closest relatives. In such a case the patient often denies his delusions when speaking to the doctor. In other cases the patient is quite willing to talk about his delusions and has no objection to discussing them at great length. The patient who is cautious in expressing his delusions has obviously a better preserved personality than the one who will talk about his delusions to all

* Strictly speaking, the word 'paranoid' refers to a disturbance of the individual's relationship to the world, so that both delusions of grandeur and delusions of persecution are paranoid delusions. There is, however, a tendency in the English literature to use the term 'paranoid' as an equivalent of 'persecutory'.

and sundry. The first type of patient is acting as if his delusions were true, while the second is virtually undisturbed by his ideas of persecution and has dissociated them from his everyday life. This relative indifference towards paranoid delusions is seen in most chronic defect states, but a few of these patients continue to react vigorously against their alleged persecutors throughout the whole of their illness.

In the past much stress has been laid on the degree of systematization of the paranoid delusions and it has been suggested that the greater the systematization the worse the prognosis. This is not true, since acute paranoid psychoses with fairly well systematized delusions may recover. The older psychiatrists put forward the idea that in some paranoid patients one could understand the paranoid delusions as the logical elaboration of a single false premise. Practical experience demonstrates that a completely systematized set of delusions does not occur. When a detailed discussion of allegedly systematized delusions is possible, it always becomes obvious that the patient is illogical when dealing with his delusions and it becomes apparent that minor delusions which are not closely connected with the main theme are present, but not very obtrusive. Patients with fairly well systematized delusions usually have only a slight personality defect. It may well be that because they retain sufficient judgement, they systematize their delusions. There is also a good deal of drive and affect behind their delusions. Apart from their delusions they are usually able to think clearly and their general behaviour is good, so that the delusions appear to be encapsulated.

Before leaving this discussion of paranoid delusions it is necessary to consider the attitude of self-reference. Ideas of self-reference are very common and may become marked in any psychosis. In acute schizophrenia a patient may feel that people are watching him and talking about him. This may be due to the beginning of a delusional experience or to a sense of change induced in the patient by the illness as such or by an associated depression. When a persecutory delusion is well established it may lead to marked self-reference when every event is misinterpreted as a hostile act. Some patients believe that everything around them is organized for their benefit, prefabricated as it were, in order to test them in some undefined way. Many of these patients are unable to specify their persecutors or to give any reason for such behaviour.

Delusions of grandeur are not uncommon in schizophrenia, and with the decline of general paresis the commonest cause of grandiose delusions in British mental hospitals today is schizophrenia. These patients believe that they are God, Jesus, the Virgin Mary, Napoleon, and so on. In some cases there is an attitude of superiority, but in most cases the patients talk of their elevated status in an indifferent sort of way and are prepared to carry out menial tasks. Grandiose delusions are usually associated with other fantastic delusions, but in a few patients the self-elevation is not very marked and the patient's claims are not utterly ridiculous. These patients become self-appointed prophets and reformers and have an attitude of superiority, believing firmly in their status and mission so that they are able to persuade others of their beliefs and gather round themselves a group of converts. It is not possible to explain schizophrenic delusions of grandeur except to say that in acute states they appear to be based on delusional experiences and in chronic states they can be understood as arising from a combination of thought disorder and hallucinations.

The theory of the older French psychiatrists that delusions of grandeur are due to a rationalization of delusions of persecution is still repeated in many textbooks. According to this the patient explains his persecution by assuming that he is an important person, since if he were so important he could expect to have so many enemies. There does not appear to be any justification for this view, since grandiose delusions can, in fact, occur at the onset of a schizophrenic illness and in the presence of a few ill-held persecutory delusions. On the other hand, many patients with well-held affect-laden delusions of persecution never develop grandiose delusions.

Hypochondriacal delusions are extremely common in schizophrenia. In the acute stage such delusions may be partly due to depression, but in both acute and chronic patients sensations of bodily change form the basis for the bulk of these delusions. The hallucinatory basis of the hypochondriasis is, of course, diagnostic of schizophrenia. Some schizophrenics present with marked hypochondriasis which steadily progresses and finally the hallucinatory basis of the condition becomes obvious. These patients should not be confused with others who suffer from chronic hypochondriasis of unknown aetiology. This is a condition of incurable insistent hypochondriasis which is not schizophrenic because the complaints are not based on bodily hallucinations, that is, the patient does not experience a bodily sensation which he knows is produced by outside agencies in the absence of any real external stimulus. The bizarre nature of hypochondriacal complaints cannot be considered to be diagnostic of schizophrenia since it depends so much on the patient's cultural background and intelligence: thus, for example, a depressed mental defective may have very bizarre hypochondriacal complaints.

Although delusions are nearly always present at some stage in a schizophrenic illness there is no special delusional content which is diagnostic. Paranoid delusions, although common in schizophrenia, may in fact occur in many different psychiatric conditions. The delusion that the end of the world is at hand has been claimed as characteristic of schizophrenia by some workers. This delusion is by no means uncommon in acute schizophrenia, where it is often based on apophanous experiences of the nature of delusional perception. In these cases, however, it is the delusional experience and not the content which is diagnostic. In fact, the delusion that the end of the world is at hand is not in itself diagnostic of schizophrenia and can occur in other illnesses, such as in a depression in a very religious person.

Perceptual Disorders

The disorders of perception, i.e. illusions and hallucinations, can be grouped together as sense deceptions. An illusion is a misinterpretation of an external stimulus, while a hallucination is a perception in the absence of an external stimulus. Illusions are quite common in paranoid schizophrenia since the increased suspiciousness leads the patient to misinterpret his environment. Sometimes it is difficult to be sure whether a patient with a marked degree of self-reference has illusions or verbal hallucinations. A careful discussion of what the patient believes other people are saying about him may allow the examiner to decide whether the patient is mishearing scraps of other people's conversation or whether he is hearing verbal hallucinations which he is attributing to the people around him.

Some psychiatrists distinguish between hallucinations and pseudo-hallucinations, but the literature on the subject is confused (Taylor, 1981). In some cases, the descriptions of pseudo-hallucinations are clearly those of true hallucinations. A pseudo-hallucination is said to be a mental image which occurs in full consciousness, is clear and vivid, though lacking the substantiality of a perception, and is not located in outer space but in 'subjective' space. The patient knows that they are not real perceptions, i.e. has insight. The pseudo-hallucination is purely of academic interest and has no prognostic or diagnostic value in schizophrenia.

Hallucinations, like all other schizophrenic symptoms, do not occur in isolation but in connexion with other symptoms. Many years ago Schröder (1926a, b) pointed out that the hallucinatory syndromes themselves should be studied and not just the hallucinations. He described four common hallucinatory syndromes: confusional hallucinosis, self-reference hallucinosis, verbal hallucinosis, and fantastic hallucinosis. The prominent features of confusional hallucinosis are clouding of consciousness and visual hallucinations, while auditory hallucinations, if they occur, consist of noises or odd words, and it is extremely rare for hallucinations to consist of sentences. The patient with self-reference hallucinosis hears voices talking about him and it may be difficult to decide to what extent he is hearing hallucinations and to what extent he is misinterpreting and mishearing remarks which he overhears. The patient cannot reproduce the actual words which the voices are saying, but he is able to give a general idea of what is being said. In verbal hallucinosis the patient hears clear hallucinatory voices talking to him or talking about him, and he is able to repeat what they say accurately. The patient with fantastic hallucinosis produces a strange fantastic set of ideas which is based on auditory hallucinations, visual hallucinations, bodily hallucinations, and delusions. It is usually impossible to be certain how much an experience described by such a patient is to be attributed to hallucinations in any one perceptual field and also how much the delusions depend on hallucinations. The first of these hallucinatory syndromes is due to coarse brain disease, but the last three are frequently seen in schizophrenia.

Auditory hallucinations in the form of voices are the commonest schizophrenic symptom and are often diagnostic of the condition. There is evidence that the equivalent of 'voices' may be experienced even by schizophrenics who have been profoundly deaf since early infancy (Critchley et al., 1981). This being so, it is strange that many investigators have not given much weight to this symptom and that little has been done to investigate it experimentally. Elementary hallucinations are not so prominent, but patients may hear buzzing, whistling, and other noises which are often attributed to the machinations of the persecutors. Some chronic patients with fantastic hallucinosis hear noises like screaming and complain that hundreds of people are being murdered in the cellars. Sometimes these massacres are seen as well as heard. However, the hallucinatory voice is characteristically schizophrenic, so that if in a state of clear consciousness a patient hears well-organized voices consisting of more than one sentence he should be diagnosed as suffering from schizophrenia unless it can be proved otherwise. Or to put it in another way, continuous auditory hallucinosis in the absence of coarse brain disease is due to schizophrenia. Of course, some depressive patients do hear voices, but the voices consist of short isolated phrases or sentences which revile the patient or tell him to commit suicide. Thus he may hear such things as 'rotten sod!', 'kill yourself!', and so on, but not continuous connected abuse.

The hallucinatory voices in schizophrenia vary considerably in duration, in content, and in the effect they have on the patient's thought, behaviour, and emotion. It is difficult to describe the detailed differences since there is a marked overlap in the variations of different qualities of the phenomenon. The intensity of the voices can be considered from the point of view of the duration of the phenomenon, the degree of interference with mental activity, or the effect of attention or distraction on the severity of symptoms. They may be continuous, but may cease when the patient talks to someone or concentrates on a mental or physical task. Alternatively, the voices may be continuous and obtrusive so that the patient may become incoherent because the voices continuously interfere with all directed thinking. Thus this kind of hallucination is associated with severe thought disorder. When auditory hallucinations are as severe as this, the patient tends to turn away from the examiner and whisper or talk in reply to the voices. This hallucinatory aversion has to be differentiated from negativism. The patient whose voices cease when his attention is directed to a task shows very little thought disorder and is usually able to carry out fairly responsible work and take care of himself. The incoherent patient not only shows marked intellectual impairment, but usually is dirty and untidy and may even be incontinent of urine or faeces. The intensity of the voices usually varies, but in many patients sudden increases in intensity which occur from time to time for no apparent reason lead to outbursts of shouting, swearing, scolding, and general excitement. These hallucinatory excitements are easily distinguished from catatonic excitements. A few patients find that shouting at the hallucinatory voices may lead to some relief for a short period.

The clarity of the voices varies from patient to patient. In some cases the voices are quite clear, can be recognized as coming from a particular place and even from a particular individual; they therefore have the same quality as ordinary voices, while in others the voices are different from normal and can be distinguished from reality. In yet other patients the voices are indistinct and vague, so that some chronic patients describe their voices as if coming from a great distance. Clarity is only one factor which determines the ability of the patient to reproduce the content of the voices. The organization of the content of the voices also helps the patient to reproduce them. At times the voices talk disjointedly and mention odd phrases which are strange and foreign to the patient, and in some cases the voices show gross formal thought disorder, while in other patients the content is well organized and clearly expressed. The relation of the voices to the patient's 'own' thoughts and feelings is very variable. The voices may talk about the patient's private thoughts and innermost secrets, so that the content deals with affect-laden topics and the patient believes the privacy of his thoughts has been invaded. Other patients are not troubled very much by the content of the voices, but are troubled by the phenomenon itself, which is experienced as unpleasant and irritating. The content of such troublesome hallucinations may be nonsensical and apparently irrelevant; thus, for example, one patient frequently heard the words 'sausage and chips'. In chronic defect states the content of the voices may be stereotyped, and this particularly happens to abusive voices, for example, one chronic schizophrenic continuously heard the words 'Gorgie* masturbator', while another heard the words 'Wanker's* doom'. This leads us to the attitude of the voices towards the patient. Usually the voices are hostile and abusive, but occasionally they are neutral in attitude and, rarely, they are reassuring. It is interesting that both delusions and hallucinatory voices in schizophrenia are usually concerned with hostility towards the patient. Apart from the attitude towards the patient there is also a difference in mode of address, so that the voices may talk about the patient, they may talk to him, or they may actually instruct him. Hallucinatory conversations about the patient are diagnostic of schizophrenia. These sometimes take the form of a running commentary in which every act carried out by the patient is commented on. Voices which talk to the patient are usually abusive, often obscene, and make reference to sexual topics such as masturbation, fornication, and homosexuality. In England the voices frequently call female patients 'whores' or 'prostitutes' and male patients 'poufs' or 'masturbators'. This is obviously related to traditional social attitudes. Women feel that it is much worse to be accused of promiscuity than homosexuality, and vice versa for men. Nevertheless, sexual themes are much less common than they used to be, and this reflects the changes in cultural traditions.

Occasionally the voices talk to the patient, reassuring and encouraging him. Voices which instruct the patient are not very common and the response of the patient to these instructions is very variable. Thus some patients have no difficulty in refusing to carry out the instructions, others have difficulty in deciding what to do, while a few are compelled to carry out the instructions no matter how unpleasant they are. This may lead to suicidal and homicidal actions in response to hallucinatory instructions. The attitude of the patient towards the voices is very variable, and many chronic paranoid schizophrenics are fairly indifferent to their voices and treat them as old friends. Some patients complain about the hallucinations as such or their content, while others seem to realize the abnormality of the voices and refuse to talk about them. Such patients may talk about their voices only when they become friendly with the examiner, but when they are observed over a long period they may be seen to be talking to their voices. The sudden onset of hallucinations may lead to severe distress, so that the patient becomes extremely depressed and anxious. He may develop a painful insight into the abnormal significance of the symptom and attempt suicide. The acute distress of these patients is often extremely disturbing to the observer.

---

* 'Gorgie' is a district in Edinburgh and 'Wanker' is a slang term for masturbator.

The attitude of the patient towards his voices is also related to his ideas about their source. He may be able to give no explanation of their origin or he may attribute them to spirits, witches, telepathy, hypnosis, machines, radio, television, X-rays, atomic radiations, and so on. Some patients experience their voices as arising from different parts of their body such as their tongue, chest, abdomen, arms, or legs. Thus one patient had the Crown Prince of Germany and two staff nurses in her chest, and these people were continually talking to her! At times the patient attributes all the voices to real people in his environment and this leads him to deny that he hears voices since they appear to him to be real voices from people around him. Such patients usually admit that other people talk about them and when they describe what is being said it becomes obvious that they are hearing voices. It is not possible to determine what it is that makes these patients attribute the hallucinations to their fellows; it may be the quality of the voices or their affect-laden nature. Examiners unaware of this special kind of voice may miss the fact that a given patient is hallucinating, and as a result fail to understand the aggressive behaviour of the patient who, believing that people around him are making unpleasant remarks, attacks some of his fellow patients.

Certain special types of auditory hallucinations may occur in schizophrenia. Firstly, there is *Gedankenlautwerden* or *écho de pensée*, which is diagnostic of schizophrenia. Unfortunately, there is no English technical term for this interesting symptom which consists of the patient hearing his own thoughts spoken aloud. In the chronic stage of the disease the patient may hear his thoughts spoken aloud by people around him while he is thinking, or he may hear people around him reply to his thoughts, or talk about his thoughts before he has spoken them. The other special kind of hallucinatory voice is the functional hallucination, when the patient hallucinates only as long as he receives a stimulus in the perceptual field concerned. Thus in the case of voices the patients hear them when some noise is occurring, such as the noise of a train, the rustling of leaves, or the sound of running water when a tap is turned on. This is, of course, not an illusion, since the noise and the voices are both heard so that there is no question of a misinterpretation of the noise.

Very few experimental investigations of verbal hallucinations have been carried out. It has been claimed by some workers that action potentials can be detected in the speech musculature of schizophrenics hearing voices. Even actual faint whispering has been recorded (Green and Preston, 1981). Since verbal hallucinosis appears to be a central feature of schizophrenia it is possible that experimental investigations of this phenomenon could lead to a better understanding of the nature of the illness. It has already been suggested that there is some central interfering process which may manifest itself in auditory hallucinosis and in thought disorder. This idea is supported by the fact that sensory deprivation has less effect on schizophrenics than normals, since this central interfering process would lead to a decreased dependence on incoming stimuli. Conrad (1958a) has tried to correlate the primary delusional phenomena, thought disorder, and auditory hallucinations. His views will be outlined in a later chapter of this book.

In contrast to auditory hallucinations, visual ones are very uncommon in schizophrenia; so much so, that their presence should be regarded as throwing doubt on the diagnosis. When they do occur they usually do not play much part in moulding the clinical picture. Careful interrogation about the visual hallucinations usually demonstrates that the patient is talking in metaphorical language, but sometimes he is talking about pseudo-hallucinations; often the patients refer to them as visions. They may occur in the acute stages of the illness or in the chronic defect state, especially in the fantastic form of chronic schizophrenia. In these chronic patients it may be difficult to decide whether the patient is talking about hallucinatory experiences or about dreams. As pointed out before, some chronic patients have mass hallucinations in which they both see and hear large numbers of people being murdered or tortured.

Bodily hallucinations are quite common in schizophrenia so that the patients may complain of induced sensations of heat, cold, pain, or electric shock. The psycho-analysts have suggested that the electrical hallucinations are disguised sexual sensations, but it is difficult to understand this explanation since many of these patients also have frank sexual sensations. Thus the male patients complain that erections and orgasms are induced by some external means and also that seminal fluid is extracted from them, while female patients complain that they are being raped by known or unknown persons. In acute patients the complaints are usually straightforward so that the patients may complain of severe pains or unpleasant sensations which are attributed to external sources and to disease. In the chronic patients, however, the complaints are usually bizarre and are attributed to peculiar sources. Thus, for example, the patients may complain that their flesh is torn away, they are flayed alive, their bowels are torn out, animals and machines are inserted into their bodies, and so on. In patients with this kind of hallucination it is not easy to determine what is due to visual, auditory, or bodily hallucinations. Machines, radio waves, X-rays, atomic radiation, and so on, may be claimed to be the source of bodily hallucinations. Occasionally, reflex hallucinations occur when the patient has a hallucinatory experience in one perceptual field due to a stimulus in quite another perceptual field; for example, the patient may feel pain in his chest when he sees the doctor turning a key in the lock of the ward door.

Hallucinations of smell are not uncommon, so that patients may complain of gas, odours of decomposition, chemical smells, and so on, and the hallucinatory smell is woven into their paranoid delusions. Sometimes it seems that the abnormal smell is really an illusion based on delusional misinterpretation. The patient feels tired, lethargic, and strange and, since he is unable to understand that this experience is due to a natural bodily change, he comes to the conclusion that he is being drugged or doped. This leads him to fasten on any unusual smell or taste which he experiences. Hallucinations of taste do occur, but it is never easy to be sure that the abnormal taste is based on a hallucination or the delusion.

There is a rare disorder in which the patient complains of only one symptom: that he emits an unpleasant odour. It is difficult to decide whether this is an hallucination or a delusion and, in any case, the relation of this condition to schizophrenia is uncertain.

Emotional Disorders

Although disorders of emotion always occur in schizophrenia the characteristic emotional disorders may not be clearly present until the illness has been going on for some time. These disorders can be classified into two main groups: disorders of mood and disorders of emotional expression. The common mood disorders in schizophrenia are elevated mood, depression, anxiety, and perplexity. Elevated mood of the hypomanic variety is not common in schizophrenia, although some chronic fantastic schizophrenics have a hypomanic mood. These patients are cheerful, with marked pressure of talk, but the fantastic content of their speech makes the diagnosis obvious. The elevated mood in schizophrenia usually has none of the infectious gaiety of true mania, but is one of exaltation and ecstasy. The patient has an ecstatic transfigured look and the examiner is impressed by the lack of rapport. Often the patient is not willing to talk about his feelings, but if he does so he will talk about being in a state of grace, of an indescribable happiness, or even use the word 'ecstasy'. Usually he believes that he has been in a special type of association with the Almighty and may express this by saying that God has spoken to him. Ecstatic states are not diagnostic of schizophrenia since they occur in epileptics and hysterics. In some religious sects ecstasy is expected of the true believer. Mania is not usually associated with ecstasy, but the symptom can occur in mixed affective states which are short-lived and usually occur when the patient is passing from mania to depression or vice versa.

Depression is extremely common in the early stages of schizophrenia. Helmchen and Hippius (1967) found it in as many as half of new admissions. Sometimes a classical melancholia ushers in the illness and this is not uncommon in the so-called paraphrenias in middle age. In depressives with marked persecutory ideas it may be very difficult to differentiate the clinical picture from that of schizophrenia, but the presence of apophanous symptoms and the continuous auditory hallucinosis make the diagnosis of schizophrenia obvious. Delusions of persecution occurring in a depressive setting are not diagnostic of schizophrenia and it may be some time before unequivocal schizophrenic symptoms occur. In some cases treatment with electroconvulsive therapy relieves the depressive mood and the underlying schizophrenic symptoms then become obvious. Sometimes the depression seems to be a natural reaction to the distress caused by schizophrenic symptoms. Since some intelligent young schizophrenics have a painful realization of the inner change which is taking place, they may justifiably be afraid that they are going mad, and may attempt suicide. In other patients the sudden onset of auditory hallucinations seems to produce marked depression and anxiety. Although disorders of emotional expression rather than disorders of mood are prominent in chronic schizophrenics, nevertheless depressive moods are met with in chronic schizophrenia, so that some hebephrenics appear to be depressed and patients with marked bodily hallucinations are usually depressed and morose.

Since the depot neuroleptics came into extensive use, it has been noticed that depressive symptoms are much more common than had been realized. At first it was suspected that the drugs produced the depression but it has now been shown that the acute symptoms mask the depression, which is revealed when the patient improves (Knights and Hirsch, 1981).

Although anxiety is usually associated with persecutory delusions and hallucinations in acute shifts, severe anxiety states may occur before the appearance of schizophrenic symptoms. The patient with self-reference hallucinosis is usually very anxious and frightened. While anxiety is common at the onset of the illness and in acute shifts, it does not occur in chronic defect states. The perplexity which often occurs at the onset of the illness in young people is probably partly due to anxiety. These patients are puzzled and bewildered and unable to describe their experiences, and their replies to questions are frequently disjointed and desultory. The intravenous administration of sodium amylobarbitone often relieves the perplexity and allows the patient to talk about his schizophrenic experiences. Perplexity in itself is not diagnostic of schizophrenia as it can be produced by severe anxiety.

Although some disorders of emotional expression are diagnostic of schizophrenia, it is not necessary to assume that they are primary and cannot be understood as arising from other disorders. The schizophrenic is bound to appear to have an abnormal expression of emotion since he thinks about things and experiences things in a way which is totally foreign to the normal observer. One of the earliest indications of the illness is that the patient loses his finer feelings for those nearest and dearest to him, so that he may become coarse, brutal, or unfeeling towards his family. Occasionally there are senseless outbursts of rage which are short-lived and almost without any cause. However, it is well to remember that difficult, awkward, rather unfeeling behaviour may occur in adolescent crises.

The characteristic schizophrenic disorders of affective expression are flattening, incongruity, and stiffening of affect. In flattening of affect there is a gross lack of emotional response to the given situation. For example, a patient when told of the death of a parent or sibling shows no emotion. Incongruity of affect occurs when the emotion expressed is quite out of keeping with the situation. In stiffening of affect there is a retardation of changes in emotional expression, so that affective expression changes more slowly than in normals and any given affect is maintained for too long a period. Flattening and incongruity of affect are frequently used to establish the diagnosis of schizophrenia. It is, of course, impossible for an observer to estimate the severity of any one symptom in a psychiatric clinical picture without being influenced consciously or unconsciously by other symptoms. The diagnosis of schizophrenia is usually, and quite justifiably, made on the total impression given by the patient, and the examiner then brings forward symptoms in order to support the diagnosis. Since abnormalities of emotional expression have for many years been considered to be diagnostic of schizophrenia, the average British psychiatrist is likely to look particularly carefully for this symptom in order to establish a diagnosis, which has really been made on other grounds. Because the normal range of emotional expression is extremely wide, mild degrees of flattening or incongruity of affect can only be used cautiously as diagnostic symptoms. Thus some non-schizophrenic persons smile when they are anxious, worried, or bewildered and others smile when they fail to understand what is said to them. This is the placatory smile and does not indicate pleasure. Some abnormal persons rarely show any emotion, while others are amused by brutal and horrible events. Many criminals who have committed violent crimes show absolutely no emotion when they discuss the horrifying details of their offences. It would seem that such a person is able to tolerate the knowledge of his crime only by separating all affect from it. This dissociation of affect in persons who have recently committed a crime of violence should not be mistaken for schizophrenic flattening of affect. Although lack of affective expression on the part of the schizophrenic may lead to a failure of rapport it must be remembered that the hostility of the patient and the unpleasant features of the interview situation may also prevent the establishment of good rapport. Nevertheless, faulty rapport is sometimes due to a failure on the part of the psychiatrist.

While it is easy to understand that a failure to establish good rapport with the patient may lead to a false diagnosis, it is not so obvious that the establishment of a good rapport may also have the same result. A kindly, understanding interviewer may make a great effort to understand the patient and feel his way into the patient's life situation, and in doing so he may understand too much and overlook important schizophrenic symptoms.

Nearly all patients in the chronic stage of the disease show blunting of affect. Thus chronic paranoid patients frequently produce their paranoid delusions without much affect and are not disturbed if their beliefs are treated lightly. There is a dissociation between their delusions and the real world; for example, the self-styled Queen of Heaven scrubs the floors. One should not make too much of this. Human beings can become accustomed to almost any way of life; even ex-kings become used to being business executives. Some chronic patients may be upset for a very short period when their delusions and hallucinatory experiences are discussed, and in a few patients the delusions continue to have a marked affective loading. These patients become angry when their beliefs are treated lightly and may shout and scream at the examiner if they feel that their views are being treated with scorn.

The symptom of ambivalence includes more than affective disorders, but it is convenient to deal with it here. Bleuler used this term to designate the contemporaneous presence of a negative and positive attitude towards a person, an action, or an idea. He therefore talked of affective ambivalence, ambivalence of the will, and intellectual ambivalence. In affective ambivalence the subject loves and hates the same person at the same time. This occurs in normals, but usually the negative or positive attitude is completely or almost completely denied, whereas in schizophrenic affective ambivalence both attitudes are clearly present. Ambivalence of the will, or ambitendency, is really a catatonic symptom and occurs when the patient wishes and does not wish to carry out a given action. For example, when an examiner offers his hand to some catatonic patient, the patient may begin to move his hand, then stops, then starts again, and so on, until he finally stops moving his hand altogether. Intellectual ambivalence, or the assertion and denial of the same idea, occurs in normals, but is never completely conscious as it is in schizophrenia. Bleuler considered that ambivalence was one of the fundamental symptoms of schizophrenia.

It is difficult to allot the strange experience of depersonalization to any of the main group of symptoms. It is probably best to consider it as an emotional disorder. The depersonalized patient has a strange, unpleasant, subjective sense of internal change and this may be associated with a sense of environmental change or derealization, when the external world appears strange or unreal. Despite the definite feeling of internal or external change, there is no delusional interpretation of this change and the patient has complete understanding of its psychological nature. These patients often complain of a loss of affective responsiveness, so that a mother may complain that she has no emotion for her children, and a breadwinner may complain that he is not as upset as he should be about the financial difficulties due to his illness.

Depersonalization is common in acute schizophrenics, but it soon develops into clear delusional experiences. It is unfortunate that the Scandinavian authors tend to use the term 'depersonalization' to designate delusional experiences of passivity and control from outside. It is said that some schizoid personalities may develop severe depersonalization during psychogenic reactions or in depressive illnesses. Since this symptom is difficult to describe, these patients often give the examiner a rather odd impression and at times may lead the inexperienced to diagnose schizophrenia.

Behaviour Disorders

Disorders of behaviour occur in all forms of schizophrenia, but they are more striking in catatonic schizophrenia because in that type of illness they are often bizarre and cannot be easily understood as arising from the patient's abnormal ideas. Attempts have been made to understand all catatonic symptoms as motor expressions of psychological conflicts, but it is, of course, just as possible that the content of consciousness which is associated with the motor disorder is a rationalization of a symptom which is produced by some neurophysiological disorder. In this connexion it is interesting that symptoms similar to catatonia in humans can be produced in monkeys by the administration of bulbocapnine. Catatonic symptoms will therefore be discussed in this chapter as motor symptoms in their own right, and the symbolic significance of symptoms will be discussed later on when the psychological theories of schizophrenia are considered.

Before considering objective changes in motor activity it is necessary to discuss the important schizophrenic symptom of loss of control over one's own voluntary acts. Many schizophrenics have passivity feelings and experience some or all of their voluntary acts as being controlled from outside. We have already discussed loss of control of thought, which is, in fact, only a special case of this more general disorder. This experience of being controlled may puzzle the patient so that he is unable to say how it is being done and who is responsible for it, but in other cases he may attribute the control to machines, radio waves, and so on. The belief that any part of one's own voluntary activity is controlled from without is typically schizophrenic, but in evaluating this symptom the patient's educational standard and cultural background must be borne in mind. Some non-psychotic people in Western civilization believe in telepathy, telekinesis, and spirit control. Thus a depression or psychogenic reaction in a spiritualist may be associated with bizarre ideas of passivity. In passing, it is worth noting that devout Catholics when depressed may believe that they are possessed by the Devil or devils.

It is not easy to deal with the schizophrenic motor and behaviour disorders in a systematic way, because there is some degree of overlap of the different phenomena. The individual disorders of movement, posture, and speech will be dealt with first and then the more complicated disordered patterns of behaviour. Catatonic disorders of movement can be classified as simple disorders of the execution of movements, abnormal spontaneous movements, and abnormally induced movements.

Any motor act can be carried out in a faulty way in catatonic schizophrenia and this may be due to ambitendency, obstruction, or mannerism. The peculiar starting and stopping of a motor act due to ambitendency has been discussed in a previous section. In obstruction or blocking a movement is carried out correctly at first, but suddenly stops before it is completed and the body returns to the neutral position or the movement is completed after a little time. This can be considered to be the motor equivalent of thought blocking. A mannerism occurs when a normal goal-directed movement is carried out in an abnormal stilted manner and, although the purpose of such a movement can be understood by the observer, the manner of execution is abnormal. The mannerism may affect the associated movements more than the essential motor act itself.

The abnormal spontaneous catatonic movements consist of non-goal-directed movements which are carried out without the intervention of an examiner although they may be accentuated by examination. These symptoms are stereotypy, parakinesia, handling, and intertwining. It is not always easy to distinguish between a stereotypy and a mannerism. A stereotypy is a movement which is not goal-directed and which is carried out in a uniform way, but some mannerisms which are abnormal exaggerations of expresssive movements may be confused with stereotypies; however, they are not executed in such a rigid way. Some authors have described bizarre acts as a symptom in schizophrenia, but these are really odd and peculiar mannerisms. Parakinesia consists of a continuous irregular movement of the musculature so that patients with this symptom grimace, twitch, and jerk continuously. The clinical picture may not be dissimilar from that of Sydenham's chorea, but usually the movements are not as violent as those in Huntington's chorea. If the movements are most marked in the face and neck they have a superficial resemblance to tics. Since parakinesia causes voluntary movements to be carried out in a jerky way, speech is also affected, so that the patient speaks in short sharp bursts and his speech is disjointed and desultory. Handling is an odd variety of behaviour in which the patient touches and handles everything within reach. This symptom is usually associated with intertwining, when the patient continuously intertwines his fingers or grasps his clothes with his fingers and kneads a small piece of cloth.

Most abnormally induced movements appear to be due to an excessive compliance on the part of the patient. The following symptoms are of this variety: automatic obedience, echopraxia, perseveration, forced grasping, *Mitgehen*, co-operation, and opposition. In automatic obedience the patient carries out every command which is given to him. This symptom has also been called 'command automatism', but this term has been used to designate a syndrome consisting of flexibilitas cerea, echolalia, and echopraxia. Echopraxia occurs when a patient repeats every action of someone in his immediate environment. Perseveration consists in continuing to carry out a goal-directed activity after the need for this activity has ceased. It may take the form of repetition of an act or word, but in this case it is different from a stereotypy because it has been initiated by a goal-directed activity. Perseveration of a posture or a mental set may occur at times, and perseveration of the theme of thought which has already been discussed is a special variety of the latter. Forced grasping and *Mitgehen* usually occur together. In *Mitgehen* the patient moves his body in response to a light pressure by the examiner. Thus, for example, when one presses lightly with one finger on the undersurface of the forearm the arm rises smoothly as if one were moving an 'anglepoise' lamp. The patient moves his body in the direction of the light pressure, so that if it is applied to the back of the head one can cause the patient to bend over and often fall forward. In order to elicit this symptom the examiner instructs the patient to resist the pressure, then talks to him to distract his attention, and while doing so exerts gentle pressure on a limb or part of the body, and as he continues to talk to the patient the *Mitgehen* begins. It is important to instruct the patient to resist, since many catatonic patients are easily influenced. Forced grasping occurs when, despite instructions to the contrary, the patient presents his hand whenever the examiner presents his hand for a handshake. Occasionally this kind of forced responsiveness is so marked that the patient's hand follows the movements of the examiner's presented hand like a piece of iron follows a magnet, the so-called 'magnet reaction' (Kleist). *Mitmachen*, or co-operation, occurs when the patient acquiesces in every passive movement of the body made by the examiner, but as soon as the examiner lets go the body returns to its resting position. Opposition (*Gegenhalten*), which also can be considered to be a disorder of posture, is precisely the opposite of co-operation, because the patient resists all passive movements of his body to precisely the same degree as the pressure exerted by the examiner. In mild cases of this disorder the patient may allow gentle, slow, passive movements, but opposition sets in when the movements are made forcibly and abruptly.

Disorders of posture consist of stereotyped postures, manneristic postures, psychological pillow, and waxy flexibility. Stereotyped and manneristic postures are often seen in catatonia, and odd, bizarre, stereotyped postures may be maintained for hours and may alternate with stereotyped actions. Manneristic postures are stilted and odd but are not rigidly maintained. Some catatonics have a posture which seems to express a turning away or withdrawal from the world. Thus some of these patients sit motionless with a bowed head and with closed eyes or with their eyes staring fixedly at the floor, while others sit in awkward constrained postures with their heads turned away from the centre of ward activity. Stereotyped and manneristic attitudes can at times be understood as symbolic expressions of the patients' conflicts. Patients with a psychological pillow lie with their heads two or three inches off the pillow and despite the uncomfortable nature of this position they maintain it for many hours. Waxy flexibility (flexibilitas cerea) figures prominently in all textbook descriptions of catatonia although it was always uncommon and is now very rare. The term 'waxy flexibility' describes the phenomenon very well. The patient allows himself to be placed in any position and then maintains this position for at least several minutes, if not longer. Some patients maintain the posture for a few seconds and then slowly return their limbs to the resting position. This is not flexibilitas cerea and there is no adequate technical term for it, although it has been called *Haltungsverharren* by German psychiatrists. False waxy flexibility may be produced in bewildered, anxious patients who believe that the doctor is carrying out a test and therefore co-operate by maintaining the imposed posture. As in elicitation of *Mitgehen* these patients should be told that they do not have to co-operate, and then an attempt should be made to elicit the phenomenon while the patient is being distracted by conversation.

Speech, like any other variety of motor activity, may be affected in catatonia, but before dealing with speech disorders it is necessary to discuss disorders of mimicry and abnormal attitudes towards the examiner. Mimic expression and, in particular, facial expression is always affected in catatonia—so much so that in mild catatonia the stiffness of facial movement may be the most striking indication of the illness. The face is usually expressionless; emotional changes, if they occur, take place slowly, are never fully developed, and fade slowly. This peculiar 'deadpan' expression may involve the expressiveness of the eye movements, but in most patients there is a contrast between the flat emotionless face and the lively expressive eye movements.

Abnormal expressive movements occur, and of these grimacing is the most common. This may be due to expressive movements accompanying a conversation with hallucinatory voices or it may be a simple catatonic symptom which is not apparently associated with a conscious attitude. Repeated grimacing, of course, occurs in general parakinesia. A not uncommon abnormal facial expression is so-called *Schnauzkrampf* (snout spasm), which consists of a marked wrinkling of the nose with pouting of the lips, so that the lips look very much like an animal's snout.

The attitude of the patient towards the questioner is very variable. Whereas some patients turn towards the examiner when he speaks to them, other patients turn away when spoken to and remain turned away. This turning towards the examiner can be called 'advertence' and is very characteristic of some varieties of catatonia. It is not surprising that *Mitgehen*, co-operation, and forced grasping occur in association with advertence. Aversion or turning away from the examiner may be explained as due to distracting voices, to negativism, or to a conscious autistic attitude.

The forced responsiveness which expresses itself in the attitude of advertence can also at the same time express itself in prosectic or prompt speech. Echolalia, which is a variety of forced responsiveness, may occur with or without marked advertence. The patient with prosectic speech turns towards the examiner when spoken to, and continues to speak in an undertone as long as the examiner speaks to him or encourages him with gestures such as nodding or smiling. In severe cases the content of speech is verbigeration, that is, it consists of senseless, incomprehensible sounds which are frequently repeated, but sometimes a few odd words or phrases can be made out. However, in the mild cases the words can be made out, but there is frequent repetition of sentences. In echolalia the patient repeats the last few syllables which have just been said by the examiner, and this is usually associated with echopraxia. Many patients with prosectic speech have some degree of echolalia. Advertence also occurs in association with prompt speech, but here the answers are intelligible, though the patient seems to say the first thing that comes into his head. If asked about simple things in which there is little involvement of the personality, accurate answers are usually given, but as soon as questions involve such affect-laden topics as the length of stay in hospital the answers become inaccurate. *Vorbeireden* is always associated with this symptom, but it is difficult to determine how far it is due to a forced responsiveness, formal thought disorder, or to an attitude of deliberate refusal to answer questions accurately. These patients never tire of being questioned and will answer the most ridiculous questions.

Stereotypies and mannerisms frequently occur in speech so that the patients tend to speak in a strange way, use strange words, or repeat words and phrases. Some patients speak in an odd stilted way, others adopt accents of various kinds, while others repeat a word or phrase in a stereotyped way. With the passage of time the word or phrase may become so distorted that the original words cannot be recognized. For example, one female patient repeatedly said 'Eseamarrider', which was a corruption of 'He's a married man', and related to an unfortunate liaison before the onset of her illness. Verbigeration, which has already been mentioned, is really a special case of verbal stereotypy in which the stereotyped material is unrecognizable. Perseveration of words or phrases may also occur in catatonia.

The last speech disorder to be considered is muteness or the refusal or inability to reply to questions. Some patients do not answer questions, but can be seen continuously whispering to themselves; in this case it appears that the refusal is due to aversion induced by hallucinatory voices. Other patients do not reply to questions and show no speech activity. This is occasionally due to a mannerism, in which case the patient will give some indication of his wants and he may write at request although he refuses to speak. Mute patients may turn away when spoken to or may turn towards the examiner and look at him with an empty, blank facial expression. Most stuporous patients are completely mute and it may in some cases be possible to abolish the stupor for a short time by the intravenous administration of sodium amylobarbitone. This may allow the patient to talk about the experiences which he has had during the stupor and he may attribute his behaviour to a delusional belief or he may be quite unable to explain it.

Apart from these catatonic speech disorders, non-specific speech disorders may be found, so that flight of ideas or retardation of speech may occur in schizophrenia. Some paranoid patients, especially fantastic paraphrenics, have a marked pressure of speech and are importunate garrulous persons. However, the content of their speech becomes increasingly muddled as the flood of fantastic delusions is poured out. Writing may also be affected in catatonia, so that stereotypies and mannerisms show up well in written material. These include distorted individual letters, elaboration of letters, additional twirls and lines, repetition of words and letters, and patterns of words. Some paranoid schizophrenics never stop writing and handing notes to the nurses and doctors. These patients may expect no reply or they may be querulous petitioners who insist on a reply. The letters themselves may be well written and well laid out or quite disjointed. Many of these chronic paranoid schizophrenic letter-writers write a normal letter with the usual margins, but then write longitudinally in the margins. One cannot be certain if this is because of pressure of writing or a shortage of paper, or both. It is also interesting that the degree of formal thought disorder in written material does not correspond to the degree of thought disorder in speech. Thus some patients with very slight formal thought disorder in speech may show marked disorder of conceptual thought in their letters: the reverse is also not uncommon.

Many complicated abnormal patterns of behaviour are seen in schizophrenia, but the common catatonic patterns are excitement, stupor, impulsive behaviour, and negativism. Excitements due to a marked increase in verbal hallucinations have already been discussed. While some of the excitements which occur in catatonia are due to voices, others are catatonic and cannot be derived psychologically from some other phenomenon. These excitements consist of senseless violence and over-activity in which the patient gives a strange, odd impression to the observer. The excited manic may be markedly over-active, but the mood is cheerful and somewhat infectious. The manic is in good contact with his environment and can make unpleasant apposite remarks, but the excited catatonic is out of contact with his surroundings and often behaves in a brutal inconsiderate manner. These patients destroy clothes, fittings, and furniture, and they may make violent senseless assaults on their fellow patients, nurses, and doctors. If not treated these excitements may last for a few weeks, a few days, or a few hours. The intramuscular administration of phenothiazines and similar compounds will usually cut short these excitements. Sometimes the excitement consists of continuous over-activity in which the patient runs up and down, wanders incessantly, bangs things, talks, shouts, or moans continuously, handles everything within reach, or rocks and moves his body continuously. Excitements may alternate with stupor and, sometimes, before the introduction of tranquillizers, the patient often passed into stupor, then back into excitement, and so on, many times. Occasionally mild excitements take the form of clownlike over-activity, and the patient jumps up and down, dances, turns somersaults, laughs and sings, and generally plays the fool in an exaggerated way.

In stupor the patient sits or lies motionless and does not respond to speech or react to other stimuli. No emotional response occurs when he is questioned about affect-laden topics such as his family and so on. The face is expressionless, but from time to time a sly grin may flit across it. The eyes often show a liveliness which contrasts markedly with the flat unemotional facies. A psychological pillow is usually present and sometimes *Schnauzkrampf* occurs. The muscles may be normal in tone, may be flaccid, or may show increased tone or opposition. Waxy flexibility or co-operation is often present. Saliva often dribbles from the mouth, incontinence of urine usually occurs, sometimes retention is also present, and incontinence of faeces is common. A sudden impulsive act may interrupt the stupor; for example, a patient may lash out at someone or hurl a cup or plate and then relapse into stupor. In milder cases the patient may be completely motionless but can be pushed into action. For example, if he is taken to the toilet and placed on the seat he will micturate or defaecate, and when food is placed in front of him he will eat, but he will not go to the dining table spontaneously. This mild type of stupor can be called 'akinesia'. Some patients in catatonic stupor will eat if hand fed, while others will not chew or swallow the food which is placed in their mouths. Stupor occurs in severe depressions, but here the patient looks miserable, shows some response to affectively charged questions, has no catatonic postural or motor disorders, and is not incontinent of urine or faeces. This differential diagnosis of stupor is to some degree purely academic, since electroconvulsive therapy will relieve both catatonic and depressive stupor. Some catatonic patients, when they recover, are unable to describe their experiences during stupor, while others can describe fearful delusional beliefs and hallucinations. Most patients in catatonic stupor will come out of it when 0·25–0·5 g of sodium amylobarbitone is injected slowly intravenously, but a few stuporous patients do not respond.

Impulsive actions are common in catatonics, so that these patients often suddenly attack someone, smash a window, throw a plate or other object, and are then perfectly calm. In mild cases where the patient is accessible he is usually unable to explain why he committed this act, but occasionally he will say that he did it in reponse to a hallucinatory command.

The term 'negativism' is often used very loosely to mean any refusal on the part of the patient to do something. Kleist (1927) has described negativism as an active striving by the patient against all attempts to make contact with him or influence his behaviour, so that the negativistic patient actively resists all intervention. When the examiner offers his hand the patient withdraws his and when the examiner approaches him he turns away. All passive movements are vigorously resisted and any attempt to force the patient to do something leads to increasing resistance. Severe excitements may result from attempts to force the patient to do something or to prevent him from carrying out a spontaneous act.

Collecting and hoarding form a common abnormal behaviour pattern and can be considered to be a mannerism. The pockets of male chronic patients and the handbags of female chronic patients are often found to be full of rubbish. These patients frequently resist all attempts to remove the rubbish and become very angry and abusive when the nursing staff takes away their hoard. Usually useless rubbish is collected, such as old newspapers, pieces of stale food, especially bread, wood, matchsticks, grass, stones, dead insects, pieces of string, pieces of toilet paper, and scraps of soap. In milder cases the collecting may be more selective and only special objects are collected. Occasionally this gives rise to repeated thefts of objects which are useless to the patient; for example, Leonhard had a patient who stole bicycles although he could not ride them.

Other manneristic behaviour patterns are not uncommon. Sometimes they are simple refusals such as a refusal to eat or to speak, but often they are complicated behaviour patterns which are quite senseless. For example, one patient always went to bed in the usual way, but every morning was found sleeping under the bed. If she was put into bed during the night she did not resist, but as soon as the nurses went elsewhere she crawled under the bed again.

In catatonic and hebephrenic patients with marked ethical deterioration, all sorts of unpleasant anti-social behaviour may occur. Such patients frequently steal food and cigarettes from their fellow patients. Sometimes this is done openly, but often it is done cunningly and with great skill, so that an apparently severely deteriorated catatonic may steal the food from a fellow patient's plate with unbelievable deftness. Other patients are spiteful and play tricks on their fellow patients and on the nurses. They may trip or push others over, spit on them, snatch their chairs away, and so on. One female patient would creep up behind a nurse while she was bending over and attending to a patient in bed, run her hand up the nurse's clothes, and if possible tug at the pubic hair. Sometimes the behaviour is not as malicious as this, but the patient annoys the nurses by hiding when he is due to go to bed, wandering away whenever possible, and similar behaviour.

Deteriorated schizophrenics often behave in very degraded ways. They may neglect themselves and become very filthy, and if not carefully supervised they may be doubly incontinent. Some patients handle faeces, urine, or nasal mucus, while others smear faeces on themselves, the fittings, or other patients. Sometimes these unpleasant habits appear to have a delusional basis. For example, one patient mixed her urine with Ovaltine and smeared the mixture on her body. This, she claimed, was no longer Ovaltine, but 'Ovarltine' which would improve her body. Sometimes unpleasant behaviour has a playful, silly aspect as, for example, the male patient who smeared his head with faeces because he had always wanted bronze-coloured hair.

Hoarding can consist of collecting unpleasant things. For example, one patient killed cats and other small animals, then wrapped them in cloth and stored them in her room, while another patient caught and killed birds, then carried the dead bird tucked in her bosom. Sometimes the tricks played on others are very unpleasant. For example, a chronic schizophrenic used to wrap up her faeces into neat parcels and carry them about. At an opportune moment she would drop a parcel out of a window on to the head of someone standing below. Luckily her aim was not good!

Ethical deterioration in hebephrenics and mild catatonics may lead patients into vagrancy, prostitution, or petty crime. Usually the criminal activities of chronic schizophrenics consist of petty pilfering, but some patients with marked affective blunting may commit brutal assaults. Homicide may be committed because of delusional beliefs or hallucinatory instructions, especially in acute shifts. It has been estimated that 23 per cent of a series of 119 mass murderers were schizophrenic. However, none of the notorious British mass murderers since World War II has been clearly schizophrenic.

Suicide and attempted suicide are not uncommon in acute schizophrenic shifts. Possibly many unexplained suicides in young people are due to schizophrenia. On the whole, suicide is rare among chronic schizophrenics in mental hospitals, but occasionally it does occur.

Disorders of Consciousness

Consciousness is a state of awareness of the environment and in normal persons the degree of this awareness varies within very wide limits. For purposes of description, consciousness can be imagined as a stage on which the individual contents of consciousness come and go or as a medium in which the contents move. Using these similes, we can speak of restriction of consciousness and clouding of consciousness; in the former the number of the contents is decreased, while in the latter the clarity of the contents is diminished.

Although clouding of consciousness is not typical of schizophrenia, perplexity and anxiety in acute shifts of the illness may reduce the level of awareness, but this does not produce actual clouding. Attempts have been made to explain clouding of consciousness in schizophrenic-like illnesses as being due to intense anxiety. If this were so, one might expect that intravenous administration of sodium amylobarbitone would relieve such clouding and this would distinguish the condition from similar states due to coarse brain disease which are, of course, made worse by such treatment. Acute schizophrenic illnesses with dream-like changes of consciousness have been called 'oneiroid states' or 'oneirophrenia', and will be described below.

In general, it can be said that obvious clouding of consciousness or any other sign of coarse brain disease is incompatible with a diagnosis of schizophrenia. However, it is not always easy to be sure that a patient's orientation is adequate, and twilight states can occur in acute schizophrenic shifts. In these states the patient may have a completely false orientation for time and space which exists side by side with the correct orientation, so that he is living in a real world and in a delusional world at one and the same time; this was called a system of 'double book-keeping' by Bleuler. In such a condition it may not be easy to establish the fact that the patient is correctly orientated. Some chronic patients in mental hospitals, because of their lack of interest, can give only a very approximate temporal orientation and many, because of delusional ideas, may not be able to give the name of the hospital correctly. Other patients refuse to give the correct date on request, but subsequent conversation reveals that they are talking past the point. This may be due to an attempt to shorten the interview, to playful silliness, or to speech promptness. Thus a patient may give the date inaccurately, but later when asked for the date of a historical event, such as the outbreak of World War I, may give the current date.

Consciousness has been used by some authors to include attention and the consciousness of one's self. Attention includes the directed nature of consciousness, the selection of contents of consciousness, and the degree of the clarity of the contents of consciousness. Schizophrenic symptoms which consist of disorders of attention and consciousness of one's self have already been discussed to some degree. In this work, consciousness, when used without any qualification, will be used to signify the level of awareness.

Disorders of Memory

In ordinary tests of memory schizophrenic patients do not show any abnormality, but disorders of memory may be caused by schizophrenic delusions. *Déjà vu* and *déjà vécu** experiences occur in normals and may be more pronounced in many different neuropsychiatric disorders, including schizophrenia. Thus a schizophrenic may believe that he has previously experienced a part or whole of his current experiences, or he may believe that a part or whole of his current experience has been previously known, forecast, or prophesied. These are delusional modifications of the *déjà vu* experiences which are seen in normals. Another quite different type of *déjà vécu*

* These are strange experiences that a given situation has been seen or experienced in the past. In normals this does not usually go beyond the idea that the situation has been experienced before.

experience may occur in schizophrenia, when the patient asserts that his delusional ideas had been present long before the onset of his illness, so that delusional events which never happened are remembered with a sense of complete certainty. In normal persons thoughts unconnected with previous perceptions do not have the same quality as percepts, but in this disorder under discussion they acquire a hallucinatory perceptual quality. This is not necessarily the same as memory falsification. Some degree of falsification of memory occurs in all of us, since we all modify some memories and omit others in order to accentuate the pleasant memories and to soften the unpleasant ones. Schizophrenics with over-valued ideas and delusions often distort their memories in order to produce support for the ideas and delusions. Thus one could say that there are two different varieties of memory falsification in schizophrenia: memory distortion, in which real memories are distorted by a delusional attitude, and memory falsification, in which delusional ideas acquire the characteristics of memories. Both these disorders may play a part in the back-dating of delusions, which is so common in paranoid schizophrenia.

The confabulations which occur in some chronic schizophrenics are a special variety of memory falsification. The most fantastic stories about world travel, journeys to the moon, visits to heaven, giving birth to thousands of children, and so on, may be produced by these patients. It seems that free-rising fantastic ideas acquire the quality which usually belongs to things which have been experienced. Delusional misidentifications are very common in paranoid schizophrenia and may be expressions of different phenomena. In acute shifts, delusional perception may take the form of misidentification, when the perceptual image of a given person acquires a special significance for the patient. In other acute cases and some chronic cases the misidentification is due to a delusional set and the environment is misinterpreted in order to fit in with the delusional ideas. A patient may insist that a familiar person has been replaced by a substitute (Capgras syndrome) or that various strangers are really one and the same person (Fregoli syndrome). Sometimes in chronic schizophrenia the patient persistently identifies every one in his environment as someone from his previous life. These patients can usually be persuaded to misidentify all newcomers, and misidentifications may be well held and repeated every time the given person is presented to the patient. It is as if all perceptions of human beings immediately acquire the quality which goes with a previous percept. It is possible that in these cases a fragmentation of perception allows certain properties of the perceived object to emerge and to be organized by the patient's fantasy. In some cases a negative misidentification occurs and the patients deny that they have ever seen the given person before, although they may have seen him many times. For example, they may deny that their wives or parents are in fact their wives or parents. Sometimes the same person is misidentified differently each time he is presented to the patient. It could be that both these phenomena are due to a marked concretization of memory images, so that the memory image of a given person is maintained in all its individual detail and this does not correspond exactly with the subsequent perceptual image. The difference between the memory image and the perceptual image leads the patient to misidentify the same person in a different way every time he appears.

Delusional memories are, of course, varieties of primary delusional experiences. Schneider has claimed that some delusional memories can be classified as delusional perceptions. He gives the example of the patient who remembered that there was a crown on the fork he used as a boy and then claimed that this indicated his connexion with a princely family. For Schneider, this experience is two-membered, like a delusional perception, since one link connects the patient to the memory image and a second link connects the memory image to the abnormal signification. He cites another case of a man who remembered being told at the age of 10 years that he was the heir apparent. In this case the abnormal signification is contained within the memory image and the phenomenon is one-membered like a sudden delusional idea, and is therefore not diagnostic of schizophrenia.

Thus two major memory disorders occur in schizophrenia. Nonperceptual images may acquire the quality of memories, or current perceptual images may be falsely associated with an unshakeable sense of recognition or of non-recognition.

Chapter 4

The classification of schizophrenia

In 1899 Kraepelin classified schizophrenia into hebephrenic, catatonic, and paranoid groups, and later E. Bleuler (1911) added simple schizophrenia as a fourth group, so that it is now customary to divide schizophrenia into hebephrenia, catatonia, paranoid schizophrenia, and simple schizophrenia. It is generally agreed that the boundaries between these groups are not hard and fast, so that the clinical features in any given case may change rapidly in the acute shifts of the illness, and also during the course of the years the symptomatology may change so much that the illness may have to be reclassified in its later stages.

In paranoid schizophrenia the paranoid symptoms, i.e. delusions and hallucinations, determine the clinical picture. Mild affective disorders may occur, but are not prominent and, while excitements and odd catatonic symptoms can occur, the motor symptoms are never very important for any length of time. Paranoid schizophrenia usually begins over the age of 25 years, and it seems that the personality must be well established before this variety of schizophrenia can occur. Gross deterioration of the personality is not common in this group. Since paranoid symptoms are prominent in other psychoses and attempts have been made to set aside all functional psychoses as paranoid states, a separate chapter will be devoted to paranoid psychoses.

Catatonic schizophrenia is dominated by the presence of motor disorders. Hallucinations, delusions, thought disorder, and disorder of affect are also usually present to some degree, but they are much less prominent than the motor symptoms. This illness tends to occur in adolescence and early adult life, but occasionally occurs in the fourth decade or even later. It is often acute in onset and runs a shifting course. Recovery from the first attack of catatonia is fairly common, but if the illness is progressive, the personality deterioration which occurs is usually severe in the late stages.

In hebephrenia disorders of abstract thinking and affect are the outstanding clinical features. The affect is much shallower than in normals and many of these patients are silly and childish in their behaviour. The formal thought disorder is usually of the negative kind and the delusions are poorly organized and ill held. Catatonic symptoms are rare and when they occur are transient. Hallucinations, especially auditory ones, are present, but do not seem to have much effect on the patient. Kraepelin called this variety 'silly dementia' and this term sums up the clinical picture very well. The illness usually begins insidiously in adolescence or early adult life and the prognosis is poor.

Diem described a simple dementing form of schizophrenia in 1903. A little later E. Bleuler used the term 'simple schizophrenia' to designate those patients with gross formal thought disorder and flattening of affect in the absence of delusions, hallucinations, or catatonic symptoms. This illness develops slowly, with gradual deterioration, the patient slowly goes downhill socially, and it is difficult to determine the exact point of onset. The men often become tramps, beggars, or petty thieves, while the women may become prostitutes. It is often difficult to distinguish simple schizophrenia from inadequate psychopathy. However, in schizophrenia there is a history of a change in social adjustment, while in psychopathy the person concerned has always been very poorly adjusted.

There is a tendency, especially among Swiss psychiatrists, to diagnose simple schizophrenia rather freely. This is well seen in a recent follow-up study of 27 simple schizophrenics in which it was shown that 4 patients had completely recovered, 5 had developed a different form of schizophrenia, and 18 were still suffering from simple schizophrenia, but 5 of these had only slight impairment. From the protocols of these cases it is difficult to see why some of them were diagnosed as suffering from simple schizophrenia; for example 1 patient had an acute illness in which a delusional mood occurred.

Cameron (1947) has classified schizophrenia in accordance with behaviouristic concepts and has described three main groups, the terms for which are self-explanatory: the aggressive, the submissive, and the detached. He has divided each of his three groups into subgroups, so that the aggressive group is subdivided into persecuted, grandiose, and self-punitive, the submissive group into compliant, dedicated, and transformed, and the detached group into avoidant and adient. The word 'adience' is used in psychological literature to signify the making of an approach to others. Thus 'adience' and 'adient' are somewhat similar to the terms 'advertence' and 'advertent' used in this text. Cameron's classification is interesting, but does not add very much to our understanding. He seems to have dispensed with simple schizophrenia and to have renamed paranoid, catatonic, and hebephrenic schizophrenia as aggressive, submissive, and detached forms respectively.

An interesting approach has been made by C. Schneider (1942), who has described three symptom-complexes in schizophrenia and claimed that these syndromes could occur either in pure form or in combinations. He believed that there was no psychological connexion between the individual symptoms of each syndrome, but assumed that the three syndromes corresponded to three normal groups of functions which were closely interrelated, but which could be separately affected by the schizophrenic process. Thus schizophrenia was held to cause the isolation and disorder of complexes of functions within the nervous system. Schneider claimed that these views were supported by the occurrence of pure examples of these syndromes and by the fact that in each syndrome the symptoms tended to occur in a regular sequence.

The three syndromes are the thought withdrawal syndrome, the desultory syndrome, and the drivelling syndrome. Naturally, thought withdrawal is experienced in the first syndrome, but this is associated with a fragmentation of thought, verbal derailment, and blocking. Inspirations or sudden delusional ideas which appear to come from natural sources are also a part of this syndrome. These patients have cosmic, universal, or religious experiences. The experience of loss of personal control over one's actions frequently occurs so that the patients experience their own actions as being made or forced upon them from outside. The outstanding affective disorder in this syndrome is perplexity.

The desultory syndrome is characterized by desultory thinking, i.e. thought makes jumps and therefore proceeds in an irregular way. There is a lack of inner drive and these patients are unable to react quickly and adequately to environmental changes. The affect is flattened and the patients are unable to feel happy or sad, but may pass into states of anger, anxiety, whining, or despair. These patients feel changed in themselves and have bodily hallucinations.

Vague drivelling thinking is the outstanding feature of the drivelling syndrome. There is no gross grammatical disorder and, although speech and thinking are superficially integrated, the content is drivel. Delusions of significance and primary delusional experiences also occur. The affect is inadequate and there is a lack of interest in real things and values.

Schneider claimed that a special variety of experience is characteristic of each syndrome. The thought withdrawal syndrome is associated with the experience of alienation of one's own acts and *Gedankenlautwerden,* disorders of social feeling, and bodily hallucinations are associated with the desultory syndrome, whereas the drivelling syndrome is associated with primary delusions.

This is an interesting approach, which unfortunately was formulated during World War II and has not yet been tested to any extent. Two different investigators have used Schneider's classification in follow-up studies and have found it useful.

No discussion of the classification of schizophrenia is complete without a presentation of the views of the Frankfurt school. Kleist regards schizophrenia as a disease of the nervous system which may be confined to one neurological system or which may affect many different systems within the central nervous system. The first group of system illnesses, typical schizophrenia, is made up of many subgroups which are due to different neurological system illnesses. Occasionally two neurological systems are affected and this gives rise to a combined typical form of schizophrenia. On the other hand, the atypical schizophrenias are due to disorders of many different neurological systems. Kleist believes that the disorders of the nervous system in these atypical schizophrenias may be caused by some agent from outside the nervous system, such as a hormone produced by an endocrine disorder. The symptomatology in the atypical forms is much more variable than in the typical forms and the course of the illness is more episodic, marked remissions being much more common. Typical schizophrenias tend to have a more insidious onset and a more steadily progressive course than the atypical varieties. Finally, the atypical variety has a much greater genetic loading than the typical.

Kleist divides schizophrenia into four major groups: paranoid, catatonic, hebephrenic, and confused. Confused schizophrenia consists of clinical pictures in which there is severe disorder of speech or thought which gives rise to grossly muddled expressions. The term 'hebephrenia' is used to include all patients in whom the outstanding symptom is a disorder of affect without any severe catatonic symptoms being present and with only mild or transient paranoid symptoms. Kleist has divided paranoid schizophrenia into seven typical and one atypical form, catatonia into seven typical and one atypical form, confused schizophrenia into three typical and two atypical forms, and hebephrenia into four typical forms.

Leonhard (1936), who made a careful study of chronic schizophrenia in a mental hospital, later joined Kleist and took part in the follow-up studies of the Frankfurt school. He has classified chronic schizophrenia in a slightly different way. He divides schizophrenia into systematic and non-systematic types which correspond to Kleist's typical and atypical forms. He describes three varieties of atypical schizophrenia: affect-laden paraphrenia, schizophasia, and periodic catatonia. Like Kleist, he has separated from schizophrenia a group of non-affective functional psychoses which have a favourable outcome. These psychoses have been designated 'cycloid psychoses' and are anxiety-elation psychosis, excited-inhibited confused psychosis, and hyperkinetic-akinetic motility psychosis (*see* Chapter 6). Leonhard (1959) considers that the non-systematic schizophrenias are more closely related to the cycloid psychoses than to the systematic schizophrenias.

Since it is possible that Leonhard's classification could be a useful framework for further investigation of chronic schizophrenia, a brief description of the Leonhard sub-types of schizophrenia will now be given.

NON-SYSTEMATIC SCHIZOPHRENIAS

Affect-laden Paraphrenia

This illness is distinguished by the affective loading of the paranoid delusions, so that these patients talk about their delusions with irritation or enthusiasm. In the systemic paranoid schizophrenias the delusions have no such affective loading, and often the patient does not become upset when one laughs at his delusions, or if he does become emotionally disturbed it is only for a short time and the disturbance soon passes away. This does not occur in affect-laden paraphrenia where the more one denies the patient's delusions the more upset he will become. These patients may shout, scold, and threaten when they feel that their beliefs are being treated discourteously.

At the onset of the illness severe affective swings into anxiety or ecstasy often occur and may continue as the psychosis progresses. These affective changes are always associated with the formation of delusional ideas. In anxiety, ideas of self-reference occur, together with auditory hallucinations, while in ecstasy ideas of happiness occur in association with visions and auditory hallucinations. The abnormal body sensations in affect-laden paraphrenia have a completely hallucinatory character because they are connected with outside influences. On the other hand, in anxiety elation psychosis these sensations can be understood as arising from the abnormal affective state. The clinical picture at the onset of affect-laden paraphrenia is that of anxiety with ideas of reference, but sometimes one finds a more hostile attitude to the environment when the patient is irritable and aggressive.

The degree of systematization of delusions varies from case to case; sometimes they may be so well systematized that the clinical picture is one of paranoia. Because of the bipolar nature of the affect, delusions of persecution and happiness may occur together. Often delusions become progressively more illogical and finally a fantastic delusional system occurs, in which there are extravagent grandiose ideas, misidentifications of people, memory falsifications, absurd ideas, and hallucinations in all sensory fields. These symptoms are somewhat similar to those occurring in the systematic form known as fantastic paraphrenia, but they are rarely completely expressed in affect-laden paraphrenia where some of these fantastic symptoms can be absent while others dominate the clinical picture. Apart from this, the affective loading of delusions is very obvious in affect-laden paraphrenia; and if it is not apparent at first sight it will become so when the patient is stimulated.

Catatonic and schizophasic symptoms may be found in this illness. Catatonic illnesses are sometimes found in the relatives of patients with this illness.

Schizophasia

Kraepelin (1913) described schizophasia as a variety of schizophrenia in which there was a gross confusion of speech so that the patient's speech was completely unintelligible. This gross confusion contrasted with the patient's fairly well ordered behaviour and ability to work and make social contact. In an investigation of the relatives of schizophasic patients, Leonhard found that schizophrenic illnesses in these relatives were rarely pure schizophasias, since catatonic and paraphrenic features were also frequently found.

Leonhard believes that there is a relationship between schizophasia and the confusion psychoses, but that the morbid phenomena in schizophasia are more pronounced. He claims that two forms of this disorder can be seen, one being the Kraepelinian variety and the other consisting of a disorder of speech which tends to be associated with catatonic symptoms. In the first form there is marked pressure of speech with severe confusion, many grammatical mistakes, but few neologisms. In the other form the patient has very little drive and the severe confusion is restricted, but neologisms are more common. These two forms are not genetically distinct, since they may both occur in the same family.

Periodic Catatonia

This is a catatonic illness in which remissions regularly occur and in which there is usually an admixture of hyperkinetic and akinetic symptoms. The hyperkinesia acquires a certain degree of rigidity because of the admixture of akinetic features, so that movements tend to proceed in a stiff, jerky manner and their natural grace is absent because the harmonious interplay of the individual motor acts does not occur. This distortion of motor activity leads to a loss of meaning of movements, so that reactive and expressive movements lose their significance. Thus gestures become vague, indefinite movements and facial expressions become grimaces. Excitements which occur in periodic catatonia are parakinetic because of this modification of the natural course of the motor acts. When these patients are akinetic an aimless movement of an extremity often occurs, which generally becomes uniform and may be a stereotypy or iteration. Thus stereotypy occurs despite the general postural rigidity and the rigidity of the mimic expression. In spite of the impoverishment of movement, these patients, when akinetic, often repeatedly take on definite postures and have postural stereotypies. Leonhard considers that the admixture of hyperkinetic and akinetic features can also be seen in impulsive actions and in negative behaviour in states where the patient has a poverty of movement. Leonhard believes that this illness is related to motility psychosis; in this latter disorder hyperkinesia and akinesia do not occur together, but alternate with one another and on the whole the symptoms are less severe.

Although there are remissions after the acute shifts, permanent defect finally occurs and this is likely to happen more rapidly after attacks of akinesia than after hyperkinesia. Leonhard divides these defects into mild, moderate, and severe, which he designates as states of psychic lameness, dullness, and stupidity respectively. In the severe defect of stupidity there is a degree of deterioration which is reminiscent of organic disease. In the defect states there is an impoverishment of drive, but impulsive excitements are frequent and excitements due to irritability also occur.

If the illness is mild, it may resemble a motility psychosis both in the symptomatology and in the course of the illness. Symptoms of schizophasia or affect-laden paraphrenia may be present at some stage of the illness.

SYSTEMATIC SCHIZOPHRENIAS

In the non-systematic schizophrenias the symptoms tend to be polymorphous and because of the diversity of symptoms it is difficult to outline the clinical pictures very sharply. On the other hand, in the systematic schizophrenias the symptomatology is clear-cut and the clinical picture is unequivocal. In these disorders Leonhard believes that specific circumscribed functional fields are affected, so that in each sub-form a definite higher function of the nervous system is involved. If this is so, then investigations of the systematic schizophrenia should lead to an understanding of the higher functions of the nervous system.

These sharply delimited clinical pictures of systematic schizophrenia are found in the end states. Earlier in the illness the non-specific effects of the morbid process or environmental pathoplastic factors may be intermixed with the defect symptoms so that the illness is difficult to classify. As a general rule the onset of the illness in the systematic group is gradual, whereas an acute onset is more likely in the non-systematic group, but may also be present in the combined systematic forms. Despite the difficulty in classifying the illnesses in the early stage, it is much easier to do so once the observer has learned to recognize the typical end states.

In the majority of systematic schizophrenias only one psychic system is affected, therefore the diagnosis of these varieties of schizophrenia does not depend merely on the presence of individual symptoms, but on a characteristic combination of symptoms. For example, a given case is a 'phonemic' paraphrenia not because auditory hallucinations are very prominent, but because there is a special variety of auditory hallucination, a characteristic disorder of affect, and thought disorder. Again, 'phonemic' and hypochondriacal paraphrenia differ because bodily hallucinations occur in the one and not in the other, but the fact that the basic mood is quite different is just as important. It is therefore always necessary to identify a specific combination of symptoms before a diagnosis can be made.

Systematic Catatonias

Leonhard classifies these into: (1) Parakinetic catatonia. (2) Manneristic catatonia. (3) Proskinetic catatonia. (4) Negativistic catatonia. (5) Speech-prompt catatonia. (6) Speech-inactive catatonia.

1. *Parakinetic Catatonia*

The parakinetic movements are not prominent in the early stages of this illness. As the condition progresses they become more obvious. Parakinesia in itself is not diagnostic of this condition since it may occur on the background of general motor excitement in periodic catatonia. Voluntary actions are carried out in an unnatural, awkward way and it seems that the motor activity is broken down into its constituent movements and the smooth transition from one individual movement to the next is absent. The jerky choreiform involuntary movements which occur seem to be distorted reactive and pseudo-expressive movements. Facial movements are especially affected and these patients often grimace a good deal. The motor disorder affects speech, so that these patients speak in short, sharp utterances; the words appear to be chopped up, and the sentences are usually short and agrammatical. As far as the content of speech is concerned, these patients may make remarks which are to the point, but at times their remarks seem to be fortuitous and irrelevant. In mild cases the parakinesia and hyperkinesia are not obvious until the patient has been stimulated.

2. *Manneristic Catatonia*

Mannerisms occur at the onset of the illness, but as the condition progresses all involuntary movement becomes less and less and, as a result, posture and movement become stiff. With the development of the illness motor activity becomes increasingly stereotyped and this may result in all activity being carried out in a fixed manneristic way. As the impoverishment of movement becomes more pronounced, mannerisms of commission become replaced by mannerisms of omission. Thus the patient tends to have stereotyped attitudes, a stiff facial expression, mannerisms of food refusal or refusal to go to the toilet, and so on. Opposition (*Gegenhalten*) occurs and the 'psychological pillow' is seen. In very severe cases any given posture may be maintained for some time (*Haltungsverharren*), but generally this is not so marked and usually the limbs slowly return to the rest position after the examiner has placed them in an unusual position.

3. *Proskinetic Catatonia*

Because of the readiness with which these patients turn towards the examiner when spoken to, this form was originally called 'prosectic', but Leonhard now uses the term 'proskinetic' in order to stress the abnormal readiness of these patients to begin automatic movements as a result of external stimuli. The typical prosectic speech disorder has already been described. Apart from this, these patients show intertwining movements, co-operation (*Mitmachen*), and *Mitgehen*. These patients are usually able to occupy themselves when directed, but as a rule they show marked affective flattening with an unconcerned sort of self-satisfaction. Excitements are not common in the defect stage and, when they do occur, take the form of short attacks of scolding or aggression. In the acute stage severe excitements occur, when the patient is restless, handles everything, tries to force himself through any open door, and attacks other patients.

4. *Negativistic Catatonia*

Marked negativism is seen in these patients but, if they are not irritated by the examiner, it may only show itself as a failure to carry out instructions or to answer questions. When the doctor approaches the patient in a gentle, friendly manner, ambitendency may occur. If these patients are examined brusquely and attempts are made to overcome their negativism by force, then severe excitement occurs. These patients show no indication of higher affectivity, but their basic drives are preserved, and this is seen in greediness and erotic tendencies. Despite the general lack of contact, these patients are liable to make apposite remarks when least expected.

5. *Speech-prompt Catatonia*

In this form the patient always turns towards the examiner and answers questions when spoken to. *Vorbeireden* is present and the patient seems to say what is immediately present in his mind, regardless of its suitability as an answer to the question. When spoken to, these patients turn towards the examiner with an empty, meaningless facial expression and answer all questions, even when the questioning continues for a long time.

6. *Speech-inactive Catatonia*

In the early stages of the illness these patients answer questions slowly, but later on they do not answer at all. When spoken to, they look here and there and often make whispering noises. From time to time they become very excited, when they scream and gesticulate in response to hallucinatory voices. In the early stages the patients admit to auditory hallucinations of a troublesome kind and also produce fantastic confabulations, but as the illness progresses they become so inaccessible that it is impossible to know whether these symptoms are still present. All motor reactions are slowed down and this is probably because the patients are being distracted by the auditory hallucinations and are unable to attend to stimuli from without. The only initiative, motor activity, and affect shown by these patients are in relation to their hallucinations when they are excited.

The Hebephrenias

These forms are poor in symptoms and this may lead to diagnostic difficulties, especially in mild cases. In the earlier stages the clinical picture may be obscured by non-specific symptoms, such as depressive and euphoric mood states and states of excitement or inhibition of a catatonic nature. Irritated moods occur early in the illness and often continue into the defect stage.

Leonhard has described the following four sub-groups of hebephrenia: (1) Silly hebephrenia. (2) Eccentric hebephrenia. (3) Shallow hebephrenia. (4) Autistic hebephrenia.

1. *Silly Hebephrenia*

These patients have a severe affective blunting which is associated with a contented or mildly cheerful mood, so that they smile or giggle in a characteristic way which becomes more pronounced when they are stimulated by others. There is a marked ethical blunting but, owing to their lack of drive, they only become criminals in so far as the opportunity presents itself. In the early stages these patients tend to play silly, childish tricks on others and these tricks are often spiteful and malicious. However, at times they may become ill-humoured and irritable and then act rather spitefully. Mood states of all kinds may occur in the acute stage of the illness. As the affective blunting progresses, these patients lose their drive and hang about in a happy-go-lucky way. They may even become so inactive that they give the impression of a catatonic illness, but their posture and movements are not catatonic and the silly smiling indicates the diagnosis.

2. *Eccentric Hebephrenia*

The characteristic features of this form are mannerisms and a general querulous attitude. It often begins with obsessive, compulsive symptoms which can be considered as precursors of the mannerisms. However, the mannerisms are most unlike those of manneristic catatonia, since these patients often will not talk about them and try to keep them secret, so that evidence of their existence comes from reports of the nursing staff or relatives. The manner of speaking, which is uniform and monotonous, together with the repeated querulous complaints and demands, suggests the manneristic quality of the illness. These patients produce the same grievance time and time again, irrespective of the listener's attitude, so that one has the impression that the patient is not speaking freely, but is producing material which has been learned. Collecting is a very common mannerism in this illness. These patients often collect rubbish of all kinds. Objects of value may be collected and then the mannerism appears in the guise of senseless stealing. These patients appear rather cheerless and depressed, but the main impression is one of severe affective flattening. In the defect stages no excitements occur despite the querulous attitude, but in the earlier stages ill-humoured mood states are present which are associated, irritated excitements. Mood variations do occur in the later stages, but are much milder. The affective blunting is associated with an ethical blunting, which often leads to anti-social behaviour, so that these patients frequently become beggars, tramps, and prostitutes. The thinking of these patients appears to be impoverished, but performance on intellectual tasks is not too bad and paralogia does not occur.

3. *Shallow Hebephrenia*

Flattening of affect is very marked in this form and the observer can detect no emotional response when topics which should affect the patient are touched upon. In contrast to this shallow affect, these patients are readily accessible and will carry on a reasonable conversation in a factual way. The mood state is one of indifferent satisfaction, but it is interrupted from time to time by states of ill humour when the patient may be anxious, irritated, or, very rarely, euphoric. In these mood states hallucinations and ideas of reference occur and the patient may become extremely excited and aggressive. The hallucinations may occur in all sensory fields, but most often they take the form of hallucinatory voices. In spite of the fact that these patients shout at auditory hallucinations when they are excited, they have a clear understanding of the morbid nature of these voices when the excitement dies away. Leonhard therefore suggests that they are of the nature of pseudo-hallucinations. There is a general lack of initiative in these patients, but they will take part in day-to-day activity of the mental hospital and do not have to be closely supervised.

4. *Autistic Hebephrenia*

This form is characterized by autism and a marked affective blunting. The facial expression is stiff and impenetrable and, as in speech-prompt catatonia, the observer cannot understand anything of the patient's inner life because of his enigmatic facial expression. Ill-humoured states occur in which the patient is very irritated, shouts threats or accusations at someone in the environment, and may attack this person. These states therefore differ from those in shallow hebephrenia in that here the aggression is directed against a specific person. The mood, which is reminiscent of eccentric hebephrenia, is one of rejection mixed with discontent, so that it is in marked contrast to the indifferent satisfaction of the silly and shallow hebephrenics. Usually these patients give short off-putting answers to intelligence test questions, but where they do answer it seems that the defect in intelligence is not very great. Initiative is, of course, deficient, but these patients can frequently be trained to carry out work requiring some independence of action. They do their work efficiently but, if they have to speak, they only say the absolute minimum required. In general, they tend to avoid others and walk past people whom they know without speaking.

The Systematic Paraphrenias

In common with many German authors, Leonhard uses the term 'paraphrenia' to designate all the paranoid schizophrenias. These illnesses are, of course, characterized by delusional ideas and sense deceptions, but thought disorder is also present and plays some part in the production of the paranoid symptoms. Leonhard believes that the disorder of the logical process of thought is a prerequisite for the setting free of some of the contents of the patient's own thinking, which are then able to appear independently as hallucinations. Apart from this, delusional ideas in paraphrenia are also connected with the formal thought disorder. Unlike Kleist, Leonhard does not separate from the other paranoid schizophrenias a group of confused schizophrenias in which thought disorder is the leading symptom. He believes that the severity of the thought disorder runs parallel with the severity of the paranoid symptoms, so that in incoherent paraphrenia one finds the most marked degree of thought disorder associated with the most insistent and troublesome type of hallucinations.

As in the other systematic schizophrenias, accessory symptoms may occur in the acute stage of the systematic paraphrenias and make accurate diagnosis difficult. Anxiety and other affective disorders may occur, perplexity is not uncommon, and ideas of reference may also appear. These symptoms may mask the specific symptoms which are usually present, but if one is familiar with the essential symptoms because of an acquaintance with advanced cases, then it is often possible to find them in the acute syndrome. On the whole, only paranoid symptoms occur in systematic paraphrenia, and catatonic or hebephrenic symptoms are very rarely present at any stage of the illness. Severe affective disorders are unusual in these illnesses, and suggest affect-laden paraphrenia. An acute onset is in favour of a non-systematic paraphrenia, since the systematic variety usually runs an insidious course.

Leonhard has described the following six sub-forms of systematic paranoid schizophrenia: (1) Hypochondriacal paraphrenia. (2) 'Phonemic' paraphrenia. (3) Incoherent paraphrenia. (4) Fantastic paraphrenia. (5) Confabulatory paraphrenia. (6) Expansive paraphrenia.

1. *Hypochondriacal Paraphrenia*

Specific bodily hallucinations, specific hallucinatory voices, and a certain mood state must all occur for this sub-form to be diagnosed. The bodily hallucinations are usually referred to internal organs and are usually described so grotesquely that it is impossible for a normal person to empathize with the patient. Often these sensations can only be described by the patient in a general way, such as 'tortures', 'misuse', and so on. The patient may produce technical neologisms in order to designate these sensations. Hallucinations of smell and taste may occur, but are not characteristic. In the early stages visual hallucinations are occasionally present, when the patient sees frightening visions, but later on they are not prominent and marked visual hallucinations contra-indicate the diagnosis of hypochondriacal paraphrenia. Hallucinatory voices consist of short phrases which are only partly connected with what the patient is thinking and do not fit in with his thoughts like the voices in 'phonemic' paraphrenia. In the early stages the voices often have a close connexion with the patient's thought, and *Gedankenlautwerden* may occur. Later on the voices are usually disconnected phrases, especially insulting words, without any real sense, so that the patient is usually unable to remember and reproduce them. The patient is more distressed by the occurrence of the voices as such than by their content. The voices and sensations are frequently attributed to devices which affect the patient from a distance, but more rarely they are attributed to people in the environment. The mood is permanently morose and dissatisfied and often develops into irritation. These patients complain bitterly about their hallucinations and are usually querulous; in particular they frequently insist in a monotonous way on their discharge from hospital. Since they easily become excited when contradicted and they maintain their interest in their home and family, it is obvious that their affectivity is fairly well preserved. These patients have thought disorder which Leonhard calls 'unconcentrated thinking'. They tend to wander from the point, talk about subjects loosely related to the task in hand, and are inclined to verbal derailments.

2. *'Phonemic' Paraphrenia*

Here the outstanding features are the hallucinatory voices. Bodily hallucinations and hallucinations of smell and taste do not occur. Leonhard considers this form to be the mildest of all the systematic paraphrenias. The voices often contradict or confirm what the patient is thinking, and are so closely related to his thinking that he treats them as real people with whom it is possible to hold a conversation. This is in contrast to hypochondriacal paraphrenia, where the patients are never seen talking to their voices but merely complain about the voices as such. *Gedankenlautwerden* occurs, and not only are the thoughts spoken aloud to the patient as he thinks, but they may also be spoken to the world at large so that the whole world knows what he is thinking. The content of the voices is also affect-laden in that the voices talk about those things which are unpleasant and disturbing to the patient, but the voices are not usually abusive. The voices are occasionally attributed to apparatus, but often they are thought to come from the radio or to be due to people in the environment who may be close to the patient or some way away. They may also be thought to be due to invisible beings such as spirits or witches, but occasionally they appear to emerge from within the body. Visual hallucinations occur from time to time, but are never important. The mood state is usually well balanced, but when the patient talks about the unpleasant things which the voices say he may become somewhat angry. In the later stages of the illness the patient usually becomes resigned to the voices and talks about them calmly, whereas the hypochondriacal paraphrenic never becomes habituated to his hallucinations and continues to complain bitterly about them even in the late stages. The affective responsiveness of the 'phonemic' paraphrenic is well preserved, so that he is usually a parole patient carrying out responsible work within the mental hospital and he may not even require hospital admission. Of course, some degree of affective blunting does occur, since these patients finally tolerate their apparently unpleasant symptoms rather patiently. In general conversation these patients show little disorder of thinking, but in problem-solving they talk about the problem indecisively and are unable to orientate themselves towards an objective of thought, while they are often successful with simple problems. Leonhard calls this variety of thought disorder 'woolly thinking'.

3. *Incoherent Paraphrenia*

Auditory hallucinations are prominent throughout the illness, but thought disorder only becomes marked later on when the hallucinations are very severe. Bodily hallucinations are commonly reported in the early state of the illness, but later on they are not present. Occasionally one can separate confabulatory remarks from among the incoherent expressions in these patients, and Leonhard believes that they are probably derived from visual hallucinations. In the later stages the patients are entirely occupied by their auditory hallucinations. Thus facial expression shows that they are not turning towards the examiner, but that their attention is directed entirely towards their inner experiences. The patient may look here and there, but does not look at the examiner very much or he may look at the examiner with a peculiar rigid gaze. The patient is obviously hallucinating during conversation, when he can often be seen whispering or talking quietly to the phonemes. Now and then he becomes excited and talks loudly or shouts abuse at the voices, often denying insults or accusations; shouting out, for example, 'You're a liar', 'You rotten swine', etc. The hallucinatory aversion and the continuous hallucinosis which cuts into all conversations occur in no other form of paraphrenia. These patients show no initiative and have no interest in anything. When asked questions their replies are short and perfunctory and are often given in a very low voice. It is obvious from what they say that they have a very severe thought disorder in which incoherence is associated with contaminations. They are usually dirty and untidy and often have incontinence of urine and faeces.

4. *Fantastic Paraphrenia*

In this illness hallucinations and delusions play an equal part. Bodily hallucinations are always marked and invariably described in a grotesque way which makes it impossible for the examiner to empathize with the patient. The description of bodily sensations resembles that of hypochondriacal paraphrenia, but this is the only symptom which is apparently qualitatively the same in the two different sub-forms of systematic schizophrenia. Hallucinatory voices are less obtrusive, but visual sense deceptions play a very important role in this sub-form. Isolated visions may be seen, but the characteristic symptom is the scenic hallucination in which scenes are visualized and accompanied by auditory and somatopsychic experiences; often these are scenes of horrible tortures and mass murders. This phenomenon partly accounts for the fantastic quality of the illness. However, this fantastic element is strengthened by the indifference with which these patients treat everyday practical experiences and by their manifestly absurd ideas. The same sort of gross illogicality also occurs in the misidentification of people in the environment, when the patient regards all people with whom he comes into contact as being different persons from those they say they are. These patients also have absurd, grandiose ideas in which they elevate themselves to an extraordinary degree and may call themselves God. However, they draw no conclusions from these fantastic, grandiose delusions and do not object to being treated as patients. Their affect is shallow and if their ideas are laughed at they may flare up somewhat, but the affect quickly dies away. However, they often maintain a definite interest in their environment, are usually interested in their family, and superficially their general attitude often appears to be quite natural. When they talk about their fantastic ideas they frequently become somewhat muddled, but if one questions them carefully, then the train of thought becomes fairly clear. Tests of intelligence show that the main feature of the formal thought disorder in this variety of paraphrenia is derailment.

5. *Confabulatory Paraphrenia*

Here the outstanding feature is falsification of memory, and these patients produce plastic, detailed descriptions of alleged events. In some cases in the early stages there may be dream-like experiences which appear to be precursors of the later confabulations, but in other cases the confabulations may clearly be present at the onset of the illness. The characteristic confabulations generally have a fantastic quality and are concerned with other parts of the world, other worlds, or even the moon and stars. It is as if visual and auditory images connected with the patient's fantasy life emerge spontaneously and acquire a sensory character, which normally is only associated with memory images. As the patients evaluate their environment correctly, Leonhard assumes that their critical sense will only allow the confabulations to be valid when they are concerned with other places and other times. Quite a number of these patients say that these fantastic events happened in dreams or trances and this can be regarded as an indication of partial preservation of the patient's critical sense. These patients also have 'perceptual falsifications' in which objects in their environment, especially people, continually appear to be different, so that the size, shape, and general appearance of things change from day to day. Leonhard explains this as an abnormally detailed concretization of memory images so that, for example, when a person is seen by the patient, he is contrasted with the detailed memory image of his appearance on the day before and the different features of his present appearance are emphasized, while the general similarity is overlooked. Grandiose ideas which are often very extravagant also occur and are always worked into the confabulations. These patients have an elevated mood which supports the grandiose delusions and partly contributes to the fantastic and sensational character of the confabulations. Leonhard considers that the formal thought disorder in this variety of paraphrenia enhances the absurdly fantastic nature of the confabulations, because the transition from concrete to abstract thought in these patients is disturbed, so that while they can maintain a critical judgement in concrete thinking, they cannot carry out abstract tasks. Thus in everyday life they are well ordered, but in intelligence tests they show a peculiar pictorial form of thinking.

6. *Expansive Paraphrenia*

Although in the early stages of this variety sense deceptions do occur, later on they are entirely absent, so that this form is quite unlike any other systematic paraphrenia and is almost entirely delusional in the later stages. The delusions are always expansive and are not associated with persecutory delusions. However, the gandiose ideas are within reasonable limits and the patient acts according to his ideas. In the fantastic and confabulatory paraphrenias, the grandiose delusions do not lead to any consistent behaviour, but in expansive paraphrenia the patients behave as if they were highly placed, so that the whole personality is much more affected by the grandiose delusions. They take on a haughty pose, adopt a superior attitude when dealing with others; thus they are familiar in a friendly way with the doctors and tend to look down on their fellow patients. They try to impress others by their style of dress, the use of high-sounding phrases, and the production of secret documents, which are written in code. Usually the expansive behaviour and productions of these patients have a very monotonous character, since the same ideas and attitudes are repeated without much variation. This is in contrast to the richness of ideas of the confabulatory and fantastic paraphrenics. These expansive paraphrenics tend to become garrulous when they speak about their grandiose delusions and they bring forward their requests and complaints with a great deal of verbosity. They carry out their expansive behaviour and activities with a certain amount of eagerness, but otherwise they show a general deficiency of initiative. The affect of these patients gradually becomes blunted and in the final stages they do not become irritated even when laughed at. A very marked disorder of thought is present which mainly affects verbal thinking, so that mistakes in grammar and word formation frequently occur. Leonhard believes that concepts are not absent in these patients, but they are very inexact, and the finer details are missing. He calls this variety of thought disorder 'coarsening of thinking'.

Astrup (1957) and Fish (1958a, b) have classified groups of chronic schizophrenics according to the schemes of Kleist and Leonhard and they both find that Leonhard's scheme is more satisfactory. Leonhard believes that his sub-groups do not overlap and he claims that those relatively rare cases which do not fit into one of his sub-groups are combinations of two different sub-groups. However, it is best to consider Leonhard's sub-groups as syndromes and to classify cases of chronic schizophrenia according to the most prominent symptoms, even if some atypical symptoms are present. Leonhard's scheme can easily be applied to chronic schizophrenics and, once sufficient skill has been acquired, it can be applied cautiously to acute and sub-acute cases.

So far, no one has been able to demonstrate a clear relationship between the acute clinical pictures and the chronic sub-groups. Some authors have, in fact, pointed out that the course of the illness in patients belonging to the same chronic sub-group has often been very different. Astrup has studied chronic cases classified according to Leonhard's scheme and has attempted to classify the acute clinical pictures by using the concepts of Carl Schneider (1942). He therefore classified acute clinical pictures into four main groups—hebephrenic and hebephrenic-paranoid psychoses, catatonic and mixed catatonic psychoses, paranoid psychoses dominated by projection symptoms, and paranoid psychoses with systematized delusions. He used the term 'hebephrenic' in the sense of severe schizophrenic affective disorder and his hebephrenic group showed marked affective blunting, autism, and the desultory syndrome. His catatonic group had marked catatonic symptoms and the desultory syndrome. The paranoid psychoses dominated by projection symptoms had the thought-

Table 7. COURSE AND OUTCOME IN RELATION TO INITIAL CLINICAL PICTURE
(*After Astrup*)

	Hebephrenia and hebephrenic–paranoid psychoses (desultory syndrome)	*Catatonia*	*Paranoid psychosis with projection symptoms (thought-withdrawal syndrome)*	*Paranoid psychosis with systematized delusions (drivelling syndrome)*
Number of cases	40	44	51	43
Social remissions	9	18	16	14
Progressive course	31	26	22	29
Full remission	Nil	Nil	13	Nil
Slight paranoid defect	4	1	Not stated	25
Severe paranoid defect	Nil	3	Not stated	4
Slight hebephrenic defect	8			
Severe hebephrenic defect	19			
Systematic catatonia	3	3		
Non-systematic catatonic defect state	4	19		

withdrawal syndrome and projection symptoms, while the paranoid psychoses with systematized delusions had the drivelling syndrome. The relation between the acute and chronic clinical pictures in Astrup's series is shown in *Table 7*.

Astrup has also ranked the sub-groups in each of Leonhard's major groups according to the severity of the average clinical picture which he has estimated on the basis of the level of social integration. Thus he considers that the paranoid group ranges from the mildest to the most severe as follows: affect-laden paraphrenia, schizophasia, 'phonemic' paraphrenia, hypochondriacal paraphrenia, expansive and confabulatory paraphrenia, fantastic paraphrenia, incoherent paraphrenia. He ranks the hebephrenias from the mildest to the most severe as autistic, eccentric, shallow, and silly. This investigator also carried out conditioned reflex and other physiological experimental investigations on his series of chronic schizophrenics and found that the severity of the clinical condition was roughly inversely related to the performance on the tests used.

It may be that Leonhard's scheme is a useful research tool and that investigation of the differences between the different sub-groups may lead to the isolation of pathoplastic factors, and thus clear the way for the identification of the basic neurophysiological disorder or disorders which form the essential lesion in schizophrenia. That it has not yet achieved much is not necessarily the fault of the system. In the end, all research on schizophrenia must be guided by and be based upon clinical phenomena and their differentiation.

Chapter 5

Paranoid states

History of 'Paranoid States'

In British psychiatry, the term 'paranoid states' tends to be used to cover all conditions in which the predominant symptoms are those of paranoid delusions. Within this category are to be found, more or less, all those conditions variously known as 'paranoia', 'paraphrenia', 'paranoid schizophrenia', 'paranoid depression', and 'paranoid personality'. A classification of disorders in terms of symptoms, whether a single one or a closely linked few, is never satisfactory, neither in medicine—dyspnoeic states—nor in psychiatry—paranoid states. In order to understand the classification of paranoid illnesses, it will be necessary first to consider the historical development of the concepts of schizophrenia, paraphrenia, and paranoia.

The Greek word 'paranoia' was revived in the eighteenth century, but the first stage in the development of its use in modern psychiatry can best be dated to 1818 when Heinroth described delusional states as 'disorders of intellect' (*Verrücktheit*) not fundamentally involving the other faculties of the mind, i.e. feeling and will, although he recognized that some admixture was usually present. In its time this was an important contribution to the notion of partial insanity. In 1845 Griesinger described the same conditions, but regarded them as secondary to a preceding disorder of feeling. In 1863 Kahlbaum used the term 'paranoia' for chronic fixed delusions of persecution and grandeur. He considered this condition to be a disorder of intellect and distinguished it from those disorders which passed through this stage onto a final one. This became generally accepted. In 1893 Kraepelin made a great step forward when he suggested that all those functional psychoses which lead to mental deterioration should be grouped together as a disease entity. Since these disorders appeared to stand in close relation to adolescence, in 1899 he decided to call them 'dementia praecox', a term which had already been used by Morel. However, he did not consider that the disorder was entirely a disease of young people, and in the 8th edition of his textbook, in 1913, he wrote:

> It has become evident that the assumptions on which the chosen name was based were at least doubtful. As will be discussed in more detail later on, the possibility that in a certain number of cases of dementia praecox a complete and lasting recovery occurs cannot be denied in the present state of our knowledge, also the relations to adolescence

do not appear to be absolute: I admit that I do not consider that the facts in both these directions are yet by any means settled.

Kraepelin considered that dementia praecox was fundamentally a disorder of emotion and volition. He therefore regarded it as distinct from paranoia and paraphrenia. The latter was characterized by hallucinations and delusions, but did not show deterioration, and concerning the former he wrote: 'If, with the help of these explanations, the attempt is made to define the concept of paranoia as it forms the foundations of the following exposition, stress would be laid on these features of it, the insidious development of a permanent and unshakeable delusional system resulting from internal causes, which is accompanied by perfect preservation of clear and orderly thinking, willing and acting.'

Mayer (1921) followed up the 78 cases which Kraepelin had used to establish his concept of paraphrenia. He found that 40 per cent of these patients showed obvious signs of dementia praecox within a few years. In the group of patients who corresponded to Kraepelin's clinical picture of paraphrenia, Mayer found a family history of schizophrenia in some cases. Apart from this, he found that the original clinical picture in patients who finally showed signs of schizophrenia could not be distinguished from that which occurred in those who remained paraphrenic. Mayer concluded that paraphrenia was not a disease entity which could be sharply distinguished from schizophrenia. This view was adopted by most German-speaking psychiatrists.

E. Bleuler (1911) showed that dementia praecox did not necessarily end in deterioration and that it could begin later in life. He introduced the term 'schizophrenia' in order to get away from the idea that this disorder was necessarily an adolescent mental deterioration. M. Bleuler (1943) studied the schizophrenias which occurred later in life. He defined 'late schizophrenia' as:

1. Schizophrenia occurring for the first time after the age of 40 years.
2. The symptomatology should not differ from that of schizophrenia occurring earlier in life or if it did differ it should not do so in a clear and radical way.
3. It should not be possible to attribute the illness to a neuropathological disorder, because of the presence of an amnestic syndrome or associated signs of organic nervous disease.

In one series of mental hospital schizophrenics, he found that 15 per cent were late schizophrenics and in another series 17 per cent. Among them 68 per cent began in the fifth decade, 28 per cent in the sixth, and 4 per cent after the age of 60 years. Angst et al. (1973) found that 35 per cent of paranoid schizophrenia began after the age of 40 years and 13 per cent after 50 years.

A series of 110 chronic schizophrenics (Fish, 1958a) was reviewed from the standpoint of the clinical features in relation to the age of onset. A fairly reasonable estimate of the age of onset could be obtained in all but one case and this hebephrenic patient was not included in the analysis. The incidence of the three different forms of schizophrenia in the different age-groups is shown in *Table 8*.

Table 8. AGE OF ONSET OF DIFFERENT TYPES OF SCHIZOPHRENIA IN A SERIES OF 110 CHRONIC PATIENTS

Age-group (years)	*Hebephrenic schizophrenia*	*Catatonic schizophrenia*	*Paranoid schizophrenia*	*Total*
19 and under	4	7	—	11
20–24	2	7	8	17
25–29	7	8	10	25
30–34	4	7	7	18
35–39	—	5	11	16
40–44	—	1	7	8
45–49	1	—	4	5
50–54	—	—	6	6
55–59	—	—	3	3
Over 60	—	—	1	1
Total	18	35	57	110

The mean age of the hebephrenics is 26 years, of the catatonics 27 years, and of the paranoid group 37 years. The difference between them is statistically very highly significant, obviously due to the late onset of the paranoid cases. For what it is worth, the frequency distribution of all these cases, when plotted on probability paper, is seen to approximate closely to a normal distribution, which suggests that the paranoid schizophrenics, including those of late onset, can be regarded as being drawn from the same 'population' as the others.

As the patients in this series all had illnesses of more than 10 years' duration and as no patients in the geriatric ward were included in this series, there is no doubt that this series was biased in favour of the younger schizophrenics.

Although it was once believed that schizophrenic clinical pictures occurring in and after middle age were related to organic disease of the brain, this is not now accepted. Such changes as are found in the brain can be ascribed more plausibly to chronic malnutrition or intercurrent disease. Kay and Roth (1961), in their study of 99 'late paraphrenics' (mean age 70 years), found that only 9 per cent showed signs of focal cerebral disease, including isolated seizures, and a further 12 per cent finally ended up resembling cases of senile dementia.

Kolle (1931) described his investigations on 19 of Kraepelin's patients, on which the definition of paranoia had been based, and 47 additional cases. In 62 of them he found primary delusions, i.e. delusions which could not be 'understood' as arising rationally or emotionally from the given state of the patient. He found also an increased incidence of schizophrenia among the relatives of these patients, six times higher among the children and three times higher among the siblings, than in the general population, but still one which was less than among the relatives of schizophrenics. It would appear, therefore, that paranoia must be regarded as a variety of schizophrenia; a milder condition than the paranoid form since it does not often end in deterioration but nevertheless one in which the prognosis for recovery is poor.

There has been much criticism of Kraepelin's concept of paranoia, including doubts as to its existence. Kolle (1957) reported that one of his students examined the case notes of all admissions to the Munich Neuropsychiatric Clinic for the years 1953–55 inclusive. Out of 13 531 cases he found 920 (6·8 per cent) with a diagnosis of schizophrenia or paranoid psychosis. Of these, 8 (0·9 per cent) corresponded to the classic Kraepelinian paranoia. As a syndrome it can be found, but the rarity explains the doubts!

If paranoia is regarded as including all disorders characterized by delusions and little else, it is then much more common than thought. It would cover monosymptomatic hypochondriacal delusions, erotomania, and delusions of jealousy, disfigurement, infestation, and of emitting an odour (Munro, 1982).

Diagnostic Criteria of Schizophrenia

This does not completely settle the question of the classification of paranoia. Several problems remain, of which the first is concerned with the criteria for diagnosing schizophrenia. The criterion of age of onset is now regarded as of little value and can be ignored.

The notion that schizophrenia always leads to deterioration is one which was abandoned even by Kraepelin and the work of Bleuler should have killed it completely. Nevertheless, some psychiatrists are still unwilling to diagnose schizophrenia in the absence of signs of mental deterioration. This is equivalent to refusing to make a diagnosis of a particular disorder until it is in an advanced state.

Such a viewpoint does not take sufficient account of the relationship between deterioration of personality and age of onset of illness. Simple schizophrenia, which begins very early, produces most deterioration of personality and late onset paranoid forms produce least change. It could well be that the immature and relatively undeveloped personality succumbs easily to the schizophrenic process, but as it becomes more and more rigid with increasing age is better able to resist the destructive effects. An opposite viewpoint would suggest that a rigid personality delays the onset of the schizophrenic process and thereby changes the clinical picture.

Both Kraepelin and Bleuler defined schizophrenia and gave exhaustive descriptions of schizophrenic symptoms, but if their definitions are considered carefully, no clear-cut diagnostic criteria are found. In advanced cases of schizophrenia with severe formal thought disorder, affective disorder in the form of blunting or incongruity, or marked catatonic phenomena, there are few diagnostic difficulties. However, in acute illnesses these signs may be absent or equivocal and then diagnosis often depends more on the observer's personal attitude than on an evaluation of the signs and symptoms.

It has previously been pointed out that one way of overcoming this difficulty is to use the concepts of *verstehende* psychology which were introduced into psychiatry by Jaspers. One can then designate a symptom as schizophrenic if it is not 'understandable'. The understandability of a symptom is assessed by the observer feeling himself into the situation of the patient, and assessing whether the symptom can be understood rationally or emotionally as arising from the situation and the changes in the patient due to the situation and his emotions. Thus one can understand that a depressed patient might hear reproachful voices, but one cannot understand his hearing his own thoughts spoken aloud. The difficulty of this approach is the subjective nature of the criterion of 'understandability'. In Jaspers' sense there is no doubt that there are some symptoms which are clearly non-understandable and therefore schizophrenic. Since schizophrenic symptoms can be caused by coarse brain disease, schizophrenia can only be diagnosed in the presence of schizophrenic symptoms if there is no evidence of coarse brain disease.

It is against this background that one can appreciate Schneider's views on schizophrenic symptoms of the first and second rank. This worker considers that in the absence of coarse brain disease certain symptoms are diagnostic of schizophrenia; these are symptoms of the first rank.

They are as follows:

1. Hearing one's own thoughts spoken aloud (*Gedankenlautwerden*).
2. Hallucinatory voices in the form of statement and reply, so that the patient hears voices speaking about him in the third person.
3. Hallucinatory voices in the form of a running commentary.
4. Bodily hallucinations, that is the patient has sensations in his body which he knows are produced by external agencies.

5. Thought withdrawal, thought insertion, and other influences on thought.
6. Thought broadcasting.
7. Delusional perception.
8. All events in the spheres of feeling, drive, and volition which are experienced as made or influenced by others.

Although important these symptoms are not essential. Other symptoms which occur in schizophrenia are designated as symptoms of the second rank and are not considered to be diagnostic in themselves, but several of them occurring together may form a clinical picture which when considered as a whole may have to be diagnosed as schizophrenia.

Because the first-rank symptoms can be so easily identified, they have been extensively studied and it would now appear that they are not as useful diagnostically as was at first thought. Thus, in the International Pilot Study of Schizophrenia organized by the World Health Organization (1973), it was found that 58 per cent of 817 schizophrenics showed first-rank symptoms, but these were also found in 22 per cent of 72 manics, 14 per cent of 142 depressives, and even in 4 per cent of 126 patients with neurotic and personality disorders (Strauss and Carpenter, 1974).

If only two groups of non-organic* psychoses, namely schizophrenia and manic-depressive insanity, are recognized, then no objection can be made to the diagnostic value of Schneider's symptoms of the first rank, since it is difficult to understand how such symptoms could arise on the basis of an uncomplicated disorder of affect. Some workers, such as Kleist and his pupils, reject this simple division of the non-organic psychoses and isolate a group of marginal psychoses which are neither schizophrenic nor manic depressive. These marginal psychoses, which will be described later, are considered by many authors to be schizophrenias which recover with minimal or undetectable defect, but there is no doubt that this concept has a heuristic value. However, whether the marginal psychoses are accepted or not, it is reasonable to consider that the presence of any one of Schneider's symptoms of the first rank makes the diagnosis of an uncomplicated affective disorder much less likely.

Relation to Affective Disorders

The second problem is concerned with the relation between paranoid symptoms and affective disorders. Although there is little doubt that paranoid symptoms can occur in affective disorders, no one today

* By 'non-organic' is meant the absence of coarse brain disease detectable by present-day methods.

would attempt to follow Specht (1905) and derive all paranoid psychoses from an abnormal affect. Thus some patients suffering from mania may have very paranoid attitudes, partly due to previous personality traits and partly to a misinterpretation of the justified reaction which their manic behaviour provokes, but these cases seldom give rise to diagnostic difficulties, since the paranoid ideas are rarely well-held delusions.

Discussion on the relation between paranoid symptoms and depressive states is confused by lack of clarity of definitions. The patient who says, 'I have committed terrible crimes and deserve to be punished', is said to be suffering from delusions of guilt. When he says, 'I have committed terrible crimes and I am going to be punished', or even, 'The police are pursuing me and will hang me for my crimes', he is not then suffering from delusions of persecution. The 'paranoid' delusions can be understood as being due to the basic mood disorder and are still related to guilt. If this distinction is borne in mind, it becomes clear that persecutory delusions are indeed rare in the depressions.

Kraepelin (1921) described a syndrome which he called 'paranoid depression'. It was a severe illness characterized by marked depression and agitation, paranoid ideas, and auditory hallucinations, and he stressed the frequency of suicide in this type of depression. However, he did not explain how the severe persecutory delusions, in the absence of marked delusions of guilt, could be understood as due to the depressive mood. From Kraepelin's description of paranoid depression it appears that some of his cases were severely agitated depressions with a complicating organic disorder such as dehydration, exhaustion, intercurrent illness, or over-dosage with sedative drugs, while other cases were paranoid schizophrenics with a marked depressive mood. However, there is a group of patients with moderately severe or very severe anxious depressions in whom marked delusions of persecution occur, but which are not considered to be justified by the patient. These persecutory delusions are very prominent, the patient protests bitterly about the persecution, and frequently attributes his depressive symptoms to its disturbing character. These patients are always very anxious, often agitated, and frequently attempt suicide. Leonhard (1959) has described this illness and called it *Argwöhnische* depression. There is no adequate description of this illness in English, but it has been recognized as an affective disorder by many British psychiatrists, particularly by Lewis (1934) and other pupils of Mapother.

It is difficult to give any adequate explanation of these severe persecutory delusions occurring in a depressive illness. In some cases they may be an exaggeration of lifelong paranoid ideas. Thus the quiet, introverted, sensitive, paranoid personality keeps his paranoid ideas to himself, but under the influence of an anxious depression these ideas become much more pronounced and come into the open, to the surprise and astonishment of his friends and relatives. Many of these patients appear to have anankastic rather than sensitive personalities, and it could be argued that many anankastic personalities have paranoid attitudes in that they feel unappreciated or deliberately upset by their fellows. They frequently are unable to understand the justified irritation and annoyance which are a direct result of their behaviour. Apart from this uncovering of paranoid attitudes by the affective disorder, it is possible that anxiety itself may play a part in the production of persecutory delusions. Anxiety may cause or exacerbate ideas of reference and then, because of its effect on goal-directed thinking, it may prevent the patient from thinking out the inaccuracy of his beliefs.

Despite all these psychological explanations of the persecutory delusions, there is no doubt that these delusions pass beyond what can be 'understood' or empathized by a sympathetic observer. However, no other 'non-understandable' symptoms are found in this illness, and the presence of continuous auditory hallucinosis or any of the symptoms of the first rank is not compatible with the diagnosis of paranoid depression. The classification of this rare disorder as a primary disturbance of affect must be regarded as doubtful, even though the depressive symptoms, the good prognosis, and the good response to electroconvulsive therapy distinguish this illness from other paranoid illnesses. Nevertheless, many clear-cut paraphrenics respond well to such treatment and although many ultimately deteriorate their prognosis is, on the whole, quite good. It would therefore be better to regard 'paranoid depressions' as being a form of schizophrenia. Of course, marked depressive symptoms may occur at the onset of a paranoid schizophrenia, but in these cases symptoms of the first rank are often present or the total clinical picture is not 'understandable'. In these cases clear schizophrenic symptoms usually appear during the course of electroconvulsive therapy.

Paranoid Personalities and Reactions

The third problem concerns the relation between paranoid personalities and paranoia as a clinical entity. The psycho-biology of Adolf Meyer regards all mental illness as the reactions of the personality to the stresses of life, i.e. as an understandable development of the personality. Kraepelin did not accept this. He considered paranoia to be different from the querulous paranoid state where the patient is litigious and is stimulated to take up a querulous attitude by some injustice. For Kraepelin, paranoia was an endogenous illness and the querulous paranoid state was a result of the interaction of an abnormal personality with a stressful environment.

Others in Germany have disagreed. Thus Kretschmer (1950) has described the syndrome of the *sensitive Beziehungswahn*—the delusions of self-reference of the sensitive person. This latter is a psychopathic personality who is shy and who feels inadequate, but side by side with his sense of inadequacy is a feeling that he is worthy of better things. He attributes his failure to achieve his true status in life to some physical, social, or psychological defect, such as physical deformity, illegitimacy, or abnormal sexual behaviour. He nurses this sense of inferiority and attributes his lack of success to his inferiority and the machinations of others, but he does not talk about these ideas. Kretschmer points out that in these sensitive personalities there is a tension between the feeling of self-importance and the humiliating environment. After many years of self-torturing ruminations, some key experience may lead to the sudden appearance of a paranoid psychosis. This experience is one which exposes the sensitive person's secret defect or which causes a sudden increase in his humiliating position. Thus, according to Kretschmer, a full-blown paranoid psychosis with ideas of reference and persecution emerges from this understandable interaction of personality and environment. While some paranoid states are due to such a sequence of events and can be described as psychogenic reactions, this does not account for all cases of so-called *sensitive Beziehungswahn.* In some cases, the paranoid psychosis emerges in a depressive illness, while in others a chronic debilitating illness or the aftermath of an acute physical illness may act as a releasing agent. In these latter cases the paranoid state improves with the improvement of the physical condition. Finally, some of these patients are really suffering from schizophrenia and the pre-morbid personality happens to be of the sensitive variety. When such a radical change of a personality as the emergence of a severe paranoid psychosis occurs, most observers feel unable to 'understand' it as a simple psychological development, and consider that the change is due to a process caused by a bodily disease rather than a development of a personality.

We have now to consider the querulous paranoid personality and the querulous delusional patient. The querulous personality is one who is always spoiling for a fight and is ready to react sharply to any real or supposed injury. Some of these patients are mildly hypomanic or hyperthymic personalities, but not all. Some querulous personalities may react to real or imaginary wrong by litigation, which is carried from one court to another. The patient then becomes deluded about the justice of his case and the lack of fairness of the judges and his opponents. He accuses the opposing witnesses of perjury and the judge of double dealing, so that frequently he is punished for contempt of court. The patient's knowledge of the law is often extensive, but he is unable to see the flaws in his own case. He may be able to convince other lay people of the justice of his case and surround himself with a group of supporters. This type of patient is not often seen in Britain and Mayer-Gross has suggested that this is due to the difference between the English and German legal systems.

In order to clarify this distinction between the paranoid personality and the paranoid state due to psychological illness, Jaspers (1910) introduced the concept of psychic process. He pointed out that new psychological symptoms may emerge in patients with no coarse brain disease, and when such symptoms occur and are permanent, then a 'psychic process' must be postulated, if these symptoms cannot be 'understood' as arising from the previous personality. Thus in the absence of coarse brain disease a definite irreversible 'non-understandable' change of the personality is caused by the psychic process. This process is analogous to the physical psychotic process due to organic brain disease which also produces an irreversible change in the personality. Although he did not express it clearly in these terms, it seems that Jaspers considered the psychic process as due to a disorder of the complicated neuro-physiological processes which run parallel with psychic events. This is in contrast to the physical psychotic process of coarse brain disease which affects the neuro-physiological parallel processes in an indirect, coarse, and haphazard way.

If the change in a person was understandable as a development of the previous personality, Jaspers called this a 'development' of the personality and thus contrasted 'process' and 'development' in paranoid states. He realized, however, that such a differentiation was not always possible in any given case, but, despite this, the distinction between the two different types of paranoid state seems to be reasonable. It must be noted, however, that Jaspers did not say that the psychic process was synonymous with schizophrenia, although in a later work he pointed out that in a large number of cases where there was a process, the psychological changes of schizophrenia were present. As the only psychological illness in which a psychic process in Jaspers' sense occurs is schizophrenia, it is therefore justifiable, until proved otherwise, to assume that where a psychic process can be demonstrated the underlying illness is schizophrenic. The differences between psychic process, physical psychotic process, and personality development are shown in *Table 9*.

It should be clear now that the term 'paranoid state' is purely a label and not a diagnosis. 'Paraphrenia' is a convenient short description for schizophrenia, usually of later onset, with marked hallucinations, sometimes with delusions, and usually with depressive symptoms which may be severe, and may even dominate the

Table 9. DIFFERENCES BETWEEN PSYCHIC PROCESS AND PERSONALITY DEVELOPMENT (*After Jaspers*)

Personality development	*Psychic process*	*Physical psychotic process*
Slow gradual change analogous to the development of a child	A new development which begins at a definite point in time	
Acute events do not signify a lasting change. The *status quo ante* is restored again	The acute process signifies a change which is not reversible. (If an acute change is followed by a complete cure and is not due to a physical psychotic process then it is considered to be a 'reaction' or a 'periodic' event)	Whether the change is transient or permanent depends on the basic physical process and not on the characteristics of the direct parallel processes
One can derive the whole course of life from the predisposition of the personality	When an attempt is made to derive the changes from the personality a limit is found at a given point in time where something new appeared, i.e. a heterogeneous change occurred	The delimitaton of the illness is in the last analysis a result of the special nature of the physical process
	There is a definite regularity of development and course of changed personality, which can be understood in the same way as the normal events of psychic life, and which possesses a new unity and a full rational and understandable coherence	There is an indiscriminate irregularity of the symptoms and course of the illness. All the phenomena succeed one another in an underivable confusion, since they are only secondarily dependent on the direct parallel process, but much more dependent on the physical brain process

clinical picture. Many of these patients eventually deteriorate and become typical paranoid schizophrenics. 'Paranoia', if it is to be used at all, should imply no more than a clinical picture of delusions, usually persecutory and sometimes also grandiose, with no current deterioration of personality. Paranoid states can be divided into the following groups: (1) Schizophrenia, (2) Personality disorders and psychogenic reactions, (3) Organic psychiatric states, and, possibly, (4) Affective disorders.

These groups are, of course, not mutually exclusive. For example, a patient with a paranoid personality may have an affective disorder which produces a severe paranoid illness, or coarse brain disease may bring to light the paranoid beliefs of a sensitive personality. Here it is worth noting that transient paranoid states without clouding of consciousness can occur as a result of acute organic disease which affects the brain directly or indirectly. Such short-lived illnesses are not infrequent in general hospitals following major operations, coronary thrombosis, and similar acute conditions.

If this classification of paranoid states is accepted, then one cannot give a prognosis for paranoid states in general, and it is not true to say that paranoid states have a better prognosis than schizophrenia. The prognosis in 'paranoid depressions' is, of course, usually very good, and those organic paranoid states which are likely to cause difficulty in differential diagnosis also tend to recover quickly. In a personality disorder, the paranoid state usually fluctuates in severity and may become quiescent for long periods. Paranoid psychogenic reactions usually disappear with environmental readjustment and general supportive measures. The prognosis of schizophrenic paranoid states will depend on the concept of schizophrenia used by the examiner.

If one accepts the definition of schizophrenia previously given, then one must say that the prognosis of schizophrenic paranoid states is poor. However, most experienced psychiatrists would agree that, while the chance of recovery is low in paranoid schizophrenia occurring in middle life, the possibility of severe deterioration is negligible and the personality is usually well preserved throughout the illness.

It may be suggested that the whole of this discussion is a waste of time because only an understanding of the psychodynamics can help in a given case. Unfortunately, while Freudian theories can often give some explanation of the content, they cannot explain the form of the symptoms. Alternatively, it can be argued that diagnostic labels are not very important because, although an observer may use one diagnostic label differently from the customary usage, his treatment and prognostic assessment in any given case will not differ radically from those of other workers.

Although the classification of paranoid states suggested here is neither new nor revolutionary, it is a framework within which experimental investigation can be carried out. The psychopathological approach to diagnosis cannot produce very refined results, since the evaluation of psychological symptoms is difficult. Mood, set, intelligence, education, and many other factors may make it difficult for a patient to describe his symptoms in detail and, unfortunately, symptoms which are superficially similar may be produced by very different disorders. All we can hope to do, therefore, is to produce as precise clinical groupings as are possible with the means at our disposal and submit these groups to physiological, pharmacological, and psychological investigations.

Chapter 6

Special varieties of schizophrenia

Mixed Psychoses

The term 'mixed state' has been used to designate a mixture of manic and depressive symptoms, whereas 'mixed psychosis' is used to designate a mixture of schizophrenia with another functional psychosis. In Anglo-American literature the term 'schizo-affective psychosis' is often used instead of 'mixed psychosis'. Disorders of this type have received various names, such as 'marginal psychosis', expressing the borderline nature, 'degeneration psychosis', indicating the familial tendency, 'reactive psychosis', which emphasizes the great incidence of precipitating stresses and is used particularly in Scandinavia, and 'cycloid psychosis', which stresses the cyclical course and its resemblance to manic-depressive disease. According to Perris (1973), this group could also include the 'schizophreniform psychosis' of Langfeldt, 'oneirophrenia' of Meduna, 'psychogenic psychosis' of Strömgren, and 'bouffée délirante' of Magnan.

Schizo-affective Psychoses

These disorders have aroused increasing interest, not only in terms of their diagnosis and classification but also because of their response to treatment (*see* Chapter 8). Unfortunately, definitions differ widely. Kasanin, who introduced the term in 1933, emphasized in his original description the acute onset in the third and fourth decades, usually after precipitating stresses, occurring in a previously normal personality. The illness lasted at most for a few months and was followed by recovery. Often there was a previous attack late in adolescence. Kendell's definition requires that the symptoms of the illness should be clearly schizophrenic or paranoid and also clearly manic or depressive. Welner et al. (1979) emphasize the acute onset, the florid symptoms including delusions, hallucinations, formal thought disorder, and perplexity, together with depression, mania, or both.

Angst (1966) includes not only those illnesses in which manic-depressive symptoms appear together with others which are regarded as typical of schizophrenia, but also those illnesses which show schizophrenic phases (often with marked affective symptoms) besides manic or pure depressive ones. He does not include 'motility' and 'confusional' psychoses (*see* p. 116) which he regards as schizophrenia. It had been commonly accepted that the illness usually started with a depressive phase, but he found that in a large proportion of cases it began with a catatonic attack, developing later into a phasic, full remitting pure depressive or manic-depressive psychosis. In the 2-year follow-up of the patients seen in the International Pilot Study of Schizophrenia, 422 of the 570 schizophrenics were remitting. Of these, 171 had relapses during those 2 years, and 39 of them showed changes in their symptoms, 29 of them (3 per cent of the total and 17 per cent of those with remission and relapse) developing at least one unequivocal affective episode after a clear period of remission. Scheldrick et al. (1977), in their very much longer follow-up, found that none of their cases reverted to schizophrenia after a relapse with affective symptoms.

Some definitions include outcome and others do not. Brockington and Leff (1979) compared 8 different definitions and found very little agreement on how patients should be classified. Procci (1976) complained about the diagnostic disagreement and pointed out that in selecting a group of young schizophrenic patients with good premorbid personality, who became acutely ill after experiencing stress and showing marked affective symptoms in addition to their schizophrenic ones, it was to be expected that they would experience remissions and have a good prognosis. He considered that schizo-affectives were a mixed group, some related to schizophrenia and others a variant of affective disorders.

Those who agree would probably argue that 'schizo-affective' was an umbrella term to cover paranoid depressions, depressions with unclear or possible schizophrenic symptoms, schizophrenia with marked depressive features, atypical phasic psychoses, and atypical paranoid manias. It could also include affective disorders complicated by undetected organic conditions, such as urinary infections, malnutrition, dehydration, and even some drug intoxications, e.g. from bromides or hysocine, all of which can give rise to persecutory delusions and hallucinations. In addition, mild confusion is frequently present in puerperal affective psychoses. In such a collection of disorders all that would be found would indicate that they are intermediate between schizophrenia and manic-depressive disorder.

Brockington et al. (1980) carefully selected patients according to various systems of diagnosis and also used a discriminant function which distinguished between manic depression and schizophrenia, but could not find any clear lines of demarcation between the two opposite poles. This was particularly true for outcome, despite the fact that 30 out of the sample of 76 patients were finally diagnosed as schizophrenic. A poor outcome was predicted by an onset of illness against a background of psychotic symptoms, together with a family history of schizophrenia, poor pre-morbid personality, poor work record, and a longer history. In other words, the more the symptoms and background resembled typical schizophrenia, the worse the outcome, and the more like an affective disorder the better the outcome.

Others consider that these patients form a distinct group. Tsuang et al. (1976) found that of 85 such patients, 71 per cent were female. This proportion is much higher than that found in the two major groupings. The mean age at admission was 28·9 years, which is about the same as that for schizophrenics (28·6 years) but significantly lower than that of primary affective disorder (40·8) and even of bipolar (43·2) and unipolar (48·7) sub-types. Precipitating stresses in this group were common (61 per cent); in a later paper (Tsuang et al., 1977), they were found in 78·4 per cent, compared with 35·4 per cent in affectives and 11·0 per cent in schizophrenics. In these three groups, complete or social recovery occurred in 46·2 per cent, 57·8 per cent and 7·7 per cent respectively. The conclusion was that this group of 'atypical' schizophrenics most closely resembled bipolar affectives. A similar conclusion was reached by Reich et al. (1975) on the basis of EEG sleep records. Their schizo-affectives had a much shorter REM latency (time asleep until the first bout of REM sleep) than acute or 'latent' schizophrenics, resembling depressives in this respect.

Welner et al. (1977) came to an opposite conclusion from their follow-up study of 114 schizo-affectives. Of these, 71 per cent had a chronic course, 10 per cent an episodic course, and 19 per cent lost their symptoms with neuroleptic medication. Deterioration developed in 81 per cent of the chronic type, in 39 per cent of the symptom-free cases, and in none of the episodic type. It was therefore concluded that these patients resembled schizophrenics rather than affectives.

Whether this condition is distinct from the two main classificatory divisions, or whether it is just a mixture of fringe groups, cannot be decided by purely clinical criteria, even when strengthened by psychometric and statistical methods. Investigators have therefore turned to family and twin studies. Mitsuda (1967) found more schizo-affectives than schizophrenics in the families of 'atypical' schizophrenics, and vice versa in the families of schizophrenics. Welner et al. (1979) found that the clinical picture, as well as course and outcome, in first-degree relatives was the same as that of their patients.

Genetic studies have not helped so far. Cohen et al. (1972) found that among monozygotic twins, the concordance was 7 out of 14 (50 per cent) for schizo-affectives, significantly higher than the 19 out of 81 (23·5 per cent) for schizophrenics, but not for the 5 out of 13 (38·5 per cent) of affectives. Tsuang (1979) found a deficiency of schizo-affective pairs among psychotic sib pairs. Scharfetter (1981) did not find a tendency for the relatives of his index cases to have the same diagnosis. All these workers agreed that there was no evidence for genetic homogeneity in this group.

Within the broad group of schizo-affective disorders a more narrowly defined group has been studied in particular detail by Kleist (1921) and his pupils. Leonhard (1959) has given a careful description of these psychoses (*see below*), using the name given by Schröder—'cycloid psychoses'. Since then, further extensive work has been carried out by Perris (1974), whose definition requires a characteristic psychotic episode followed by a complete resolution. The symptoms consist of mood swings and at least two of the following:

1. Confusion (from slight perplexity to gross disorientation).
2. Paranoia-like symptoms (delusions of reference, influence, persecution, etc. or hallucinations not syntonic with levels of mood or both).
3. Motility disturbances (hypo- or hyperkinesia).
4. Ecstasy.
5. Pan-anxiety.

In agreement with others he found that a high proportion of patients are female. The prevalence of schizophrenic and affective disorders among the relatives was no greater than in the general population, but 38 per cent of the patients had first-degree relatives and 60 per cent had more distant relatives with the same condition. Perris therefore concluded that it was not a mixture but a nosological entity.

Brockington et al. (1982) found that out of 108 schizo-affective patients only 20 could be diagnosed as cycloids, using the criteria of Perris (with emphasis on an acute onset, a labile clinical picture, and 'confusion'). The two diagnoses were therefore not synonymous. Most of these patients would have been diagnosed as schizophrenic by British psychiatrists and as schizo-affective by American psychiatrists. The remission rate was nearly twice as great in the cycloids as in the schizo-affectives. Compared with the latter, the cycloids had less delusions, especially of a persecutory type, less defect, and more affective symptoms. The authors concluded that cycloid psychoses differed from schizophrenia, but believed that they might be a mixed group and suggested that confusion over the boundary between schizophrenia and manic-depressive psychosis arose from this group, with its florid symptoms but with a natural history similar to that of manic-depressive psychosis.

Cutting et al. (1978) examined their case records and found that cycloids comprised 3 per cent of their admissions, compared with 16 per cent for schizophrenics, 2 per cent for schizo-affectives, and 18 per cent for depressive psychoses. They compared 73 cycloids (using the clinical criteria of Perris) with 73 schizophrenics, 73 depressive psychoses, and 49 schizo-affectives. All cycloids had delusions or hallucinations and, in decreasing frequency, perplexity, motility disturbances, pan-anxiety, and ecstasy. Thought disorder was more common than in any other group. Females comprised 90 per cent of the cycloids, but less than 56 per cent of the other disorders. During follow-up, the cycloids had more admissions than any other group, but a shorter time in hospital than schizophrenics and schizo-affectives. The family history of mental illness was intermediate in type betwen those of affectives and schizophrenics. The familial psychiatric illness for the schizo-affectives was the lowest of all groups and psychological factors highest. This suggested a weak genetic predisposition and prominent psychogenesis.

Cycloids were more likely to have been diagnosed as schizo-affective or atypical psychosis, and in subsequent episodes almost half were diagnosed as affective psychosis on one admission and schizophrenic on another. They would have been excluded from schizophrenia by Feighner's criteria (because of affective symptoms and history less than 6 months) which rely heavily on the Kraepelinian course of the illness. The WHO criteria (Wing et al., 1974) give great weight to Schneider's first-rank symptoms and would have included them in nuclear schizophrenia. The authors concluded that the data available did not support the idea that cycloids were an atypical form of affective disorder.

Leonhard divides the cycloid psychoses into three main groups—anxiety–elation psychosis, confusion psychosis, and motility psychosis. He insists that these illnesses, like manic-depressive illnesses, are bipolar in that two extreme clinical pictures may occur, but features of these two extremes do not occur usually at the same time. The bipolar nature of the illness is shown in the alternation of the extreme clinical pictures during a given phase or the occurrence of each pole of the illness in pure form in different phases of the illness. His descriptions of confusion psychosis and motility psychosis coincide with the descriptions of motility and confused psychoses by Kleist and Fünfgeld. He claims that the anxiety psychoses and the expansive autopsychoses described by Wernicke in 1906 and by Kleist are the two poles of anxiety–elation psychosis.

In the following brief account, it must be pointed out that the major credit for the careful description and delineation of the marginal psychoses must go to Kleist, who first described motility psychosis in 1909 and has collected and analysed the atypical functional psychoses for over 50 years.

The Anxiety–Elation Psychosis

In this illness the basic disorder is a mood change either of anxiety or of ecstasy. The anxiety is associated with typical ideas of reference and sometimes with illusions and hallucinations, but all these paranoid symptoms can be understood as arising from the mood. These patients often complain of bodily sensations, and it may not be easy to determine whether these hallucinations are being attributed to some external agency. Ideas of guilt, inferiority, and self-reproach are usually present to some extent. Occasionally depersonalization, derealization, and even mild ideas of passivity may occur. The alternative mood state is one of enthusiastic euphoria which often has an ecstatic character and in which desires to make other people happy nearly always occur. Pseudo-hallucinations of hearing and vision are usually present and these may be associated with confabulations which concern the exalted experiences. Ideas of reference of a mildly grandiose kind may also be present. These patients sometimes complain of hypochondriacal hallucinations which they usually attribute to a higher power. The symptomatology of this illness is very diverse, and symptoms characteristic of manic-depressive illness, confusion psychosis, or motility psychosis may also be found. Rapid oscillations between anxious and ecstatic mood states are very common. The individual attacks of psychosis usually last about the same length of time as attacks of manic-depressive disease. The pre-psychotic personality is often anxious or somewhat hypomanic, with a mildly enthusiastic outlook, but depressive personalities are also found.

The Confusion Psychosis

In this variety of psychosis, thinking is disordered, while affectivity and psychomotor activity are not. In the excited state the most outstanding symptom is the incoherent pressure of speech, the content of which is out of keeping with the situation. Playful, transient misidentifications of persons occur and fleeting ideas of reference and auditory hallucinations are common. On the other hand, in the inhibited state there is a poverty of speech which may even amount to mutism. Perplexity, ideas of reference, ideas of significance, illusions, and hallucinations are often found in the inhibited state. The commonest variety of hallucinations is auditory, but visual and somatic hallucinations can occur. As with all cycloid psychoses, features of manic-depressive and other cycloid psychoses may be present. The duration of an individual attack is similar to that of a manic-depressive illness. The common types of pre-morbid personality are excited and reserved personalities.

The Motility Psychosis

The outstanding disorder in this psychosis is one of psychomotor activity, either hyperkinesia or akinesia. The hyperkinetic state is characterized by a motor restlessness, which is made up of expressive and reactive movements. Inarticulate screaming, often with an expressive character such as anger, may occur in hyperkinetic excitement. The hyperkinesia may also interrupt speech. If it is severe it may prevent speech altogether. At the opposite pole, the inhibited state, all forms of movement are restricted, but reactive and expressive movements are affected earlier than voluntary movements, so that in mild cases, although voluntary movements can be performed, the illness can be recognized because of the rigidity of the posture and mimicry and the absence of reactive movements. Thus the patient is unable to perform automatic actions and cannot change uncomfortable postures. Symptoms characteristic of the other bipolar psychoses may also occur, in particular incoherent pressure of speech may be present. Incoherence due to the irregular utterance of disconnected expressions of speech is characteristic of motility psychosis, but pressure of speech is typical of confusion psychosis. In this illness the clinical picture frequently swings from one pole to the other. On the whole, pure akinesia is much rarer than pure hyperkinesia. Hyperkinetic attacks usually only last a few weeks, but akinesia often lasts several months. The cycloid personality seems to be the commonest type of pre-morbid personality.

It can be seen from this outline that the cycloid psychoses cannot be sharply delimited from one another or from manic-depressive disease. Both Kleist and Leonhard consider that these illnesses have some relationship with manic-depressive disease, but Leonhard also considers that they are related to his non-systematic schizophrenias. Whether one agrees with the views of these workers or not, the fact remains that a group of marginal psychoses exists. This is supported by Pauleikhoff's investigation of 1000 male and 1000 female psychiatric admissions to the Heidelberg Clinic in 1949 and the first part of 1950. In 3 male and 32 female patients the differential diagnosis lay between schizophrenia and cyclothymia. Of the 32 female patients, 5 presented a manic excited picture and the remainder a depressed paranoid illness. Pauleikhoff (1957) considered that the clinical picture of the manic excited patients was similar to Kleist's motility psychosis. He found a few patients in whom schizophrenic symptoms appeared in the course of an illness which had presented as a typical depression, and another small group of patients who had had a typical manic-depressive illness at one time and a schizophrenic illness at another time. Unfortunately, this author does not give case summaries or a detailed analysis of the 35 atypical endogenous psychoses. His concept of schizophrenia is obviously a very broad one; thus, for example, in 1 case delusional perception is stated to have occurred, but in the case summary there is nothing which goes beyond a delusion-like reaction. Pauleikhoff gives the ratio of schizophrenic to cyclothymic admissions to the Heidelberg Clinic in the years 1946–49 as 1·6 : 1, and this would suggest that schizophrenia is diagnosed more readily in that clinic than in many others. It is interesting that even with such a broad concept of schizophrenia there is still a small group of marginal psychoses (0·5 per cent of the total schizophrenic and cyclothymic patients in Pauleikhoff's series).

Schizophreniform Psychoses

Langfeldt (1939) introduced the concept of schizophreniform psychoses on the basis of a study of patients diagnosed as 'schizophrenic' or 'schizophrenic?' who were admitted to the Oslo University Psychiatric Clinic in the years 1926–33. In a follow-up study of 100 cases diagnosed as 'schizophrenic?', he found that 55 had not developed typical schizophrenic defect states or subsequently shown typical schizophrenic process symptoms. Twenty-eight of these cases were considered to be reactions in psychopathic personalities, 10 psychogenic reactions of a neurotic kind, 7 exogenous reactions, 9 manic depressives, and 1 atypical schizophrenia. From a study of the protocols of illustrative cases, which Langfeldt cites in his monograph, it would appear that at least 3 of his reactions in psychopathic personalities and 3 of his manic depressives fit the descriptions of cycloid psychoses given by Leonhard. Three cases appear to be anxiety–elation psychosis, 2 cases motility psychosis, and 1 confusion psychosis.

The concept of a schizophreniform psychosis due to a psychogenic reaction in a psychopathic personality is widely held among Scandinavian psychiatrists. Certain objections to this idea immediately spring to mind. In the first place, if one uses Schneider's concept of psychopathic personality, then manic-depressive psychoses are often reactions in psychopathic personalities. Secondly, psychopathic personalities are quite common, but psychotic schizophrenic-like reactions in psychopaths are not very common. This would suggest that some special constitutional predisposition is necessary before such psychoses can occur. Thus we have come back once again to the concept of a third, possibly a fourth or functional psychosis or marginal psychosis.

The idea that there is a group of true or nuclear schizophrenias and a group of false or pseudoschizophrenias is firmly held by many different clinical psychiatrists. Rümke (1957) has differentiated between these two groups and subdivided the pseudoschizophrenias into endogenous, exogenous toxic, characterogenic, developmental, cerebral organic, pseudoschizophrenia, and unclassifiable cases. The endogenous pseudoschizophrenias are atypical manic-depressive psychoses, degeneration psychoses, paranoid psychoses, and obsessive compulsive psychoses. In these patients the accessory symptoms of schizophrenia are present, but the schizophrenic colouring is missing. In the diagnosis of schizophrenia, Rümke lays great stress on the 'praecox feeling', by which he means the feeling of lack of contact which the experienced observer has when he examines a typical schizophrenic. The terms 'exogenous', 'toxic', and 'cerebral' organic pseudoschizophrenia are, of course, self-explanatory. Charactero-genic pseudoschizophrenia includes the severe schizoid personality who has the psychogenic reactions and also many paranoid personality developments. Developmental pseudoschizophrenia is a severe hysterical illness which occurs in adolescence, and Rümke considers that this is reminiscent of the introverted type of the severe variety of degenerative hysteria. He believes that psycho-analysis can help in the understanding and treatment of all cases of functional pseudo-schizophrenia, but it cannot explain the nature of true schizophrenia. The essential feature of a true schizophrenic symptom is that it cannot be explained by means of the theory of the abolition of defence mechanisms.

Oneiroid States (Oneirophrenia)

In 1924 Mayer-Gross described psychotic states in which a dreamlike change of consciousness was present. He called these 'oneiroid states' and pointed out that several different factors could be responsible for the presence of an apparent confusion in acute schizophrenia. Thus there may be some difficulty in establishing that the orientation is correct in some patients with ecstatic states, since the mind is flooded with emotion. Similar difficulties may arise in patients with marked autism associated with well-marked wish-fulfilling delusional experiences. Marked perplexity with the false impression of disorientation may occur in severely hallucinated patients with hallucinatory aversion. Occasionally severe formal thought disorder occurs in acute schizophrenia and gives rise to apparent confusion. Some deluded patients have a system of 'double book-keeping', in that they are in contact with the real world, but they are more interested in their delusional experiences. Such patients may appear to be disorientated when, in fact, they have a double orientation.

Mayer-Gross believed that ecstatic states, marked wish-fulfilling delusional experiences, and severe hallucinosis were responsible for the oneiroid form of experience. In this state the patient experiences a wealth of romantic scenes, which follow each other in rapid succession, so that he lives through such adventures as earthquakes, volcanic eruptions, fires, floods, being frozen in ice, battles, bombardments, shipwrecks, and so on. Such experiences are based partly on hallucinations and partly on illusionary misrepresentations of the environment. The patient actively participates in these events, has compassion for the victims, and has a sense of responsibility for his own actions. There is a permanent state of tension which is partly due to the nature of the delusional experiences, but also to the inconclusiveness of them, and the patient lives in expectation of a turning point which never comes.

Acute hebephrenic and catatonic clinical pictures are seen in which dreamlike experiences occur. Thus, for example, a patient in an acute catatonic stupor was given sodium amylobarbitone intravenously. His stupor disappeared and he spoke in a slow, tired way. When asked why he spoke like this, he pointed out rather testily that he was tired, which was only to be expected since he had been travelling in a space ship for several days.

Meduna and McCulloch (1945) grouped together all acute schizophrenic clinical pictures in which clouding of consciousness occurred and called them 'oneirophrenia'. They claimed that an anti-insulin factor was present in the blood of these patients, but this has not been confirmed by other investigators.

Latent Schizophrenia

The term 'latent schizophrenia' was introduced by Bleuler (1911) to designate a group of patients with odd, distorted personalities, which he believed were due to a schizophrenic process which had not been acute and had ceased to be active. This concept is not very helpful and is beyond proof or disproof. It is, of course, well known that some abnormal personalities suffer from atypical phasic psychoses, but this does not allow us to suppose that either the personality or the psychosis has anything in common with schizophrenia. Many British and German psychiatrists would regard latent schizophrenics as psychopathic personalities.

Pseudoneurotic Schizophrenia

Hoch and Polatin (1949) have described a variety of schizophrenia which presents as a neurosis, but the withdrawal from reality is much greater than in a neurosis. Ambivalence is not localized, but is diffuse and widespread, and emotions are either inappropriate or cold. Quite often there is an overt hatred of one member of the family. Anxiety is present and it affects the whole of the psychic life, and the symptoms of different neurotic illness may be present at the same time, so that there is pan-anxiety and a pan-neurosis. All varieties of sexual perversion may be found in the same patient. Short-lived psychotic episodes occur which are followed by a reintegration of the personality. Ideas of reference, hypochondriacal ideas, and depersonalization feelings are present in these psychoses.

The diagnosis of pseudoneurotic schizophrenia is fairly popular in the United States, and this is to be expected, since psycho-analytic theory forms the basis of this concept. Despite the fact that Freudian theory has sharply delimited the different neurotic clinical pictures and sexual perversions, it is well known that different kinds of symptoms and perversions may occur in the same abnormal person, so that their presence is not diagnostic of schizophrenia. Apart from this, psychotic episodes are quite common in abnormal personalities. If one takes these facts into account, it would appear that pseudoneurotic schizophrenia is, in fact, neurotic pseudoschizophrenia. Its prevalence in the United States may be partly due to the prevalence of psycho-analytically orientated psychotherapy in that country. Very bizarre clinical pictures may be seen in analysands who have been upset by a personal analysis. The acute disturbance produced by the psycho-analysis is highly coloured by the unconscious material, and the set of free association which has been acquired in the analysis makes the patient continue to produce such material for some time after the cessation of the analysis. These post-analytic pseudoschizophrenias usually subside rapidly with supportive treatment. It seems likely, therefore, that some pseudoneurotic schizophrenias are basically iatrogenic disorders produced by deep psychotherapy.

Pfropf Schizophrenia or Grafted Schizophrenia

This is schizophrenia occurring in a mental defective, and it was originally suggested that the schizophrenia was grafted on to the mental defect, but some workers have insisted that this illness is really a shift in a childhood schizophrenic who has been incorrectly diagnosed as a mental defective. Since the high-grade mental defective can be considered as being at the lower end of the normal distribution curve for intelligence, there is no reason why the high-grade defective with an I.Q. of 70 should not be just as liable to develop schizophrenia as the highly intelligent person with an I.Q. of 130, so that grafted schizophrenia probably does occur.

It has been suggested that childhood schizophrenia is an important cause of mental defect. If this is so, then many cases of grafted schizophrenia have been incorrectly diagnosed and are really shifts of a childhood schizophrenia occurring in adolescence and adult life. However, phasic psychoses with bizarre symptoms do occur in mental defectives, and these illnesses often resemble schizophrenia. The response to electroconvulsive therapy is good, but recovery usually occurs spontaneously within a few weeks or months. Some of these psychoses are probably atypical affective illnesses which have a rather bizarre symptomatology owing to the release of the primitive ideas of the mental defective.

Periodic Catatonia

Gjessing (1932a, b) studied periodic catatonias and in some patients he found a diphasic course of metabolism which was related to psychiatric symptoms. The reaction phase, which consisted of stupor or excitement, began at a fairly sharply defined point during the metabolic changes. Gjessing called these catatonias with an associated metabolic change the 'syntonic synchronous' or 's.s. reaction' type of catatonia. The metabolic changes consisted of nitrogen retention followed by excretion, and Gjessing described three types of 's.s.' catatonia, A, B, and C, in which the reaction phase began at different points on the nitrogen balance curves, as shown in *Fig*. 1. In Type A

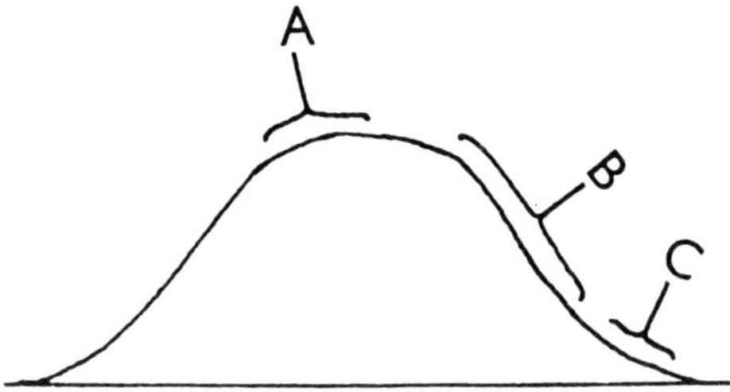

Fig. 1. Nitrogen balance in periodic catatonia. (*After Gjessing*.)

the reaction phase began just before the end of nitrogen retention, while in Type B the illness occurred after the onset of negative nitrogen balance and before the point half-way between the onset and the end of negative balance. The illness in Type C occurred towards the end of the negative balance. The reaction phase in Type A was an akinetic stupor, but in Types B and C it was a psychomotor excitement which was more violent the later it began in the phase of negative nitrogen balance. With increasing age and duration of the illness, the time of onset of the reaction phase in the negative phase of nitrogen balance became later, so that Type B finally became Type C.

Gjessing found that certain factors tended to modify the nature of the illness. Thus a special diet of 30–40 per cent fat tended to make the psychomotor excitement less severe. In some cases cold fronts and warm–cold air exchanges could retard or hasten the onset of a reaction phase. Psychological upsets could also bring about a premature onset of a reaction phase in some cases. Gjessing believed that phasic variations of thyroid function between hypo- and hyper-function occur in step with the clinical features, and claimed that the illness could be cured with large doses of thyroid, but other investigators have not found this treatment very useful. The patients do respond to neuroleptic drugs. Electro-encephalographic changes occur in this illness, and Rowntree and Kay (1952) found in 2 cases that the slow activity increased when the reaction phase began, was most marked at the height of the attack, and decreased as the attack subsided. In one of their cases the activity was as slow as 2 c/s.

Pernicious Catatonia

This illness begins suddenly, but there is a prodromal period for a few weeks before the onset of the severe symptoms, and during this time the patient may be dejected, lost in thought, or may complain of headache and constipation. This is followed by a sudden onset of senseless excitement which is often associated with some degree of self-mutilation. These patients do not speak, they beat wildly at everything around them, and they may bang their hands or heads on the wall or on the floor. Sometimes they tear their hair out in handfuls and bite their own arms and hands. It is quite impossible to make contact with these patients because of this senseless violence, so that it is not possible to know if thought disorder, sense deceptions, anxiety, and other symptoms of that kind are present. If electro-convulsive therapy is not given, death occurs in 1½–14 days following the onset of the illness. This is due to inter-current disease and exhaustion, and usually takes place on the third or fourth day. In 50 per cent of cases there is a family history of schizophrenia, and the pre-morbid personality is extroverted and sociable in 75 per cent of cases.

Senile Schizophrenia—Late Paraphrenia

There is no doubt that schizophrenia can occur after the age of 60 years, but it is not very common. Thus, in a series of 264 senile patients from the city of Edinburgh who were admitted to psychiatric institutions in the year 1957, 7 were found to be suffering from schizophrenia which had begun after the age of 60 years. Huber et al. (1975) found that of schizophrenics admitted to the Bonn University mental hospital, the disorder had begun after 40 years in 14 per cent, and of these after 50 years in 24·3 per cent and after 60 years in 3·1 per cent. The commonest clinical features were paranoid delusions in 23·2 per cent, and together with hallucinations in 55·4 per cent. Clinically, there does not appear to be any obvious difference between late paraphrenia and paraphrenia of earlier onset. Both are a particular syndrome of schizophrenia.

Post (1966) described three forms:

1. Paranoid states with auditory hallucinations (the most common).
2. Paranoid delusions of extensive conspiracy accompanied by auditory hallucinations.
3. Delusions and hallucinations of bodily influence with voices talking about the patient, commenting on the patient's behaviour, and repeating or anticipating the patient's thoughts. Erotic delusions were sometimes also present.

Roth (1955) has described a senile paranoid psychosis and called it late paraphrenia. This illness is commoner in females than in males and usually occurs in widows or spinsters living alone. Social isolation is an important factor in leading to the final breakdown, though it may sometimes be a consequence of an asocial schizoid personality (Kay and Roth, 1961). One-quarter of these patients have some defect of sight or hearing. There are no signs of dementia despite the presence of a florid paranoid state. These patients complain of being raped and gassed and that strangers enter their rooms and interfere with their belongings. Hallucinations of all kinds occur, such as voices, elementary auditory hallucinations, smells, and lights. Intelligence and judgement on matters not concerned with the paranoid symptoms are extremely good. Since these patients may believe that they are being poisoned, they may eat very little and develop a confusional state due to malnutrition. Roth's patients had marked longevity, so that only 5 per cent were dead within 6 months of admission, and 2 years after admission only 20 per cent were dead despite the fact that the mean age on admission was high. However, recovery was uncommon and only 20 per cent were discharged from hospital within 2 years from admission.

Childhood Schizophrenia

Severe behaviour disorders in childhood may be very odd, and the imprecise use of the term 'psychotic' or 'schizophrenic' by psychoanalytically orientated authors makes the situation even more difficult. In 1933 Potter suggested that the following clinical features occurred in childhood schizophrenia: withdrawal of interest from the environment, dereistic patterns of thinking, feeling, and action, diminution or deficiency in emotional rapport, diminution, distortion, or rigidity of affect, variation in motility, either increased or decreased, or bizarre or stereotyped behaviour, and regression.

Cameron (1958) points out that three different schizophrenic clinical pictures have been described in children by various authors. These are Heller's 'dementia infantilis', de Sanctis's 'dementia precocissima', and Kanner's 'infantile autism'. In Heller's disease the child develops normally for 2–3 years and then a speech disorder occurs, which leads to a decrease in the vocabulary and the production of neologisms. As the illness progresses speech ceases to be intelligible and is replaced by incoherent sounds. At the same time there is a loss of all skills, so that the child becomes wet and dirty and behaves like an imbecile. Motor disorders occur and the child grimaces and may have mannerisms. Heller stressed the bright appearance of these children which distinguished them from ordinary mental defectives. This disease was originally attributed to cerebral degeneration, but Cameron has described a typical case in which no abnormality was found in the brain at post-mortem.

De Sanctis described speech disorders and catatonic disorders in children of 2 to 3 years of age. Alternating states of excitement and catatonic stupor were present, and in the latter rigidity and waxy flexibility occurred. In his wide experience, Cameron has not yet seen a case conforming to this description.

Kanner (1948) described infantile autism in 1943, in which the child turns away from the world and shows lack of affective rapport. This disorder usually occurs in the first 5 years of life. The child either does not speak or uses words in an idiosyncratic way. In the latter case, stereotyped utterances, which are only partly apposite, may be used, or the child may speak in a stilted, pedantic way. These children try hard to maintain a rigid routine in their environment and, like obsessional personalities, they resist all change. They show very little desire to make contact with people, but are very interested in inanimate objects and shapes. There is no evidence to suggest that infantile autism is related to schizophrenia in any way.

Cameron (1958) reported on 25 childhood psychotics (21 boys and 4 girls). He found that 15 conformed to Potter's criteria. Although in these cases the parents showed no uniform characteristics, hardly any of them could be described as affectionate or warm hearted. The training methods used by one or both parents had been rigid and restrictive or impersonal and cold, with undue emphasis on education. In only 4 cases had delivery been normal and at full term, and in only 5 had early development been normal. Eating, bowel and bladder control, sleeping, and motor activity had frequently been disordered and the subject of conflict with the parents before the onset of the illness. In some cases abnormal behaviour had occurred from some months to one year before the alleged time of onset. This behaviour consisted of odd flapping movements of the hands, attacks of screaming and laughter at night, acute anxiety, phobias, fears of the dark, and short-lived difficulties in walking. In about 50 per cent of cases some traumatic episode occurred before the illness began, such as the mother becoming pregnant, a sibling being born, or the father returning home from the Armed Forces. The illness usually began between $2\frac{1}{2}$ and 4 years with a loss of interest in the environment, withdrawal, deterioration of speech, skills, and habits, autism, and motor disorders.

In his total group of 25 patients, Cameron found 5 with a clear primary mental defect and 3 who had been grossly retarded from birth. Another patient had juvenile general paresis of the insane, but the family background and the symptoms were similar to true infantile schizophrenia. Cameron concluded that childhood schizophrenia can occur in association with any degree of intelligence and also in patients suffering from coarse brain disease.

There is not much reliable evidence about the prognosis and treatment of childhood schizophrenia. There is no doubt that some cases become arrested and may have a further shift in adolescence or even in adult life. It seems likely that many cases are admitted to mental defective institutions both before and after diagnosis. Electroconvulsive therapy is valueless and the only treatment is psychotherapy and tranquillizers.

It has been suggested that childhood schizophrenia is different from post-pubertal schizophrenia, but this does not accord with genetic and clinical findings. Leonhard has shown that the catatonic clinical pictures in childhood are the same as those in adolescence and adult life.

Chapter 7

Course and prognosis

Age of Onset

This has been briefly considered (*see* p. 100), but merits more attention. In a multi-centred study based on a large number of cases, Angst et al. (1973) found that the peak incidence of catatonia and hebephrenia (which the authors tend to assimilate into one group) is in the third decade, as is also that of schizo-affective disorders. The peak incidence for paranoid schizophrenia is a decade later. In other words, before the age of 30 the first attack has appeared in 65 per cent of catatonics, 33 per cent of paranoids, and 56 per cent of schizo-affectives. For the last two groups, the first attack in women is significantly later than in men. The age of onset of schizo-affective illness tends to be under-estimated in cross-sectional studies, because in about 7 per cent of patients the illness starts with pure affective symptoms (unipolar or bipolar) and only later does the full syndrome appear. Longitudinal studies, e.g. Angst (1980), show a later age of onset at 32 years (S.D. 12·9 years).

Mode of Onset

Some authors have claimed that the onset of schizophrenia is always ingravescent and that careful history-taking will show that minor abnormalities have been present for many years before the acute onset. Thus Eugen Bleuler wrote: 'However, whenever we have a thorough case history, it is the exception if we are not able to detect the previous earlier signs of disease whether it be nervous symptoms, character changes or even direct overt schizophrenic manifestations.' It has previously been pointed out that it is easy to be wise after the event. Since adolescent crises and difficulties are much commoner than schizophrenia, it does not seem reasonable to attribute all the psychological difficulties before the apparent onset of the schizophrenic illness to schizophrenia. Sometimes depression or neurosis occurs in a patient before the onset of classical schizophrenic illness. Usually such illnesses do not last long and are followed by apparently complete recovery, but some time later a typical schizophrenic illness occurs. The original illness is then often regarded as a manifestation of schizophrenia, but there is, in fact, no way of proving this. In some cases the onset of the illness is at a definite point in time, although some prodromal symptoms are usually present for days, weeks, or months before the unequivocal schizophrenic symptoms appear. Depression, anxiety, suspiciousness, mild hypochondriasis, lack of concentration, and restlessness are the usual prodromal symptoms. Conrad (1958a) has called the first stage of the schizophrenic illness the *trema*, which is the German theatrical slang for stagefright before the performance begins. The *trema* precedes the apophanous stage of the illness and is characterized by senseless actions, depression, and suspiciousness. The change in the patient may lead to conflicts with the environment, and the resultant difficulties may be incorrectly considered to be reactive factors in the causation of the schizophrenic illness. Conrad believes that in some cases the shift does not pass beyond the *trema* so that apophanous experiences do not occur, but when the shift ceases a mild defect is left behind.

In some cases the illness is slowly and insidiously progressive and the exact point of onset is uncertain. Some patients appear to have a paranoid personality development, but it gradually becomes obvious that, because of the nature of the personality change, there has been a definite break in the continuity of the personality due to a process.

Course

Before discussing the course of the illness in schizophrenia, it is necessary to define the terms 'phase', 'shift', 'exacerbation', and 'process' which are frequently used by workers who study the course of schizophrenic illnesses. A 'phase' of an illness is always followed by a complete return to the pre-morbid state, while in a 'shift' of an illness there is an acute episode, in which new symptoms occur, but which is followed by a partial recovery. An 'exacerbation' is a sudden worsening of a clinical state without the appearance of any new symptoms. The word 'process' has already been discussed, but it is often used slightly differently in connexion with the course of a schizophrenic illness. Quite a fair number of authors use the term 'process' to indicate a clinical state in which there is a steady worsening. Different characteristic process symptoms have been described by different authors, so that this term is usually used to indicate those symptoms which the particular author considers to be characteristic of an active schizophrenic illness leading to mental deterioration.

Manfred Bleuler (1972) found that 64 per cent of his patients showed a cyclic course, 28 per cent a chronic course, and the remainder an irregular fluctuating course. Ciompi (1980), reporting on a follow-up of 37 years, described 8 types of course (*see Fig.* 2). The more common ones combine the features of phasic or continuous course with favourable or unfavourable outcome. The commonest,

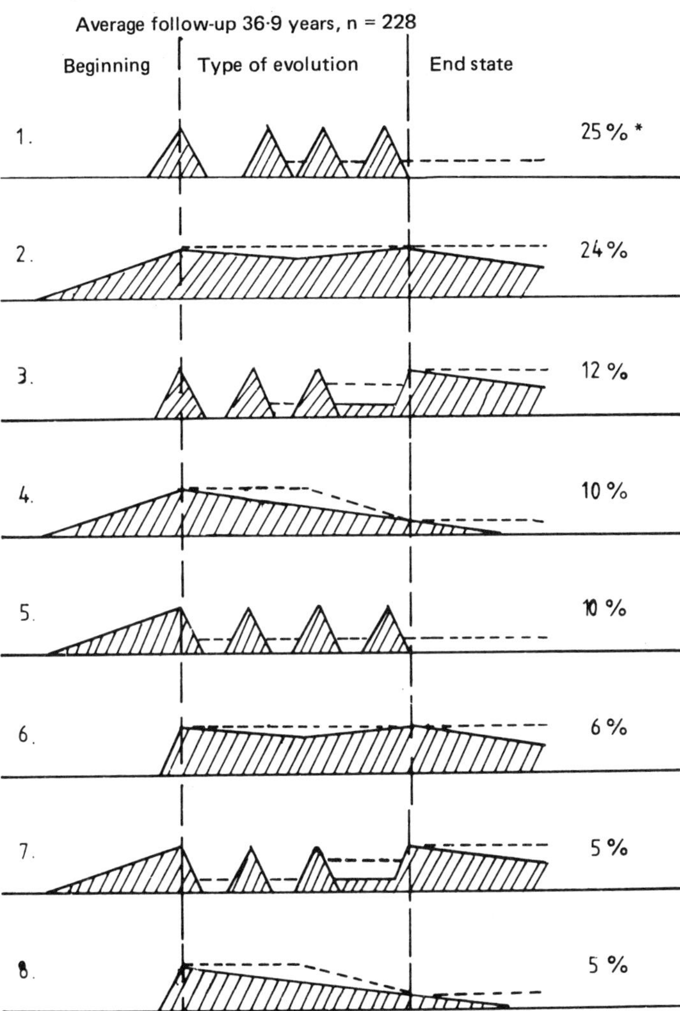

Fig. 2. Long-term evolution of schizophrenia.
(Dotted lines represent variations of the same type of course.)
* Only one single attack in 10 per cent of all cases.

occurring in 25 per cent of cases, combines an acute onset with a phasic course.

Angst et al. (1973), in an extensive multi-centred investigation, made a detailed study of the cyclical course, despite the difficulty of assessing the length of an acute phase (shift) against a background of chronic symptoms. They found that the number of phases continued to increase for about 15 years and then stabilized at 6–7. The median number of phases was 5 for schizo-affectives and 3 for other types. The frequency distribution of phases had a log-normal shape (i.e. asymmetrical with a long 'tail' to the right) so that the commonest number of phases was 2 for paranoids, 3 for other schizophrenics, and 4 for schizo-affectives (*Fig.* 3).

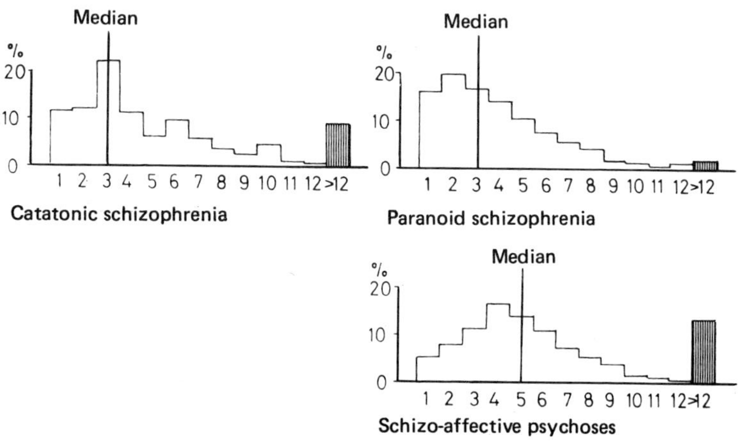

Fig. 3. Number of registered phases for paranoids, schizophrenics, and schizo-affectives.

The duration of phases also had a log-normal distribution (*Fig.* 4) which was almost identical for all groups. Most phases, 55–60 per cent, did not last longer than 3 months and 71 per cent were no longer than 6 months. Acute phases longer than 2 years were found in 6 per cent of catatonics, 14 per cent of paranoids, and only 0·8 per cent of schizo-affectives. Successive phases tended to be shorter by about 10 per cent in paranoids and by 2–3 per cent in other groups. In female schizo-affectives the phases were about 20 per cent shorter than in males.

The duration of cycles (measured from the beginning of one phase to the beginning of the next) also had a log-normal distribution and diminished with successive cycles. The first cycle had a mean duration for catatonic, paranoid, and schizo-affective groups of 25·6, 31·6, and 28·8 months respectively.

In a later paper (Angst, 1980), which is of great importance because it is based on a prospective rather than a retrospective inquiry, further information was provided for schizo-affectives diagnosed on criteria similar to those of Cutting et al. (1978), but also including depressions with paranoid symptoms. One attack only was experienced by 3 per cent of cases. The mean number of phases, based on a follow-

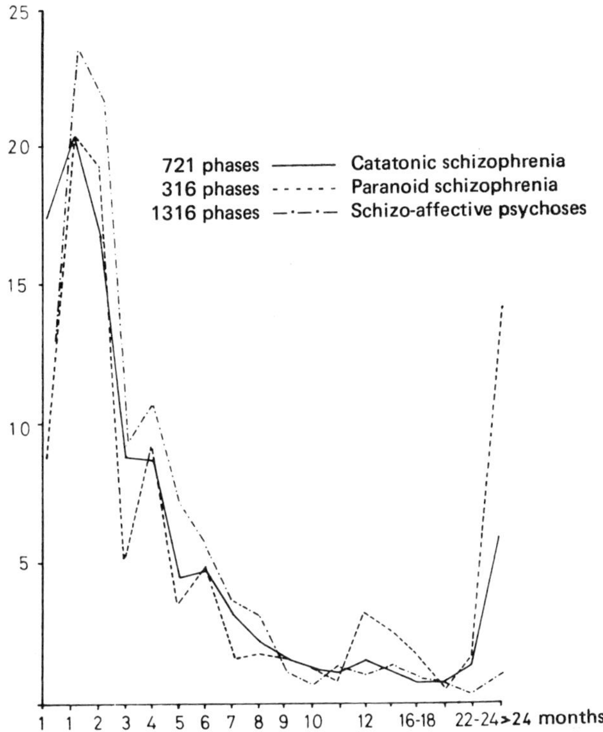

Fig. 4. Duration of phases.

up of 27 years, was 7. Their duration (geometric mean) was 4·65 months, almost the same as that of the bipolar but shorter than the unipolar affectives (also studied in this paper). The data showed that 95 per cent of phases (95 per cent confidence limits) ranged between 1·3 and 17 months. In 18 per cent of cases, the last phase had a duration of over 1 year and two-thirds of them (12 per cent of the total) lasted longer than 2 years. This gloomy outcome was counter-balanced by the finding that 'recovery' (defined as a symptom-free period of more than 5 years) occurred in 37 per cent of cases and a complete remission in 27 per cent. The duration of cycles ranged between 7 and 211 months, with a (geometric) mean of 38·8 months, and 95 per cent confidence limits of 10·1 to 149·1 months.

Arnold (1955) has published the results of follow-up studies on 500 schizophrenics in which the period of observation was 3–30 years.

His results were as follows:

1. Phasic course of illness with complete cure, 15·6 per cent.
2. Phasic course passing over into a shift-like course, 4·0 per cent.

3. Phasic course passing over into a process, 0·4 per cent.
4. Phasic course passing over into a process with exacerbations, 3·4 per cent.
5. Shift-like course, 9·6 per cent.
6. Shift-like course passing over into a process, 3·6 per cent.
7. Shift-like course passing over into a process with exacerbations, 14·0 per cent.
8. Primary process course of illness, 7·2 per cent.
9. Primary process with exacerbations, 38·0 per cent.
10. Mixed psychoses, 5·2 per cent.
11. Mixed psychoses passing over into a process, 1·4 per cent.

Outcome

There is considerable evidence that schizophrenia has become less severe during the past half-century. Many clinicians have pointed out that gross deterioration and pernicious catatonia are now never seen, and that such symptoms as waxy flexibility, *Mitmachen*, and *Mitgehen*, which were always uncommon, are now very rare indeed. Astrup (1975), for example, found that the remission rate from 1938–50 was 15 per cent, whereas for 1958–61 it had increased to 24 per cent. The corresponding figures for the rate of deterioration were 43 per cent and 24 per cent. The general outcome of schizophrenia is best considered in terms of pre- and post-neuroleptic periods, because it would appear that the use of modern treatments has had at least some effect on the course of the illness. Markowe et al. (1967) found, after a 10-year follow-up, that 45 per cent of cases showed no or few symptoms, 30 per cent had a defect state, and 25 per cent were still 'psychotic'. There was no difference between those treated with chlorpromazine or insulin (generally regarded now as ineffective).

Kraepelin (1913) found that 12·6 per cent of his cases of dementia praecox recovered from the first attack, but most of these relapsed in a few years, so that only 2·6 per cent were lasting recoveries, or if mild defects were included, 4·1 per cent were cured. However, 17 per cent of his patients had social remissions.

Ciompi and Müller (1976) followed their patients (very few of whom had received neuroleptics) for 37 years; 47 per cent had been in hospital for less than 1 year, 10 per cent for 1–3 years, and 23 per cent for over 20 years. A satisfactory social outcome was found in one-third. About one-half had a remitting and exacerbating course. With increasing age there was a decrease in severity of symptoms and by the age of 65 most patients had reached a stable end state. By this time, the different sub-types of schizophrenia had become indistinguishable.

Pritchard (1967a, b) found that the proportion of recoveries was the same before and after the introduction of the neuroleptics, but that the drugs shortened the length of stay in hospital and the patients were better on discharge.

Morrison et al. (1973) followed up 200 schizophrenic patients, diagnosed on strict criteria, for 10 years. They found that 20 per cent had never been discharged from hospital. Only 8 per cent ever recovered, most of the recoveries occurring within the first 2 or 3 years following discharge from hospital. In general, most remissions occurred within the first 2 years of illness and there were very few after 5 years. Wing (1966) found that among first admissions, half had a good 5-year follow-up prognosis and over this period required little attention from rehabilitation or after-care. One-quarter of them were still severely ill at the end of the 5 years and the rest were handicapped by less severe symptoms.

Huber et al. (1975a) followed up 502 patients for over 22 years, and found that 22·1 per cent showed a complete remission of symptoms, 43·2 per cent had 'non-characteristic' types of remission, and 34·7 per cent had typical deficiency syndromes. Only 13·3 per cent were permanently in hospital, and 55·9 per cent could be regarded as 'socially recovered'.

One of the most important investigations of schizophrenia is the International Pilot Study of Schizophrenia (IPSS) carried out under the ægis of the World Health Organization. In the 2-year follow-up (Sartorius et al., 1977) the results were:

1. 27 per cent did well, with a short illness and full recovery. In 11 per cent the illness lasted less than 6 weeks.
2. 12 per cent had a complete remission but with at least one relapse.
3. 17 per cent had a partial remission but with no relapse.
4. 18 per cent had a partial remission and at least one relapse.
5. 18 per cent remained psychotic and severely handicapped throughout.

The first two groups had a good previous personality, no family history of mental illness, early onset, and the illness had been precipitated by psychological stresses. They could therefore be regarded as schizo-affective psychoses. The second group, with its predominance of females and repeated attacks, could well be regarded as cycloid psychoses. One of the most important findings was that patients in developing countries did better than those in the developed countries. This hints at the influence of social factors on the course.

Prognosis

The prognosis is always difficult but particularly so for schizophrenia, not only because being a chronic illness it involves long-term follow-up and difficulties in tracking down patients, but also because of the different concepts of the disorder. Comparison between different reports is also made difficult by the variability of meaning of 'partial remission', 'social remission', and so on.

When one considers the prognosis in any given case, it is necessary to estimate three different aspects of the future course of the illness, i.e. the chance of recovery from the present attack, the possibility of recurrence, and the likelihood of a personality deterioration.

Family History

Vaillant (1963) found that remitting schizophrenics had a greater frequency of relatives with affective disorders than non-remitting cases. The latter had a greater incidence of schizophrenia among their relatives than the former. Winokur and Tsuang (1975) confirmed that a family history of remitting illness improves the prognosis.

Physique

It is usually held that a pyknic body build favours recovery or a mild defect, whereas the leptosomatic body build favours a worse prognosis. The dysplastic physique is usually associated with a very poor prognosis and this is summed up in the well-known phrase 'the uglier the patient the worse the prognosis'. It is interesting that Holmboe and Astrup (1957) found schizophrenic defects in 53 per cent of pyknics and 36 per cent of leptosomes in their series of 255 acute schizophrenics. However, the defect in the leptosomes was much more severe than in the pyknics.

Personality

A pre-morbid schizoid personality is associated with a poor prognosis, while a good well-integrated pre-morbid personality is usually associated with recovery or minimal defect. (*See Table* 6, p. 31.)

Intelligence

An I.Q. below the average is usually associated with a poor prognosis.

Age of Onset

Recovery is less common when the illness begins in adolescence and in early adult life or middle age, but severe defects are much commoner in the adolescents and young adults than in the middle-aged. Thus, although onset of illness at 40 years or over usually indicates that recovery is unlikely, it also indicates that severe deterioration of the personality will probably not take place.

Clinical Features

Despite the difficulties, there is good agreement between different investigators. An acute onset favours a good outcome, whereas a subacute or ingravescent onset has a very poor prognosis. The presence of clear-cut precipitating factors is indicative of recovery. Thus Holmboe and Astrup found that an onset associated with acute psychological trauma, physical illness, childbirth, and toxic disorders tended to be followed by recovery. Marked depressive features and the preservation of adequate affective expression are good prognostic signs, whereas flattening of affect and incongruity indicate a poor prognosis. Leff and Wing (1971) report that the patients less likely to relapse within a year after discharge are those with a first episode and shorter duration of illness, more auditory hallucinations, early wakening, morning depression, and guilt. Johnstone et al. (1979) found that poor outcome after an acute attack was related to previous social isolation, the presence of nuclear symptoms and residual retardation, muteness, and flattening of affect. In general, it can be said that the more atypical the clinical picture is, the better the prognosis. Thus confusion or apparent confusion (which is characteristically found in cycloid psychoses) is a good prognostic sign.

Hebephrenic clinical pictures have a poor outlook, but some hebephrenics can live outside hospital for a long time until their antisocial behaviour leads to admission. Acute catatonic illnesses with excitement have a good prognosis for the attack, but there is a high probability of recurrence. Certain catatonic clinical features, namely, negativism, stereotypies, and parakinesias, suggest an unfavourable course of the illness. The outcome of acute paranoid schizophrenia is not as good as acute catatonic illness, but is considerably better than hebephrenia. It is generally agreed that typical schizophrenic auditory hallucinations, bodily hallucinations, and sexual hallucinations are indicative of a poor prognosis.

A few examples of recent work can be given briefly. Huber et al. (1975a) found that favourable features were higher education, precipitating psychological stresses, depressive traits, perception of delusions, catatonic agitation, non-chronic thought disorders, and depersonalization at onset. Unfavourable features were low intelligence, abnormal personality, pre-morbid disturbances of social behaviour, broken homes, prolonged prodromal stages, cerebral atrophy, somatic and auditory hallucinations, and predominance of hebephrenic symptoms at onset. Ciompi and Müller (1976) found that acute onset, rich and variable psychopathology, and affective responsiveness favoured a good prognosis. Much more important were the level of personality integration before the first breakdown and the subsequent patterns of social relationships.

The development of rating scale has made it possible to use the data so obtained to predict outcome by the method of multiple regression. Astrup was the pioneer of this type of work. For example, Stephens et al. (1966), using 8 variables, were able to classify correctly 44 out of 50 recovered schizophrenics and 43 out of 50 deteriorated schizophrenics. Using a simple count of the number of symptoms with a cut-off score of 4, the numbers correctly classified were 41 and 40 respectively. The symptoms and their correlations with recovery are given in *Table 10.*

Table 10. TETRACHORIC CORRELATIONS WITH OUTCOME

Clinical feature	*2*	*3*	*4*	*5*	*6*	*7*	*8*	*Recovery*
1. Acute onset	0·40	0·42	0·40	0·34	0·54	0·29	0·60	0·66
2. Precipitating factors		0·51	0·60	0·29	0·51	0·38	0·19	0·64
3. Married			0·50	0·58	0·49	0·18	0·29	0·57
4. Pre-morbid history				0·31	0·34	0·16	0·12	0·54
5. Depression					0·31	0·13	0·16	0·52
6. Not schizoid						0·21	0·39	0·51
7. Guilt							0·26	0·53
8. Confusion								0·48

(All correlations above 0·33 are statistically significant.)

Strauss and Carpenter (1974) tried to predict outcome with the IPSS data, but found that multiple regression could account for less than half the variance. In conformity with others, they found that the best predictors were insidious onset and previous admissions, and pointed out that this was not particularly helpful: '. . . the poor prognosis of schizophrenia may not be so much a validating criterion as a tautology that chronic patients are chronic'. In other words, chronic illness remains chronic; a point not often considered by those who refuse to diagnose schizophrenia unless the patient deteriorates.

Goldberg et al. (1977) carried out a controlled trial of drug withdrawal. They found that after 2 years, 80 per cent of their patients on placebo had relapsed, compared with 48 per cent on drugs. They found that a longer time until relapse was associated with better previous personality, less time in hospital and out-patient treatment, milder illness, better relationship with relatives and others, and acceptance of medication. The patients who obtained the most benefit from drugs were those who had no disruption in early family life, whose relatives were co-operative, who took their drugs, and had had less autism before treatment. The authors pointed out that only one of these predictors concerned symptoms. The patients with these characteristics responded well to drugs; those without them were not helped by drugs as compared with placebo.

The most important findings in this work were not only that the patients with the best prognosis were those who obtained the most benefit from drugs, but they also responded best to social ('major role') therapy. Indeed, social therapy hastened the relapse of those with a poor prognosis. Although the multiple regression of the data was extremely elaborate, the authors accepted only those results which were consistent across three centres and held up on cross-validation.

Social Factors

There is no doubt that social factors play a great part in the final adjustment of the patient with a schizophrenic defect state. They may determine his discharge from hospital and his ability to live outside it, so that social recovery is often more dependent on the environment than on the clinical features of the schizophrenic illness. It has been shown, for example, that the 'possession of immediate family' is in favour of discharge from hospital. The attitude of the parents and siblings may be crucial in the patient's final adjustment. It may be impossible for the family to accept that the patient is ill, has difficulties in communication, and will have to adjust to a level of social activity which is much lower than his pre-morbid level. Some parents flatly deny their child's illness and cannot be brought to understand the need for a different approach to the patient.

Brown et al. (1972) have shown that great emotional involvement of members of the family coupled with expressed hostility is strongly associated with symptomatic relapse and indeed is the main factor. It was as deleterious when coming from the marital partner as from the parents (which argues against it being an aetiological factor in schizophrenia). Its effects could be mitigated by ensuring that the patient had adequate medication and did not have too close contact with the highly emotional relative. The authors found that other factors related to relapse were male sex, age below 45 years, more than one previous admission to hospital, decline in occupational level, low unskilled work, and failure to achieve satisfactory sexual adjustment. Typical schizophrenia had a worse prognosis than atypical forms. Hence three factors were related to outcome: previous history, clinical condition, and strongly expressed emotions.

Repeating this work and pooling the data, Vaughn and Leff (1976) showed that in 128 patients, the relapse rate was 13 per cent in those whose families showed low expressed emotion (EE) and was the same whether the patients were on drugs or not. In those with high EE the relapse rate was 51 per cent. Among them, those patients who had less than 35 hours' contact with their families had a relapse rate of 28 per cent and those with more a rate of 69 per cent. In the former group, drugs reduced the rate from 42 to 15 per cent, and in the latter from 92 to 55 per cent. A follow-up after 2 years following discharge from hospital (Leff and Vaughn, 1981) showed that the prophylactic effect of drugs in high EE homes had disappeared, but was significantly protective in the low EE homes.

In order to confirm these findings, Leff et al. (1982) carried out a controlled trial on 24 patients who had over 35 hours' contact with high EE relatives. One-half received routine out-patient care and the others received special intervention (lectures about schizophrenia, 'group' meetings with low EE relatives, and family sessions for patients with their relatives) to reduce the amount of contact with relatives and the amount of EE expressed. After 9 months, the experimental group of 11 patients had a relapse rate of 9 per cent and the 12 controls a rate of 50 per cent. Although the results were in the expected direction, the experimental group had received much more attention. This objection does not apply to the controlled trial of family therapy by Falloon et al. (1982) in which only 1 out of 17 experimental patients relapsed as against 8 of the 18 patients in the control group.

The clear evidence on the significance of family tensions and precipitating stresses on the recurrence of symptoms raises the question concerning what part they may play in the development of the first attack.

It is often difficult to persuade both the patient and his relations that a job considerably below the pre-morbid level should be tried after discharge. For example, a university graduate may not be able to understand that he is fit only for routine clerical work. In a previously dull and backward patient the schizophrenic illness may produce a defect state of such severity that the patient is virtually feeble-minded and unemployable outside a sheltered institution. Unfortunately, the lack of employment may lead to an exacerbation of the symptoms and re-admission to a mental hospital.

Acceptance by society may determine whether the patient lives outside hospital, so that the odd behaviour of the chronic schizophrenic may not be tolerated in an organized urban industrial area, whereas it may pass almost without comment in a small rural community. It is obvious that the attitude of employers, supervisors, and fellow workers may affect the employment of the arrested schizophrenic. All these social factors which have a bearing on the adjustment of the discharged patient are not readily observable or easily quantified. While it is not easy to assess the prognosis of a given schizophrenic illness on the basis of clinical features alone, it is also often difficult to assess the favourable and unfavourable social factors until the patient has been exposed to them.

Chapter 8

Treatment

It is always difficult to discuss the treatment of schizophrenia in a dispassionate way, since many psychiatrists seem to be overwhelmed by a sense of guilt when their patients fail to get well. This is understandable since, unlike the general surgeon and physician who also frequently fail to cure their patients, the psychiatrist is often forced to live with his failures. Chronic bronchitics and severely crippled patients are tolerated by society, while chronic schizophrenics are frequently rejected and remain in the mental hospital as a permanent reminder to the psychiatrist that he has failed. This seems to have caused many psychiatrists to clutch at any form of treatment which has been introduced and to become passionately devoted to some drastic form of therapy. These therapeutic enthusiasts fall into two groups—the physical therapists and the psychotherapists—and it is impossible to decide which is the most one-sided.

Fortunately, since the early 1950s we have seen the rise and development of the controlled clinical trial. This has provided a satisfactory method for determining empirically the value of a treatment and, despite rearguard opposition, it has become increasingly accepted. Until the causes of schizophrenia are discovered and lead to the development of rational methods of treatment, it behoves all those involved in the healing art and who have the care of patients to use all methods of treatment known to be effective; where such effectiveness has not been demonstrated, they should recognize that it is their responsibility to do so. Meanwhile, in the absence of specific treatments, efforts must be directed to the diminution and control of symptoms and to the maintenance of interpersonal and social relations and adjustment of the patient.

Treatment of Acute Schizophrenia

When symptoms develop rapidly or suddenly, either as a first attack or as a recurrence, it will be necessary to decide first whether the patient should be admitted to hospital or to remain at home and be treated as an out-patient. Admission to hospital is necessary if the patient is very excited and restless, threatening or abusive, or is thought to be suicidal. It is also necessary if thought disorder is so great that communication with others is almost impossible. Even if the patient is not so disturbed, but is unable to look after himself and neglects such basic activities as eating, drinking and dressing himself, it may be necessary to admit the patient if the family is unable to look after him. This may be because there is nobody available, e.g. if the patient is living on his own or because the members of the family have to go out to work. A sick husband may not be able to receive sufficient care and attention from his wife if she has to look after young children; furthermore, the presence of a very disturbed patient in the family may upset them. If the patient is the mother, she may be unable to look after them properly and in that case it is better for her and for them if she is admitted to hospital. It must be remembered that it is a devastating experience for a family when one of its members suddenly develops acute symptoms of schizophrenia and their resulting shock and anxiety may render them incapable of giving the patient the sympathy, patience, and understanding which is needed. In any case, they will not know how to cope and will be unable to give the skilled attention that the patient requires. Finally, a patient may disturb the peace sufficiently to bring himself into trouble with the law and in such circumstances it is advisable to admit him into hospital.

When the symptoms develop slowly, and particularly when they are characterized by apathy and withdrawal, then it may be quite suitable to treat the patient as an out-patient. This holds as long as the patient can give some measure of co-operation to his treatment.

The first stage of in-patient treatment is to ensure that the patient has sufficient to eat and drink, the latter being particularly important. The patient should also get sufficient sleep and rest. At this stage he needs peace and quiet and it may be helpful to nurse him in a side-room of the ward, away from its bustle of activity. If there is much excitement, restlessness, and much pressure from hallucinations and delusions, then neuroleptics should be prescribed. They are effective in controlling such symptoms as anxiety, perplexity, insomnia, withdrawal hallucinations, delusions, and affective disturbances (National Institute of Mental Health, 1964). If the patient is unwilling to take drugs and they are considered really necessary, he should be persuaded to do so; much can be achieved by patience, understanding, and encouragement. Intramuscular injections should be avoided as much as possible but they may have to be used if the patient is very excited and disturbed. They are often used to control violent and aggressive outbursts, but as these are generally the outcome of fear and panic, then the first step in coping with them is to try to find out what has frightened the patient and to deal with that. Skilled and experienced nursing is much better than intramuscular injections of drugs, which should be used only as a last resort.

As the patient becomes more relaxed and the symptoms diminish, he should be encouraged to take part in the group activities of the ward, and to occupy himself. It is at this point that the aid of the occupational therapist is invaluable. It is easy to make derogatory remarks about the 'arty-crafty' occupations provided by the occupational therapist, but it must not be forgotten that millions of people derive pleasure and satisfaction from such hobbies as basket-making, woodwork, handweaving, pottery, painting, and modelling. As long as it is recognized that these are pleasant undemanding activities, suitable for the 'convalescent' stage of an illness and that they are only a stage in the development of the patient's activities, their role in the management of patients can be properly understood. It is most unfortunate that in so many hospitals there are great difficulties in the way of ensuring that the products of occupational therapy become the property of the patient.

Visits from friends and relatives keep the patient in contact with his normal life and therefore should be encouraged as much as possible. If, as sometimes happens, the patient is very much disturbed by visitors, then it is better to decrease the length of the visits rather than the frequency. As soon as possible the patient should be encouraged to walk out in the grounds of the hospital with nurses and visitors. As the patient improves, he should go home for weekends as a preliminary to discharge from hospital. At this point, consideration should be given to reducing the dosage of drugs from the level given during the acute stage.

Discharge from in-patient treatment obviously does not depend on the complete disappearance of symptoms but on whether the patient can be given the care and attention he needs outside the setting of the hospital ward. The decision to discharge will therefore depend not only on his subjective state but also on his social and personal circumstances. When a patient has improved sufficiently for his discharge to be considered, arrangements should be made for him to receive the continued supervision and help necessary to enable him to return to normal life and activities, including work. Such arrangements should be started sufficiently early to ensure that no delays will occur in carrying them out.

Out-patient Treatment

Out-patient treatment could better be described as out-patient management. It should be based on the co-ordinated activity of the medical and social services; the psychiatrist, the general practitioner, the social worker, and community nurse working together as a team. When appropriate, the services of occupational and industrial therapists, and of the Disablement Resettlement Officer, will be called upon.

The psychiatrist should see the patient and relatives regularly even though, as time goes on, such interviews become less frequent. If the patient has just recovered from an acute attack, the main purpose of seeing the patient is to see how much the symptoms have diminished and to what extent normal feelings and contact with others have been re-established. These give an indication to what extent social and working life has been impaired. Interviews with the relatives should be concerned with the patient's behaviour at home, his working capacity, and his social activities. The problems of managing the patient should be discussed with them and appropriate advice given. The importance of these discussions cannot be over-emphasized. They should be started before the patient leaves hospital, they should be frank, realistic but encouraging, and, above all, they should be clear and practical. It is a sad commentary on much of current clinical practice that they are often grossly inadequate (Creer and Wing, 1974). It is particularly helpful to conduct an occasional interview in the patient's home and although this is usually done by the psychiatric social worker it should not be considered an invariable rule. In some clinics it has been the custom for the patient to see the psychiatrist and the relatives to see the psychiatric social worker; it is much better if all of them can see both the social worker and the psychiatrist.

If the patient has been put on drugs it will probably be necessary for him to continue with them for at least 1 year. Nevertheless, the psychiatrist should make it a rule to consider carefully every 3 months whether the patient should continue on the same dosage or whether it can be decreased. It is very easy to fall into the habit of giving routine prescriptions but it is not good clinical practice.

If the patient is not at work he should attend a day hospital for occupational therapy as an interim measure. There his condition can be assessed in order to make arrangements to move him on. He could be considered for re-training, e.g. in an Industrial Rehabilitation Unit, or he might be put on the Disabled Register and work found for him by the Disablement Resettlement Officer, or a place found for him in a sheltered workshop. The aim should be to bring him to the highest level of working of which he is capable and to keep him there. Finally, he should be encouraged to attend patients' clubs for as long as he can derive benefit from them.

Social Therapy

'Community psychiatry' is a fashionable term which can mean almost anything. At its best it signifies the management of the schizophrenic patient through the co-operation of all concerned, as described above.

Only too often it is an aim rather than an accomplishment. At its worst it can imply some sort of 'therapy' carried out possibly by nurses, psychologists, and social workers, and sometimes by 'aides' and voluntary workers, under the Olympian supervision of a psychiatrist who thereby spares himself the fatigue of personal contact with non-fee-paying patients. Much the same can be said of 'crisis intervention', which can come to the rescue of a family suddenly devastated by the sudden onset of acute schizophrenia in one of its members, but it can also be a way for a large 'team' of people to busy themselves with achieving no more than what can be done by one good social worker.

The therapeutic community is another development of social therapy. The general principle is to spread the responsibility for managing the ward, both general activities and therapeutic programme, on to all who have any function therein. In this way, the hierarchy of authority is flattened and patients are helped to become responsible for their behaviour and activity. Regular meetings are held, usually daily, in which all ward activities are planned and their progress evaluated. This covers not only the maintenance of the ward, including sometimes the planning of menus and meals, but also any other domestic problems that arise; social and recreational activities are organized and, finally, the therapeutic régime is considered. This includes consideration of the problems of individual members of the ward, which thereby makes the ward meeting a form of group psychotherapy. Despite the claims of enthusiasts, it is not possible to eliminate the hierarchy completely and the therapist who announces to a newcomer that 'we are all here to tackle our problems of living together' is likely to be asked, sooner or later, 'How long have you been here, and why have you not settled *your* problems; and, anyway, how is it that you are paid to do so and we are not?'

Attempts to evaluate the benefits of the therapeutic community are rare. Letemendia et al. (1967) carried out a controlled trial comparing wards run as a therapeutic community with traditional wards and found after 3 years that there was no significant difference in the results. Madew et al. (1966) found that the discharge rates were significantly better, but not all of the patients in their therapeutic community were schizophrenics. One of the great difficulties of the therapeutic community principle is that, in general, wards include patients suffering from many different disorders. In these circumstances it is extremely difficult to bring the schizophrenics into full co-operation because of their apathy and withdrawal. Of course, it is assumed that the acutely ill patient is not included. As with all activation programmes, schizophrenic patients should not be pushed too hard or they may relapse.

Psychotherapy

The foundation of clinical medicine, upon which rests the application of technological skill, is the personal contact between physician and patient. This is also the basis of individual psychotherapy with schizophrenic patients. The therapist should endeavour to maintain such rapport with the patient that the latter feels that the therapist is a friend to whom the patient can turn in his difficulties. This does not mean that the therapist should go along with the patient's delusions and hallucinations; on the contrary, the patient should be encouraged to ignore them as much as possible and be helped to hold on to such insight into his condition as he retains. The general aim should be to encourage him to maintain social relations and to mix with people, to develop his interests, and to keep him at work.

There is no evidence that psychotherapy along psycho-dynamic lines achieves more. The few researches that have been carried out have, on the whole, been disastrous to the claims of psychotherapists. One of the best of such investigations by May (1968) found that the most effective treatment for schizophrenic patients was a combination of drugs and psychotherapy; this, however, was no more effective than drugs alone. Electroconvulsive treatment was inferior to this and the least effective treatments were psychotherapy or milieu treatment. A follow-up after 3–5 years (May et al., 1981) showed that treatment with drugs or ECT gave the best outcome and psychotherapy the worst. The psychotherapists were not the most experienced but were the kind that would usually be treating such patients. It would be valuable to know if more experienced psychotherapists could have done better. Grinspoon et al. (1968) gave 200 hours of psychotherapy over 2 years to each of 20 chronic schizophrenics, 10 of whom also received thioridazine and the others a placebo. The former group showed some improvement but the latter group showed little sign of change. Rogers et al. (1967) found that client-centred therapy helped those patients receiving such treatment to stay out of hospital longer than a control group, but the difference was not significant. Feinsilver and Funderson (1972) reviewed a number of such trials, but ended up with a detailed consideration of why these trials had failed to demonstrate the value of psychotherapy!

Group psychotherapy seems likely to be more helpful as it encourages the patient to make contact with people and helps him to interact with others. O'Brien et al. (1972) carried out a controlled trial comparing group with individual psychotherapy on schizophrenic patients. They found that after 12 and 24 months, group psychotherapy was significantly better in terms of social effectiveness and psychiatric ratings than individual therapy, but rates of re-admission did not differ significantly. What is of interest is that when the treatment was carried out by medical students under supervision, it was not significantly worse than the results obtained by psychiatrists or social workers. This says something about the claims for proper training in psychotherapy. One of the most recent investigations is that by Nitsun et al. (1974) in which two matched groups of chronic schizophrenics were treated by group psychotherapy or movement and drama. Both groups improved and the authors suggest that this might be a generalized effect of the extra attention given to them. The group receiving movement and drama therapy did show a significantly greater decrease in restless and aimless activity and improved social behaviour, together with 'a greater acknowledgement of impulses and feelings stemming from a more primitive part of the personality'. Psychodrama is advocated by some, but it is unlikely to be particularly applicable to the acutely ill patients. For the patient who is making a good recovery and for the chronic patient, psychodrama can help him return to normal life by rehearsing his behaviour in the situations he can expect to meet.

Drug Treatments

The modern period of drug treatment of schizophrenia dates from the introduction in 1952 of chlorpromazine, the first of the phenothiazines, and reserpine. The latter is an extract from *Rauwolfia serpentina*, but it is now almost obsolete for use in psychiatry. Since then other classes of compounds of different chemical structure have been introduced but have only partially replaced the phenothiazines in current usage, although where comparative trials have been carried out they have been shown to have much the same general effect. So many drugs are now available that if the clinician is to make intelligent use of them he needs to have some understanding of the relationship between them. He will also find it useful to have some knowledge of the relationship between chemical structure and pharmacological activity. Thus, if for some reason, such as idiosyncratic response, he cannot use the drug of first choice he will know how to pick an alternative. The same will apply if he wishes to change to another drug because of changes in the patient's symptoms.

There are now 6 classes of drugs available, though the most recent introductions are still being evaluated. They are the phenothiazines, thioxanthenes, butyrophenones, diphenyl-butyl-piperidines, dibenzothiazepines, and benzamides. Within each group small changes in the molecule produce modifications in the pharmacological action of the drug. Thus each class contains two or more drugs and, not surprisingly, the oldest of all, the phenothiazines, contains the most. The thioxanthenes are closely related to the phenothiazines as shown

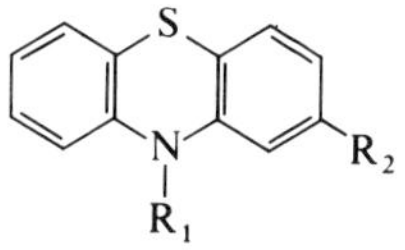

Fig. 5. Nuclei of two types of neuroleptics.

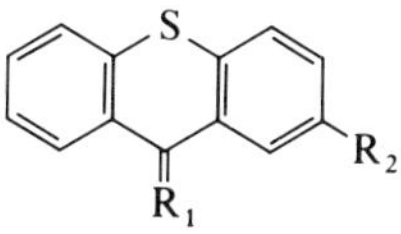

in *Fig.* 5, and are also similar in their pharmacological effects. The various members of these two groups of drugs differ chemically from each other according to the substitutions that are made at the R_1 and R_2 positions of the nucleus. Substitutions of H at the R_2 position are essential to produce an 'anti-psychotic' effect, and fluorine increases the potency much more than chlorine. The usual range of dose of the drugs (*see Table 11*) illustrates these effects.

When an aliphatic 'tail' is attached at the R_1 position, the drug tends to have sedative effects. A piperidine substitution makes little difference to the sedative effect but increases the potency. A piperazine substitution produces a 'stimulating' effect. The potency is increased but is accompanied by an increase in extra-pyramidal side-effects (*see Fig.* 6). The range of dosages shown in *Table 11* are those generally accepted, but the responsiveness of patients to these drugs varies remarkably. Some patients can take a dosage which is 10 times that which in others produces obvious side-effects. In the UK the quantities usually prescribed tend to be smaller than in the rest of Europe and those prescribed in the USA very much larger, though in recent years the use of these high dosages has tended to diminish.

The butyrophenones are a class of drugs with a structure quite different from that of the phenothiazines. The first to be introduced was haloperidol, followed by trifluperidol which is more potent in mg dosage. They have much the same action as phenothiazines though with a greater tendency to produce extra-pyramidal side-effects and akathisia. They are of particular value in patients who are intolerant of phenothiazines.

The other three classes of drugs are the most recent to be introduced. Of these the most important are pimozide and fluspirilene which are diphenyl-butyl-piperidines. It is of interest that they are selective antagonists of cerebral dopaminergic transmitters, and have a low incidence of extra-pyramidal reactions. They are 'stimulating' neuroleptics and are claimed to be of special value for schizophrenics who are apathetic and inert. The recommended dose range for pimozide is 2–10 mg per day. The dibenzothiazepines are potent neuroleptics and it has been claimed that they have minimal extra-pyramidal reactions. The benzamides, e.g. sulpiride, are said to have no sedative action and to have an anti-depressant effect as well.

Table 11. NEUROLEPTICS CURRENTLY AVAILABLE

Name	R_1	R_2	*Daily dose (mg)*
Phenothiazines			
Aliphatic series			
* Promazine	a_1	H	75–750
* Chlorpromazine	a_1	Cl	150–600
* Methotrimeprazine	a_2	OCH_3	100–700
Piperidine series			
Thioridazine	b	SCH_3	100–600
Piperazine series			
* Perphenazine	c_1	Cl	6–40
* Prochlorperazine	c_2	Cl	15–100
Thiopropazate	c_4	Cl	15–150
* Pericyazine	c_3	CN	10–90
* Trifluoperazine	c_2	CF_3	5–25
Fluphenazine	c_1	CF_3	2–10
Thioxanthenes			
Chlorprothixene	a_1	Cl	50–300
Thiothixene	c_2	$SO_2N(CH_3)_2$	10–30
Flupenthixol	c_1	CF_3	3–12
Butyrophenones			
* Haloperidol			1–12
Trifluperidol			1–3

* Available in injectable form.

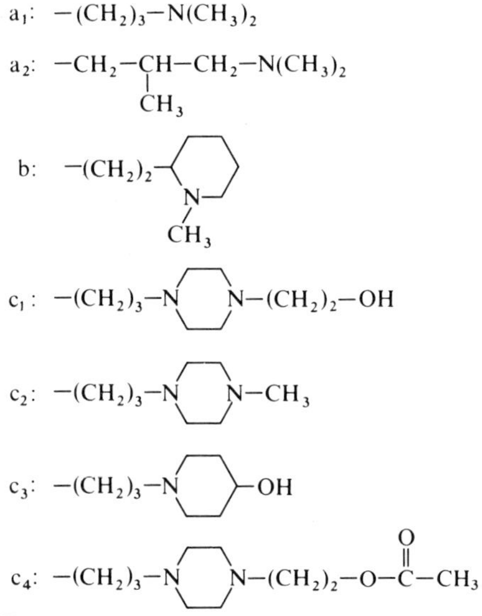

a_1: $-(CH_2)_3-N(CH_3)_2$

a_2: $-CH_2-CH(CH_3)-CH_2-N(CH_3)_2$

b: $-(CH_2)_2-$ (ring) N–CH_3

c_1: $-(CH_2)_3-N \quad N-(CH_2)_2-OH$

c_2: $-(CH_2)_3-N \quad N-CH_3$

c_3: $-(CH_2)_3-N \quad -OH$

c_4: $-(CH_2)_3-N \quad N-(CH_2)_2-O-C(=O)-CH_3$

Fig. 6. Structure of neuroleptic side-chains.

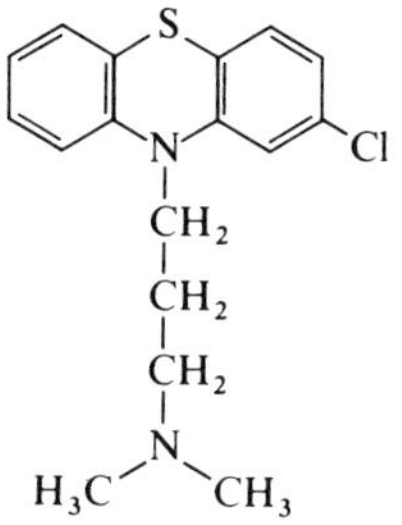

Chlorpromazine
(aliphatic
side-chain)

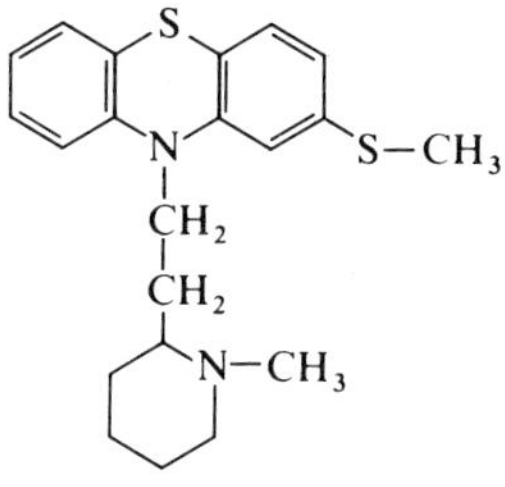

Thioridazine
(piperidine
side-chain)

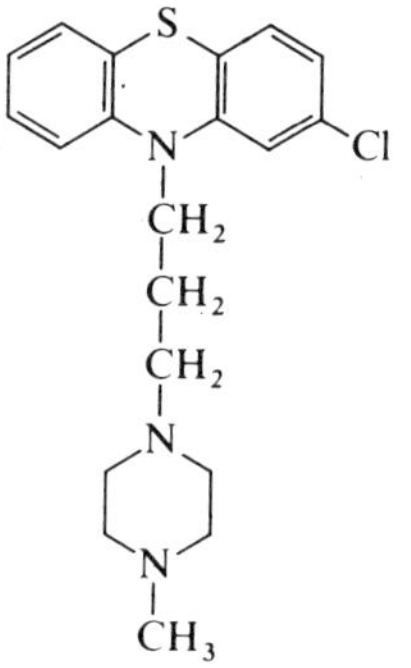

Prochlorperazine
(piperazine
side-chain)

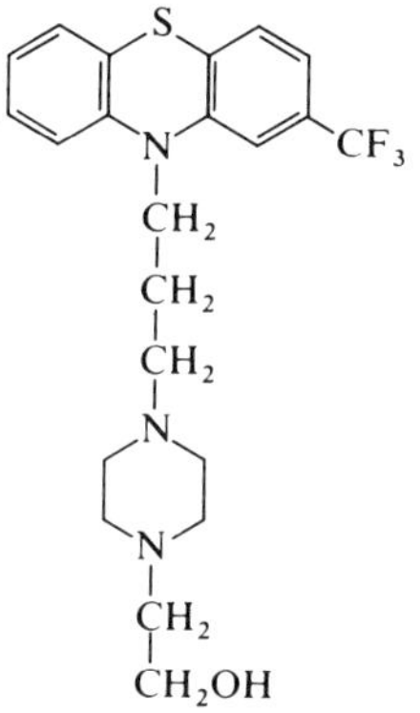

Fluphenazine
(piperazine
side-chain)

Fig. 7. Structure of four phenothiazines.

a. In Acute Schizophrenia

For the acutely ill schizophrenic, especially if he is very excited, disturbed, and agitated or has a history of severe disturbance of sleep, it may be necessary to give neuroleptic drugs by injection. One of the sedative drugs should be selected and the one most commonly used is chlorpromazine in doses of 100 mg given intramuscularly. Care must be taken over these injections as they are painful. It is sometimes recommended that a test dose of 25 mg should be given first, because of the risk of hypotension, but it is not usually necessary. If there are no difficulties the dose should be repeated thrice daily until the patient is sedated and gets some sleep. With these high doses the risk of hypotension and extra-pyramidal reactions is great and therefore the patient should be kept in bed. As has already been mentioned, he should be kept in a quiet room and given ample nursing attention. If the patient is old, frail, or dehydrated, these doses should be halved.

The patient should be given plenty to drink and encouraged to eat. As soon as possible, the injections should be replaced by an oral liquid preparation or tablets, up to 600 mg per day until the acute symptoms are controlled. If injections are not necessary, then chlorpromazine or thioridazine should be given in 100-mg doses up to 400 mg per day. If the patient does not respond to this treatment or cannot tolerate phenothiazines, then haloperidol up to 12 mg per day or chlorprothixene up to 300 mg per day should be used. With these high doses extra-pyramidal side-effects are to be expected. They can be controlled with one of the anti-parkinsonian drugs.

If the patient is not acutely disturbed but is obviously hallucinated and deluded or showing much thought disorder, smaller doses should be prescribed. If some sedation is required then chlorpromazine or thioridazine may be given up to 400 mg per day or chlorprothixene up to 300 mg per day. If sedation is not necessary then one of the other neuroleptics should be given in equivalent doses. This level of dosage should be continued for 2–3 weeks and then, once the acute phase is over, it is possible to begin reducing the dose, say by 25 per cent at a time at fortnightly intervals, and, at the same time, to reduce the frequency of administration to twice or even once a day. At this stage the aim should be to maintain the dosage at an optimal rather than a minimal level. An optimum dosage must strike a balance between control of symptoms and development of side-effects. The best way to control side-effects is to reduce the dosage of drug, but if the symptoms cannot then be controlled, anti-parkinsonian drugs will have to be given. They are often given as a routine accompaniment to the phenothiazines, but it is good clinical practice to avoid giving drugs unless they are necessary.

The prescribing of drugs should be based upon certain general fundamental principles. The physician is well advised not to try out all sorts of drugs, but to make himself thoroughly familiar with a relatively small number, say 5 or 6 among all the classes. He will thereby know how to use them and what to expect from them. He should avoid polypharmacy; if a patient is receiving several neuroleptics and difficulties arise, the physician will not be in a position to know what to do. If there is good reason for changing the patient's drug, this should be done slowly but completely. Once the patient has been started on a drug he should continue on with it for not less than 6 weeks before considering a change. Nevertheless, if there is good reason for making a change the physician should not hesitate to do so. A patient who fails to respond to one drug may respond to others. A patient may develop side-effects at low doses of one drug and yet may tolerate quite high doses of another. Above all, the prescribing of drugs should be done with common sense and sound judgement. It is absurd to expect miraculous effects from the use of neuroleptics.

Although these drugs are sometimes spoken of as 'anti-psychotics', there is no known specific disturbance underlying schizophrenia and no known specific treatment to counteract it. It would appear that in acute schizophrenia the patient is unable to cope with the influx of stimuli which overwhelm him, and there is some evidence to suggest that the neuroleptics reduce this influx. Their effect must therefore be regarded as merely a damping down of the symptoms while the normal processes of restitution take place. The Veterans' Administration studies in the USA have shown that the full effects of these drugs are not seen for at least 3 months and this is not far short of the duration of the acute phase of the illness. Patience and good nursing care are better than the over-enthusiastic prescribing of drugs and have no deleterious side-effects.

b. In Chronic Schizophrenia

It has been shown on a number of occasions that when drugs given to chronic schizophrenics are stopped, the proportion of patients who relapse varies, according to different trials, between about 30 and 70 per cent (Prien and Klett, 1972). This signifies that somewhere between 70 and 30 per cent of such patients are receiving drugs unnecessarily. This can be avoided by adhering to the rule to consider the dosage every 3 months or at least every 6 months. One suggestion that has been made is that every chronic schizophrenic on drugs should be given a 'drug holiday' every 6 months. When such proposals are made they often produce considerable alarm among the staff. The nurses fear that it may give rise to difficulties in managing the patients in the ward, but in practice this does not happen. Such relapses as do occur do not take place at the same time. The psychiatrists fear that the recurrence of symptoms in 'stabilized' chronic schizophrenics may be harmful to these patients. There is no evidence that such recurrence of symptoms has serious long-term effect but there is plenty of evidence that long-continued administration of drugs has such an effect.

The most difficult problem in the management of chronic patients on an out-patient basis is their tendency to stop taking their drugs so that they relapse and need to be re-admitted to hospital. This is partly because of the unpleasant side-effects of neuroleptics. Some of the newer drugs are better in this respect and it has been claimed that pimozide is effective for long-term maintenance, particularly in improving the sociability of patients (Pinard et al., 1972). In this respect, it has been claimed that it is better than the depot drugs (Falloon et al., 1978).

In any case, chronic schizophrenics are less reliable in taking their medication than the average patient and the introduction of depot drugs has been a valuable advance in coping with this problem.

Fluphenazine enanthate was the first to be introduced, followed by the decanoate. Flupenthixol decanoate is also now available. These drugs are in the form of an oily solution containing 25 mg per ml for the first two and 20 mg for the last. A half dose is given as a test and, if all goes well, a full dose is given about 1 week later. This is repeated every 1–3 weeks for the enanthate and every 2–4 weeks for the decanoate. If the patient has been stabilized on oral drugs beforehand the dose of tablets should be appropriately reduced. It has been stated that this treatment is liable to make the patients depressed, but Hirsch et al. (1973) in a controlled trial against placebo found that this was not so. Side-effects are common and, as they are dose-dependent, should be treated by reducing the dosage. This is most easily done by increasing the interval between injections, which should not be less than 2 weeks. With the passage of time it has been found that intervals can be increased and doses decreased. Experience has shown that the drugs should be continued for at least 4 years (Johnson, 1979).

Fluspirilene is available as an aqueous suspension of 2 mg/ml and is given intramuscularly once a week, starting with 1 ml and increasing by 1 ml weekly to an optimum level. Side-effects are less prominent than with the longer-acting depot drugs. Its resemblance to pimozide suggests that it will be particularly helpful in the social adjustment of out-patients. The introduction of these drugs gave rise at first to exaggeratedly high hopes which have been somewhat disappointed. Nevertheless, their value, still not yet adequately appreciated, will become manifest when clinical practice changes appropriately. Patients do not need to be supervised to ensure that they take their drugs, but they have to be observed carefully for the appearance of side-effects. Thus, although the management of these patients is much more effective it is neither easier nor simpler.

c. In Cycloid Psychoses

These respond well to neuroleptics, but if there is much confusion, a few ECT treatments may be required. Lithium carbonate is of prophylactic value and should be considered if two or more attacks have appeared within 4–5 years (Perris, 1978).

Treatment of Side-effects of Drugs

There are no such things as absolutely safe drugs. It is a useful assumption to make that any drug which is effective, i.e. has a 'therapeutic' effect, is bound to have unwanted side-effects. Drugs are used because the benefits they give outweigh the disadvantages.

The commonest side-effects are the extra-pyramidal reactions of pseudo-parkinsonism, i.e. rigidity, tremor, and akinesia. As they are related to the level of drug in the blood (Hausen et al., 1981), they are best treated by a temporary halt or a reduction in the dose of neuroleptic, but if this is not practicable they can be treated with anti-parkinsonian drugs. These are procyclidine 5–60 mg, benzhexol 2–10 mg, benztropine 2–6 mg, or orphenadrine 100–400 mg per day. The last two can be given intramuscularly to start with and procyclidine can even be given intravenously. They are often given as a routine accompaniment to the phenothiazines, but it is good clinical practice to avoid giving drugs unless they are necessary. It must not be forgotten that the anti-parkinsonian drugs have their own side-effects, e.g. dry mouth, blurring of vision, difficulty with micturition, and sometimes even toxic confusion. One should therefore be cautious when administering these drugs under conditions where their anti-cholinergic effects might give rise to difficulties, e.g. enlarged prostate or glaucoma. Nevertheless, after the acute phase of the schizophrenia is controlled, some patients may be 'akinetic', showing a lack of spontaneity, lethargy, and even drowsiness (Rifkin et al., 1975); all of which may respond well to anti-parkinsonian drugs. If the patient is on neuroleptics and anti-parkinsonian drugs, and it is intended to reduce the dosage, the neuroleptics should be reduced first. For patients on a stable dosage of both drugs, it is always worth trying to reduce the anti-parkinsonian drugs. Experience has shown that some patients who needed them initially do not need them later. Klett and Caffey (1972) found that when patients who had been receiving anti-parkinsonian drugs for more than 3 months, had them replaced with placebo, less than 20 per cent showed a return of extra-pyramidal symptoms.

Another side-effect is akathisia. This may begin with a peculiar crawling feeling in the legs, later developing into restless movements and swinging of the legs. Eventually the patient is unable to sit still and paces about continually. This condition is easily mistaken for agitation or even the return of schizophrenic excitement and may therefore be treated by increasing the dose of neuroleptic. The correct treatment is to reduce the dose or to switch to another drug.

Acute dystonia is fortunately an uncommon side-effect of the more potent neuroleptics. In this condition muscle spasms develop rapidly giving rise to torticollis, deviation of the jaw, and protrusion of the tongue. This frightening reaction can be stopped immediately by intravenous procyclidine. Other side-effects, such as postural hypotension, drowsiness, and dry mouth, tend to lessen in time and should be treated appropriately. Skin rashes may require switching to another phenothiazine. An increased liability to sunburn occurs in patients taking phenothiazines, especially chlorpromazine, and they should be warned about this risk. Gain in weight is common; enlargement of the breast and galactorrhoea have been described.

Obstructive jaundice was reported in the early days of the use of chlorpromazine but it has become rare. It is unrelated to a history of previous liver disease, and carrying out liver-function tests before starting with phenothiazines achieves nothing more than to satisfy idle curiosity. Agranulocytosis is an idiosyncratic reaction which may develop suddenly, especially in the first 2 months, as it can with many drugs. It is useless to try to detect its onset by means of routine white cell counts, unless these are carried out at least daily, but clinical observation of sore throat and fever is a sure warning sign. Although phenothiazines lower the epileptic threshold, convulsions are rare.

An apparently irreversible side-effect of long-term administration of large doses of phenothiazines is known as 'tardive dyskinesia'. It consists of choreiform and athetotic movements, affecting chiefly the tongue, lips, and jaw, and also the limbs and trunk. Various treatments have been proposed, e.g. thiopropazate in small doses (45 mg daily), sodium valproate, co-dergocrine mesylate (Hajioff and Wallace, 1983), and sulpiride.

Thioridazine in large doses is liable to produce retinitis pigmentosa. It should therefore be limited to below a maximum of 800 mg daily. Deposits of melanin in the skin, cornea, and lens are sometimes seen after the administration of phenothiazines in large doses over a period of years. Although no serious consequences have been described, these findings constitute another good reason for avoiding excessive prescribing of drugs.

Other Physical Treatments

Depressive symptoms are not uncommon in schizophrenia. If they are prolonged or sufficiently severe then tricyclic anti-depressant drugs should be added to the other medication. If the patient does not respond or there is a risk of suicide then the patient should receive ECT. This is especially important in out-patient treatment as there is no doubt about the high risk of suicide in such patients. ECT may also be required in the acute phase if the patient does not respond to neuroleptics. Clinical experience has shown that after one or two treatments, the patient may then respond well to the drugs. Catatonic stupor and withdrawal also respond well to ECT.

When prefrontal leucotomy (lobotomy, psycho-surgery) was first introduced it aroused great enthusiasm and many thousands of patients were given this treatment. No really well-controlled trial was ever carried out, so its value and the indications for its use are still subjects of controversy. Fortunately, the introduction of the neuroleptics has eliminated the need for this treatment in schizophrenia.

Rehabilitation

The treatment advocated above will do much to prevent patients from deteriorating and thereby becoming more or less permanent inmates of a mental hospital. Conditions being what they are, there are many schizophrenic patients in hospitals who have been there for many years and have become apathetic and withdrawn, unable to look after themselves or to live outside the care of a hospital. For well over a century enthusiastic pioneers have repeatedly demonstrated that it is possible to change this state of affairs and to replace the general atmosphere of chronic wards with an environment which at the least provides a tolerable human existence. Unfortunately, enthusiasm in therapeutics is not a substitute for knowledge and understanding, and once the pioneers had gone, conditions in mental hospitals tended to deteriorate.

There are then two kinds of chronic schizophrenic patient who require that régime of treatment known as 'rehabilitation'. The first consists of those patients who have had an acute attack, have made a good improvement, have then been discharged home, and are under some form of supervision. Instead of continuing to improve they stagnate and even begin to deteriorate and become apathetic. The family's hopes atrophy and it becomes accustomed to the presence of the apathetic and drifting member. In such circumstances, it is advisable for the patient to attend the day hospital or, if necessary, to be re-admitted so that he can be given a proper programme of activities.

The second kind of patient consists of those who have deteriorated from neglect owing to previous lack of facilities. An environment which promotes deterioration is one which provides a regular routine, lacking in variety, giving no responsibilities, and no worthwhile occupation. In such a situation, there is nothing to be gained from showing initiative and even normal individuals will quickly become torpid and apathetic. Add to this the absence of any companionship other than that of other schizophrenics and the malignant effects of the disorder on the personality, then it is easy to see why chronic schizophrenics in mental hospitals show gross 'institutionalization'.

The immediate aim of rehabilitation therefore must be not so much to reduce frustrations as to provide satisfaction from social activity and occupation. This applies just as much to patients whose discharge from hospital is very far in the future as to those who are likely to leave soon. A full programme of activities and occupation is a basic necessity in a long-stay ward. It could well be said that every such ward should have above its entrance a notice written in letters of fire: 'The condition of the patients deteriorates directly to the proportion of time they spend doing nothing.' In the old-style mental hospitals, the efforts to give the patients something to do led to their exploitation. Civil rights legislation has stopped this but at the same time, and this is particularly true in the USA, it has almost guaranteed that the patients are forced to rot in idleness.

The programme of activities must be graded so as to be suitable for the patients. Idleness leads to deterioration, but too much pressure gives rise to relapse and to aggressive outbursts. A rigid programme is no substitute for judgement and decent sympathy for handicap. For the patient on the road to recovery, it should be carried out in such a way that he feels that when the time comes to leave the hospital, it does not mean a loss of security and exposure to the struggle and competition of life but a move towards independence and freedom. In general, patients who respond best are those with minimal symptoms and affective disturbance. In those patients whose affective disturbance is high the use of drugs is likely to improve their response to rehabilitation. The first step in a programme is to assess the clinical state of the patients and their capabilities, which experience has shown are almost invariably greater than would appear. The programme should consist of graded and small steps. O'Connor et al. (1956) showed that schizophrenics are slow learners, but improve steadily for a long time. For this reason, their jobs should not be changed too soon but only after they have reached a maximum level of efficiency in them. It is most important to ensure that patients have mastered each step before going on to the next, otherwise relapse with recrudescence of symptoms may occur (Wing et al., 1964).

Industrial Therapy

When the patient is ready for it he should go into the workshop of an industrial therapy unit. Bennett and Wing (1963) have given a clear account of the aims of industrial therapy. As compared with occupational therapy it provides a realistic way of assessing the patient's capabilities; it provides the stimulus and activation that are necessary to prevent deterioration; it trains him for the discipline demanded by the requirements of earning a living, i.e. punctual and regular attendance, proper standards of work; and finally, by providing the patient with a wage which he has earned, it puts him on the road to independence. Wadsworth et al. (1962) have provided an excellent general guide to the setting-up of an industrial unit. Morgan (1974) has made clear the importance of properly designed equipment and management of the workshops. One person only should be in complete control of the running of an industrial therapy unit. Divided responsibility for the patients is a sure road to disaster. The activities of the unit should always be regarded as part of a programme which covers all the patients' needs (Ekdawi, 1972). It is very easy to slip into the tendency to regard the work and production as of prime importance so that good workers are not moved on precisely because they are good workers. The organization of an adequate system of payments is of the greatest importance and these should be at a proper level. Bennett (1970) emphasized the value of payment on a piece-work basis. Payments should be accompanied by appropriate facilities for spending the money, either in or out of the hospital. When ready, the patients should be prepared for leaving hospital either to a 'half-way house' or hostel, or to return to a home with relatives.

The change to living at home may be critical. Relatives find it difficult to tolerate the eccentricities of a patient, precisely because they are much concerned about him. A tense atmosphere, full of recrimination, may easily develop and then the patient relapses (*see* p. 137). For this reason, careful preparation of the family is needed and should be followed by continual supervision. If suitable relatives are not available, the patients may have to go to a 'nursing home' or 'half-way house'. This does not mean that they can now be left to fend for themselves. Proper supervision, occupation, and the discipline of work are still necessary. Without them, the patients may deteriorate into the same state in a 'chronic back ward' (Schmidt et al., 1977). It is greatly to be regretted that the use of 'foster homes' has not been given sufficient attention. The great example of Geel, Belgium, seems to have been largely ignored, except by Dr Adeoye Lambo at Aro, Nigeria.

Behavioural Treatment

An important development in the treatment of schizophrenia, especially in chronically deteriorated patients, is the use of behavioural techniques based on learning theory. This theory implies that whatever may have been the original basis of the appearance of abnormal behaviour, its maintenance is affected by the external environment and therefore can be changed by changing the relevant aspects of that environment. Crudely put, this means that undesirable patterns of behaviour can be 'unlearned', and replaced by new 'learned' appropriate behaviour. The methods of training used with schizophrenic patients are often based on operant conditioning, which emphasizes the active response of the patients but at the same time does not require high levels of motivation from them.

There is nothing new in the principle that rewarding good behaviour encourages it and punishing bad behaviour discourages it; indeed, society produces appropriate social behaviour largely by this method. In operant conditioning the techniques for 'reinforcing' desired behaviour have been refined on the basis of much experimental work. Many methods are being used and a valuable review has been provided by Baker (1975).

Token economies are the most elaborate development of behaviour therapy. In them, patients are rewarded with tokens for appropriate behaviour which they can then exchange for goods and privileges. Such schemes require elaborate preparation, involving the co-operation of most of the organization of the hospital, as well as changes in the routines of the ward. Hall and Baker (1973) have pointed out that unsuitable choice of patients, staff, and techniques, and lack of anticipation of difficulties, can wreck and discredit a complete programme. If not understood properly, the methods can be applied inadequately or over-rigidly, producing a hardening of the attitudes of the staff and leading to an expectation of failure. The literature contains many enthusiastic reports but there is a paucity of controlled trials. In one such trial (Baker et al., 1977) it was found after 12 months that the experimental group, which was given tokens for appropriate behaviour ('contingent reinforcement'), did not improve more than the control group, which had been given the same number of tokens regardless. The authors concluded that it was not the tokens which led to the improvement.

A number of criticisms, e.g. Davison (1969), have been made of the work using behavioural therapy for chronic schizophrenics and some of them are not unjustified. It is an old clinical tradition that chronic schizophrenics tend to deteriorate in a stagnant environment so that almost any change will halt the deterioration and sometimes even reverse it dramatically. In most of the reports the patients received more attention than in the past and, since this was often not adequately controlled for, the improvement may have been a purely non-specific effect. A controlled trial by Feitel et al. (1982) showed that increased attention by therapy aides to specific behavioural problems in patients produced significant improvement in as short a time as 3 months. There has been insufficient distinction made between the effects of chronic schizophrenia and the effects of institutionalization to which such patients are particularly vulnerable. Finally, the amount of improvement obtained by these methods is limited though there is no theoretical reason, on the basis of a psychological 'model' of schizophrenia, why this should be so. Nevertheless, behavioural therapists have shown that even severely withdrawn patients can be considerably improved and the importance of this cannot be over-emphasized in counteracting therapeutic nihilism. They have provided evidence, together with those who have worked on more traditional methods of rehabilitation, that resources of money and staff are not wasted on chronic patients in mental hospitals, but can indeed achieve considerable improvement in the patients' condition. As all rehabilitation techniques have failures, such limitation cannot be used as a criticism against any of them.

Chapter 9

Diagnosis and differential diagnosis

DIAGNOSIS

Reference was made in Chapter 1 to the difference in the proportions of patients diagnosed as schizophrenic in different countries. In 1961, the epidemiologist Morton Kramer drew attention to the great differences between the USA and the UK in first admissions diagnosed as schizophrenia, mania, and senile dementia. This took some time to penetrate, as it was still possible in 1966 for Lorr to write, '. . . in much of American psychiatry, formal diagnosis is actually ignored as relatively unimportant and outmoded, or disparaged as non-dynamic and useless'. However, several investigations were undertaken to examine the nature of these differences, culminating in a joint US–UK project (Cooper et al., 1972). In this investigation, a team of American and British psychiatrists used a structured interview and systematic recording of data, using Wing's Present State Examination and Spitzer's Mental Status Schedule, to diagnose patients in England and New York. The members of the team were largely in agreement and their diagnoses were much the same as those made in the English hospitals but very different from those made in the New York ones. It was clear that the New York concept of schizophrenia covered many conditions which were diagnosed as affective and personality disorders in the UK and by the team.

This work was extended by the International Pilot Study of Schizophrenia organized by the World Health Organization as part of its long-term programme in epidemiology (WHO, 1973). The IPSS was based on the use of the Present State Examination (PSE) (Wing et al., 1974) and the difficulties of language were dealt with by translating the PSE into other languages (Chinese, Czech, Danish, Hindi, Russian, Spanish, and Yoruba), checked by back translation. The information recorded was based on interviews only, a minor deficiency. The results showed that psychiatrists in different countries ('developed' and 'undeveloped') could make and record comparable clinical observations. It was found that schizophrenia and other disorders, defined by operational criteria, could be found and diagnosed reliably in all seven countries, the similarities across cultures being much more obvious than the differences. Only in two centres (Moscow and Washington, DC) were obvious differences in the diagnosis of schizophrenia found. The Russians placed greater emphasis on the course and less on the symptoms, and the Americans followed their characteristically broad concept.

The data were also used for making diagnoses by means of a computer program CATEGO (Wing et al., 1974), which relies heavily on the 'first-rank' symptoms of Schneider. First, the 360 PSE items were condensed into 129 Units of Analysis and then further joined together into 27 Group Units. There is room for criticism of this procedure. While one can only approve of the joining together of 'voices speak to the patient', 'voices speak thoughts', 'thoughts spoken aloud', and 'auditory hallucinations', since they are difficult to distinguish, to join hypochondriacal delusions with delusions of persecution, guilt, etc., can only lead to a blurring of important distinctions.

There was 87 per cent agreement between the psychiatrists and the program for the diagnoses of schizophrenia, mania, and depression. Among the 1202 patients interviewed, 811 were diagnosed as schizophrenic by the psychiatrists and 563 by the CATEGO program. Using also a cluster analysis, it was found that 306 patients formed a core of schizophrenics acceptable to all three systems of classification.

What are the signs and symptoms which distinguish between schizophrenia and other disorders? Carpenter et al. (1973) found that there were 24, but a multiple regression analysis showed that 12 were sufficient. Symptoms which had to be present were: restricted affect, poor insight, thoughts aloud, poor rapport, widespread delusions, incoherent speech, unreliable information, bizarre and nihilistic delusions. The following were counted only if absent: waking early, depressed facies, and elation. In the authors' 'flexible system' 5 points counted for 'probable' and 6 for 'definite' schizophrenia.

Schneider's first-rank symptoms were given great emphasis in the IPSS, both in the diagnoses of the psychiatrists and the CATEGO program, but it was found that their presence could not establish a diagnosis of schizophrenia. Wing and Nixon (1975) pointed out that they were present in 16 per cent (14 out of 79) of patients with mania, 4 per cent with depressive disorders, and 2 per cent with neuroses. Schneider himself did not claim that the symptoms were sufficiently clear-cut to be of great value in diagnosis. He also said that they did not form a coherent group, and Lewine et al. (1982) agreed when they found that the inter-correlations of these symptoms were low and that when the correlation matrix was factored, the symptoms appeared in 7 different factors. It may be added that Mellor et al. (1981), in a follow-up after 8 years, found that the diagnosis of schizophrenia was changed in 12 per cent of patients who had shown first-rank symptoms at the first admission.

In due course, a follow-up of the patients in the IPSS was carried out (WHO, 1979). Among many findings the most important is that schizophrenics have a better outcome in undeveloped countries than in developed ones. It was also possible to examine outcome in relation to diagnostic criteria and at the same time to include other diagnostic systems (including those designed for use with computers). Two such groups of diagnostic criteria have become widely accepted. The first is that of Feighner et al. (1972), which is sometimes referred to as the 'St Louis criteria'. This requires at least one of the following: delusions or hallucinations not accompanied by perplexity or disorientation, or verbal communication difficulties. In addition, at least 3 of the following 5 background characteristics are required: single, poor pre-morbid personality, family history of schizophrenia, absence of alcohol or drug abuse, and onset before the age of 40. The illness should have been present for at least 6 months and there should not have been enough affective symptoms to qualify for a diagnosis of depression or mania. The second group of criteria is that of Spitzer et al. (1975) which requires at least 2 of 8 symptoms, all involving delusions, hallucinations, or thought disorder (all are strictly defined). The episode must have lasted for at least 2 weeks continuously and depression or mania must have been excluded.

The 2-year follow-up was extended to 5 years by Hawk et al. (1975) for the American sample of the IPSS patients. They confirmed previous studies of the data that the Langfeldt and Schneider criteria had little prognostic value. Brockington et al. (1978), in their comparison of 10 definitions of schizophrenia, did not wholly agree. They found that the criteria of Spitzer, Langfeldt, the flexible system of Carpenter, and CATEGO were reasonably concordant and moderately effective as predictors. Finally, Bland and Orn (1979) compared the prognostic value of three diagnostic criteria: Feighner's, Schneider's, and the New Haven Index. Only the first were effective, but this is not surprising as they include the proviso of a duration of illness of not less than 6 months, i.e. semi-chronic patients tend to become chronic.

It would seem pointless to expect that a definition of an illness should be of prognostic value; nobody would expect that of pneumonia, appendicitis, or even multiple sclerosis. It is relevant for schizophrenia because the original definition did include prognosis, and many clinicians would refuse to make that diagnosis if the patient recovered. That attitude is not accepted here. The point of investigations on the outcome of patients chosen by research criteria is to determine if the selection has picked out a homogeneous group, and this is important in research (e.g. on treatment) because the outcome of schizophrenia is indeed extremely variable. It is not really necessary to remind practising clinicians that a diagnosis of schizophrenia can be made even if the clinical features do not fit any of the current research criteria. Schneider himself pointed out that schizophrenia could be diagnosed in the absence of first-rank symptoms and this is equally true for all the other criteria.

DIFFERENTIAL DIAGNOSIS

Some points of differentiation between schizophrenia and other mental disorders have already been discussed, notably in Chapter 5 on paranoid states, but it is now necessary to discuss differential diagnosis in detail.

Affective Disorders

In attempting to come to a decision in the case of patients suffering from atypical affective disorders, especially manias, it is always useful to consider Schneider's symptoms of the first rank, though they are usually absent in doubtful cases. Usually, if one of these first-rank symptoms is clearly present, then quite a number of the others are also. Often it is difficult to be sure that a patient has a delusional perception, *Gedankenlautwerden*, or experiences of passivity. Thus some patients have a very vivid auditory imagery which is easily mistaken for *Gedankenlautwerden*, while in others an apparent delusional perception may turn out to be a delusion-like experience, or a sudden delusional idea provoked by a perception. When asked about experiences of passivity, some patients admit such experiences, but on closer questioning it appears that they felt 'as if' they were being controlled.

Auditory hallucinations may occur in a depression, but they usually consist of odd words or brief phrases, which are heard when the patient is severely depressed. The hallucinations are voices which make odd, abusive remarks or suggest suicide, but they are fragmentary or disjointed. Continuous hallucinatory voices do not occur in uncomplicated depressions and when they appear in otherwise fairly typical depressive clinical pictures, then the possibility of dehydration, overdosage with drugs (especially hyoscine and bromide), dietary deficiencies, and other coarse brain disorders should be considered, as well as schizophrenia.

At times the depressive mood is not obvious, so that the diagnosis may have to depend on the presence of other symptoms. Depressive thought content and the typical sleep disturbance are particularly helpful. A few depressed middle-aged and elderly patients are able to put on a good front, so that they may smile and make wry self-depreciatory jokes. This 'gallows humour' may lead the untrained observer to misinterpret this apparent discrepancy between thought and affective expression as due to schizophrenia. However, skilful interrogation leads to a more obvious expression of the depressive affect.

Some manic patients are irritable and have a paranoid attitude. Often they complain about the justifiable reactions of their fellows to their troublesome behaviour, so that they may insist that they were never mentally ill, and have been wrongly committed. They may complain about the cruel acts of others when, in fact, they are describing legitimate restraint of their unruly activity. Lack of insight is quite common both during and after the manic episode, so that it is quite wrong to assume that lack of insight during an acute episode is diagnostic of schizophrenia. Chronic mania has been described, but it seems likely that, while chronic manic-depressive illnesses which are mainly manic do occur, chronic mania does not or, at best, is very rare. In every mental hospital there are a few patients who have illnesses which are mainly manic, but from time to time short-lived depressive episodes occur. A few chronic mental hospital inmates are permanently cheerful and talkative. Some of these are affect-laden paraphrenics who have ill-formulated delusions of persecutions, which are brought forward with enthusiasm but are never clearly formulated, while others are clearly cases of fantasiophrenia.

Despite all that has been said, there are some atypical affective disorders in which it is difficult to decide whether or not the illness is schizophrenia. If, after making a generous allowance for the pathoplastic effects of pre-morbid personality, idiosyncratic modes of affective expression, and so on, the total clinical picture appears to go beyond any reasonable possibility of empathy on the part of the observer, then schizophrenia must be diagnosed.

Adolescent Crises: The Crises of Identification (The 'Catcher in the Rye' Syndrome)*

Most adolescents in Western cultures have a period of mild disturbance due to difficulties in trying to change their relationship with their parents from one of dependency and love to independence and love. Many never achieve the accepted 'correct' relationship between an adult and his parents in Western cultures. In the common mild adolescent turmoil states, the adolescent may be somewhat obstinate and opinionated and on bad terms with his parents and parent surrogates. He may assert his rebellious attitude by joining minority groups and reform movements or becoming a 'drop-out'.

---

*J. D. Salinger's novel *A Catcher in the Rye* (1951, Hamish Hamilton, London) gives an excellent account of an acute episode in an adolescent crisis.

In adolescents who have had difficulties with their parents since childhood the turmoil may become severe, and the wayward behaviour of the male and the spiteful behaviour of the female adolescent may be difficult to understand. The more intelligent develop an interest in philosophy and psychology, so that they convert their personal anxieties about their own emotional relationships to others into anxieties of a general kind about the universe and the problems of mankind. Some develop an interest in esoteric beliefs, such as Zen Buddhism and the like, and this may give rise to queer intellectual productions. Often rapport is difficult to achieve, since the psychiatrist is identified with the 'establishment'.

This illness seems to be commoner in middle-class adolescents. In Britain most working-class children go to work when they are 16 years old and act out their adolescent difficulties by changing their jobs and identifying with the current craze, such as 'skin-heads' and 'bovver boys'. These teenage crazes allow many disturbed adolescents to mature with their peers and act out their difficulties. Students going to university at 18 years of age have to deal with a new world which is much less formalized. They may make their first acquaintance with heterosexual behaviour and alcohol. Many freshmen have a marked ambivalent attitude to their parents and when they have partially broken away from parental dominance by going to university they become quite upset. In addition, academic problems, in particular the discovery that they may have been bright at grammar school but that their intelligence is not outstanding in a university, add to the strain. Adolescent crises are therefore frequently seen among students.

These patients show no typical schizophrenic symptoms, but may appear strange and odd. Since schizophrenia is more likely to occur in a predisposed person who is subjected to acute or prolonged psychic trauma, it is always possible that an adolescent crisis may provoke a schizophrenic illness. Sometimes a manic-depressive illness may be provoked by an adolescent crisis, but although depression is common in adolescents, it is usually a reactive unhappiness rather than a true depressive illness.

Obsessional States

These conditions usually begin in childhood or adolescence and, although the content of an obsessional thought may be very bizarre, this does not justify the diagnosis of schizophrenia. Thus one patient ruminated continuously that as he did not believe in God, he would probably kill somebody when he was about to die because he would not be punished. One day while indulging in sexual play with his girl friend, he suddenly thought that he had a piece of faeces on the end of his glans penis. He then decided that if he inserted his uncleaned penis into his friend's vagina, this would prove that he would kill somebody when he was on the point of death. Human nature being what it is, he inserted his penis and had a satisfactory orgasm. Thereafter he ruminated on the following theme: as he did not believe in God, he would kill somebody when he was about to die, because he had inserted his penis with a piece of faeces on it into his friend's vagina, when he knew that he should have cleaned his penis in order to prove that he would not kill someone when he was about to die. Despite the bizarre quality of the content of the obsession, this patient, who had been ill for at least 12 years, showed no signs of schizophrenia and coped quite well with his job as a schoolmaster.

Obsessional states often occur in grossly abnormal personalities who are clearly psychopathic in Schneider's sense of the term. Their abnormal behaviour, especially abnormal sexual behaviour, may lead them into difficulties which give rise to psychogenic reactions and depressive illnesses. Because of the pathoplastic effect of the abnormal personality, these illnesses may show very atypical clinical pictures. However, unless clear-cut schizophrenic symptoms occur, the diagnosis of schizophrenia should not be made.

Hysteria

Some adolescent and young adult females have episodes of disturbed behaviour. Usually they have been unstable since childhood and often have had psychiatric treatment for a childhood behaviour disorder. The wild behaviour may begin abruptly or may follow a typical conversion hysteria which has been treated by a direct therapeutic attack on the hysterical symptom. In this case the symptom disappears, but is replaced by the behaviour disorder.

These patients are restless, violent, and destructive. They make repeated suicidal attempts and attempts at self-mutilation, so that the arms and legs, especially the flexor surfaces of the forearms, are slashed with razor blades, pieces of tin, broken glass, and so on. Despite the vigilance of the nursing staff, they steal and hide materials which will make good weapons and then mutilate themselves in order to create a scene. These patients sometimes describe visual hallucinations, e.g. men who threaten them, but it is advisable to be sceptical about such statements.

Despite this grossly disturbed behaviour, it is easy to make rapport with these patients. They usually develop a marked positive transference to male therapists and then act out in the transference situation. Any break in their psychological treatment is liable to lead to a recrudescence of the violent behaviour. As a rule, the illness subsides within a year, but it may last for a much longer period.

Occasionally these patients manage to commit suicide and, rarely, the illness becomes clearly schizophrenic. Psychotherapy and phenothiazine drugs are useful in the treatment of this condition, and it is important to avoid punitive measures such as seclusion or restraint, since these patients invite and enjoy punishment.

Hysterical Pseudodementia (Ganser States)

This is the syndrome of 'approximate answers', in which the patient gives answers to questions which are incorrect but which indicate that the patient knows the correct answers. The patient may also behave in a way that a lay person with no knowledge of psychiatry would consider to be mad. Despite the apparent loss of even the simplest knowledge, the patient is able to look after himself in a way which is much superior to the level which would be expected from his intellectual performance. This disorder usually occurs in psychopathic criminals who wish to avoid punishment, but it may occur in mania and early schizophrenia. Pseudodementia in a young person who has no reason to have such an illness suggests an underlying schizophrenia. As mentioned before, talking past the point occurs in some chronic schizophrenics, notably in speech-prompt catatonia.

Psychopathic Personalities

Short-lived psychotic episodes are not uncommon in psychopathic personalities when they are in severe environmental difficulties. Some psychopaths are able to live a fairly normal life for a year or two, but then they seem to become bored with their humdrum existence and begin to behave badly. They drink heavily, have extra-marital liaisons, take amphetamines or other drugs, or merely behave in a generally irresponsible way. As a result of their behaviour, they get into great social difficulties and this may precipitate a transient psychosis, following which they make a fairly adequate adjustment once again.

Many anti-social psychopaths show little emotion after very violent behaviour and most murderers, following arrest, are apparently unmoved by their crime. This dissociation of affect must not be misinterpreted as a blunting of affect and held to be diagnostic of schizophrenia. In some psychopaths, psychotherapy or Rorschach testing may reveal violent and sexually perverse fantasies, but this is not evidence of schizophrenia.

Coarse Brain Disease

Schizophrenic illnesses indistinguishable from 'endogenous' schizophrenia in symptomatology and course have been reported in a large number of different coarse brain diseases. Psychoses partly resembling schizophrenia (schizophrenic-like psychoses) are much more common than typical schizophrenia in coarse brain disease. (*See also* p. 21).

The schizophrenic-like psychosis which is most likely to cause confusion is organic hallucinosis. In this condition there are continuous auditory hallucinations in a state of clear consciousness. The hallucinatory voices are usually abusive and talk about the patient in the third person. The patient shows no personality change and his general mental activity is fairly normal. Delusions of persecution occur, but can be seen to be a logical result of the continuous hallucinatory voices. Consequently, the illness can be understood as a natural reaction to the continuous auditory hallucinosis. This condition can be produced by physical, chemical, and biological agents. Alcohol is probably the commonest cause, but physical injury, anoxia, carbon disulphide poisoning, and carbon monoxide poisoning may be responsible.

While organic hallucinosis can occur in epilepsy, a clinical picture identical with some varieties of paranoid schizophrenia is more common in this condition. In this paranoid epileptic psychosis consciousness is clear, although the patients usually appear somewhat dull and bewildered. Voices and *Gedankenlautwerden* are usually present, and delusions based on primary delusions also occur. Gruhle (1936) has pointed out that the primary delusion, in the sense of the establishment of a relationship without cause, is found only in schizophrenia and epilepsy. Experiences of control by foreign agencies and bodily hallucinations are also common. These patients have usually been epileptic for many years and have temporal lobe foci. Sometimes the sticky, slow, epileptic speech is unmistakably present, and the characteristic egocentric 'holier-than-thou' epileptic personality change can be detected by the expert. The EEG is often normal during the psychosis.

Usually there is no difficulty in distinguishing the epileptic twilight state from schizophrenia, since there is a definite disturbance of consciousness. This may be a restriction of the field of consciousness, so that the patient's thinking is dominated by a few over-valued ideas, or it may be a dream-like change of consciousness similar to delirium. Vivid visual hallucinations may be seen which are usually concerned with fire and religious topics. Conflagrations, the Crucifixion, God, Jesus, and various saints or religious reformers may be seen. These patients frequently hear the voices of God, Jesus, and the angels.

Marked restlessness, such as general over-activity, violent assaults on others, stereotyped activity, and continuous praying may occur. Sometimes there is stupor and the clinical picture resembles catatonia. The EEG usually shows abnormal rhythms which may be focal or general. These twilight states usually follow a series of fits, but if the pattern of fits is one of minor grand mal, the epileptic phenomena may not be noticed by untrained observers. Confused and odd states may occur in epileptics whose fits are so poorly controlled that they occur before the post-epileptic confusion produced by a previous fit has cleared up.

For the sake of clarity, the syndromes of organic hallucinosis, epileptic paranoid psychosis, and epileptic twilight states have been rather sharply outlined. It must be remembered that there can be some degree of overlap, so that symptoms belonging to different syndromes may occur at the same time, or one syndrome may in the course of time develop into another.

Brain Injury

The causal relationship between schizophrenia and brain injury has been considered in the chapter on aetiology (Chapter 2). Elsässer and Grünewald (1953) have pointed out that if a schizophrenic illness, which progresses to a defect state, occurs immediately after a brain injury, then the injury must be considered as causal. If there is an interval between the brain injury and the onset of the psychosis, then the injury can still be considered to be causative, if there are symptoms during this interval. The commonest bridging symptom of this kind is, of course, epilepsy. These authors point out that schizophrenic-like illnesses occur more frequently than true schizophrenia after brain injury, and these disorders take the form of organic hallucinosis or paranoid epileptic psychoses.

Feuchtwanger and Mayer-Gross (1938) in their classic paper on schizophrenia and head injury give the incidence of schizophrenic processes following head injury in a series of 1554 cases as 0·52 per cent. In a series of 1821 head injuries, Hillbom (1960) found 20 'schizophrenia-like psychoses', i.e. an incidence of 1·09 per cent. He found that these conditions were more likely to occur in association with temporal lobe lesions, while Feuchtwanger and Mayer-Gross found that schizophrenia was somewhat more frequent after frontal lobe lesions. It is, of course, difficult to estimate the site and extent of brain damage purely by clinical and radiological investigations.

There is no doubt that an illness indistinguishable from so-called endogenous schizophrenia can occur following severe brain injury.

Since the incidence of this illness is very small it has been argued that a predisposition to schizophrenia must be present. It is possible, however, that a lesion in a special part of the brain, which is usually well protected against injury, is necessary for the production of this illness, or that a special combination of focal lesions is essential. (*See* p. 21).

Toxic Psychoses

On the whole, the typical toxic confusional state or sub-acute delirious state presents no diagnostic difficulties, but some toxic psychoses, notably bromide and amphetamine psychoses, may easily be mistaken for paranoid schizophrenia.

Excessive bromide consumption may lead to a paranoid psychosis with auditory hallucinations in the absence of clouding of consciousness. The routine estimation of the blood-bromide and a routine investigation of previous medication can prevent any diagnostic error.

Amphetamine psychosis, however, presents a much more difficult problem, since most of these patients are addicts who obtain the drug illegally. Since they are dependent on the drug, they conceal the fact that they are taking it and may even continue to take it while in hospital. Thus one patient persuaded a ward cleaner to buy him an amphetamine inhaler after he had been admitted to hospital with an amphetamine psychosis. Connell (1958) has studied 42 cases of amphetamine psychoses. A few of his patients became psychotic after a single large dose of amphetamine which ranged from 75 to 975 mg in the course of 2 days. A few others took large doses of alcohol as well as amphetamine, but most of his patients were addicts taking from 50 to 325 mg per day. In only 3 cases was there any indication of disorientation, and in 2 of these there was some other complicating factor which was probably responsible for it. Twenty-five patients had ideas of reference, 36 had delusions of persecution, 29 had auditory hallucinations, 21 had visual hallucinations, 5 had tactile hallucinations, 4 had olfactory hallucinations, 6 had depression, 11 had fear, and 5 had terror. The visual hallucinations were usually of minor importance, but the hallucinatory voices, when present, dominated the clinical picture. Fear of being killed by a gang was the commonest persecutory delusion and on several occasions this led Connell to investigate the possibility of an amphetamine psychosis. In most cases the symptoms disappeared within 5 days of apparent withdrawal of the drug. In those cases where it did not, Connell suspected that the patient still had access to the drug. In view of this, not only should the urine of all acute paranoid psychotics be tested for amphetamine, but repeated tests of the urine of patients who have had amphetamine psychosis must be carried out. Six of Connell's patients had apparently normal personalities, and this contradicts the widely held view that amphetamine merely releases a constitutional predisposition to a paranoid psychosis. There is, therefore, no doubt that amphetamine is a true hallucinogen.

Morbid Jealousy (The 'Jealous Husband' Syndrome)

In this condition the patient has well-held delusions of marital infidelity; these are usually supported by a falsification of memory in which the patient claims to have had an experience which suggests that the spouse has committed adultery. For example, a miner on night shift said that he woke up during the day and through the open door of the bedroom he was able to see a mirror in which he could see his wife misbehaving with his son-in-law on the living-room settee. This belief was unshakeable despite the fact that there was clear evidence that it was physically impossible for the patient to have seen into the living-room and that the son-in-law had been 20 miles away at the relevant time. Apart from allegations of this kind, ridiculous evidence is brought forward to support the accusation of infidelity, such as undue moistness of the wife's vagina, stains on the wife's underclothes, 'bags' under the wife's eyes, and so on.

This illness occurs in both sexes, but in Britain it appears to be more common in men than in women, probably because it is more difficult for a wife to leave a jealous husband than vice versa. These jealous husbands insist on a confession and may resort to violence, or even torture, to secure one. Sometimes the harassed wife invents a story of adultery only to have it disproved by her husband, who then uses this false confession as a proof of his wife's dishonesty. Despite the grossly abnormal nature of the patient's behaviour, no clear signs of schizophrenia occur. This illness, which conforms to Kraepelin's criteria for paranoia (p. 99), is really an abnormal personality development (p. 105).

Delusions of jealousy may be the presenting symptoms in a paranoid schizophrenia, but other schizophrenic symptoms unconnected with the morbid jealousy appear sooner or later. In contrast, in the morbidly jealous patient the delusion varies in intensity for the rest of the patient's life, but no other non-understandable symptoms ever appear.

Chapter 10

Theories of schizophrenia

Before discussing the various theories of schizophrenia, we must first consider the nature of the explanations and concepts which are used in abnormal psychology. The concepts of understanding, interpretative, and explaining psychology are extremely useful in bringing clarity to a very muddled subject. In natural science we try to discover causal connexions and explain events by means of these connexions, and we therefore make experiments and observations in order to discover rules. Having discovered rules, we then look for general laws, and in many fields of physics and chemistry we are able to express these causal laws in mathematical terms. This search for causal connexions can be carried out in the field of psychopathology. Thus we can discover the connexions between localized cortical stimulation and visual hallucinations. We can at times find rules, such as the one that the same sort of psychological illness is inherited within a given family. Occasionally we find general laws, such as, for instance, that general paresis cannot occur without the presence of *Treponema pallidum*. So far we have been unable to express any of our psychopathological findings in mathematical terms.

In natural science only causal connexions can be found, but in psychology a different type of connexion occurs. This is due to the fact that psychological events can arise out of other psychological events in a way which we can 'understand'. We put ourselves into the situation and feel ourselves in the other person's shoes. Thus, for example, we can understand why a man who is ridiculed becomes angry and aggressive, or why the loss of a friend leads to depression. In this way we can understand how one psychological event arises out of another. An understandable connexion between two psychological events can be called a genetic understandable connexion, because it allows us to understand how one psychological event creates another. In psychopathology we can understand, for example, the content of dreams and delusions, the effects of suggestion, the unfolding of the life-pattern of a given person, and so on. In the individual case the decision about the reality of a given understandable connexion depends on whether or not it helps to form a coherent picture of all the objective material available to the observer, such as what the patient says, his modes of expression, his spiritual works, his style of life, his actions, and so on. The objectivity of this material is, of course, never complete. In the sense used here 'understanding' is often really 'interpreting', because it is only in a very few cases that the objective material at our disposal reaches such a high degree of completeness that it is utterly convincing. Thus 'understanding psychology' leads naturally to an 'interpretative psychology' in which knowledge gained by understanding is formulated with the help of concepts borrowed from philosophy, psychology, neurology, or folk lore. This interpretative psychology allows us to explain to some degree the behaviour of others. However, it must be stressed that the explanations of interpretative psychology are not true explanations, but merely hypothetical constructs which have been surmised and are often beyond any proof or disproof. The kind of interpretative psychology accepted by the individual psychiatrist depends on his general attitude and cultural background. Thus in the West, Freudian and neo-Freudian psychology is the common interpretative psychology, while in the Soviet Union neo-Pavlovian psychology is much more acceptable.

Causal rules are the result of inductive reasoning and can be organized into theories which correspond in some degree with that which lies at the basis of immediately given reality, so that the individual case is subsumed under these general rules. In contrast to this, understandable connexions are comprehensible connexions which are evident in themselves, and form a yardstick against which individual psychological events can be estimated and 'understood' to some degree. These 'understandable' connexions may be found time and time again and, because of their frequency, they may be mistaken for rules. However, it must be remembered that an understandable connexion may be true for an individual case, but may not apply to all cases. The frequency or occurrence of a given understandable connexion may, of course, lead to a theory which can be tested by natural scientific methods. Sometimes an understandable connexion occurs very frequently, so that it is confirmed inductively and statistically. Thus, for example, there is an understandable connexion between the high price of bread and the incidence of stealing, and this connexion is well founded both statistically and inductively. On the other hand, in some cases there is an understandable connexion between an attempt at suicide and the psychological effects of the physical discomfort produced by unpleasant winter weather conditions, so that one can understand why a certain person attempted suicide in January in the Northern Hemisphere. Despite the fact that the suicide rate is highest in the spring, this understandable connexion between the climate and a suicidal attempt may be true in an individual case.

To sum up, one can say that in psychopathology it is absolutely necessary to distinguish between those relationships which can be explained in a natural scientific way, those which can be understood by the observer trying to put himself in the situation of the patient, and those which are formulated in a special psychological jargon.*

It is unfortunate that the most popular interpretative psychology, that of Freud and his followers, has been widely used by English-speaking psychiatrists, who frequently mistake 'understandable' for 'causal' connexions. On the other hand, a different misunderstanding seems to have affected the German-speaking psychiatrists. Since some psychiatric phenomena are 'non-understandable', these psychiatrists seem to have taken the view that further psychological investigation of these is impossible. This point of view seems to be especially held among those psychiatrists who believe firmly in the organic basis of schizophrenia, and they tend to brush aside all theories based on understanding or interpretative psychology. One can sympathize with the justifiable irritation of the clinical psychiatrist when presented with esoteric theories of schizophrenia based on psycho-analytic and existentialist ideas. However, it is well to remember that beneath the almost meaningless jargon there may be some useful 'understanding' psychology which will help in the general handling and care of the schizophrenic patient.

Psychological theories of schizophrenia are useful from two points of view. In the first place, they may be heuristic and allow the construction of testable hypotheses, which will increase our knowledge of the illness and may finally lead to its causes. Secondly, such theories may have a therapeutic value when they allow the doctor to organize his ideas about the illness and make an approach to the patient. It is well known that the results of psychotherapy depend much more on the enthusiasm and special flair of the therapist than on the correctness of his psychological theories. It is therefore not possible to dismiss psycho-analytic theories of schizophrenia as inadmissible fantasy, since these theories encourage the doctor to make contact with his patients and may lead to a more humane treatment of the mentally ill.

Having dealt with some of the general psychological difficulties, it is now necessary to deal with some of the semantic and other difficulties which always arise. The first semantic problem is the use of the words 'disease' and 'illness'. It is, of course, difficult to define disease and illness, and Virchow's definition, 'life under altered conditions', is open to criticism. This could be countered if it were accepted that in illness there is some qualitative change in the organism or, in other words, there is a sharp break between the normal and the pathological, although in some cases this sharp break

* The above discussion of various types of psychology is based mainly, but not entirely, on the work of Karl Jaspers (1953).

cannot easily be demonstrated. Virchow's definition can therefore be modified to meet this objection and can be reformulated as 'disease is life under qualitatively altered conditions'.

Some English-speaking psychiatrists like to avoid using the word 'disease' and use the word 'reaction' instead. However, this word is ambiguous and can be used in at least four different ways. Thus a patient may be suffering from a mild active schizophrenic illness which may be made worse by some environmental change, for example, by attending an exorcism. This interaction of the illness and the environment can be called a reaction. A quite different state of affairs is present when a defect schizophrenic is upset by his environment, as, for example, when an eccentric hebephrenic responds to interference by others with brutal violence. This is, of course, a reaction, but is due to the interaction of the environment and the abnormal personality produced by disease. Sometimes a schizophrenic shift is provoked by severe environmental stress and this can also be considered to be a reaction. Finally, schizophrenia can be regarded as an organic reaction, or, in other words, it is a special kind of reaction of the brain to many different kinds of physical insult. There is, of course, a general objection to the use of the word 'reaction' because most illnesses are, in fact, reactions of the organism to an interference of some kind. However, it is possible that the use of the word 'reaction' may prevent some psychiatrists from regarding schizophrenia as an entirely endogenous illness.

Although Kraepelin isolated dementia praecox as a clinical entity and described its symptomatology in great detail, he did not put forward any psychological theory to account for the symptoms. He believed that disorders of emotion and volition were the characteristic features of schizophrenia, but he did not postulate that they were basic disorders and attempt to derive other symptoms from them. As C. Schneider (1942) has pointed out, once the concept of schizophrenia or dementia praecox was established, psychopathology was faced with three main tasks. These were:

1. To isolate and define the decisive signs and symptoms and to determine their incidence.
2. To find the basic psychological conditions for the formation of the specific signs and symptoms and to explain the origin of the marginal symptoms.
3. To explain the relationship between the basic symptoms and normal psychic life.

This first task proved too difficult, and most investigators took up the second task with great enthusiasm. They used the psychological theories which were current at the time, and looked for some principle which would determine the way in which different symptoms arose out of each other, or the way in which the symptoms interacted with functions which were still healthy. This principle was the 'basic disorder' of schizophrenia, from which all other symptoms were to be derived, and the search for a 'basic disorder' led, incidentally, to the most careful examination and description of schizophrenic signs and symptoms.

Weygandt (1907) used Wundt's concept of 'apperception' to explain the basic disorder. Wundt had used this term to designate the objective aspect of attention, or, in other words, the clarity of consciousness in which non-essential impressions and their accompanying motor acts are inhibited. This phenomenon is a voluntary activity, and this is shown by the presence of an idea which is recognized as the motive of the activity, by the appearance of a feeling of active participation, and by changes in the content of consciousness which appear to be the effect of the motive. Thus a weakening of apperception would lead to a thoroughgoing disturbance of psychic life, and Weygandt believed that the psychology of dementia praecox could be explained in this way, so that the psychosis was, in fact, a volitional psychosis.

Stransky (1904) divided psychic life into two major spheres, the emotional or thymopsyche, and the intellectual or noöpsyche, and held that psychological illnesses disturb the normal close relationship between noöpsychic and thymopsychic elements. In some psychological illnesses the noöpsychic and thymopsychic contents of the mind lose their early functional connexions and new ones are formed. This loss is usually only partial and takes place slowly. In dementia praecox a complete change in the relationships between the components of psychic life occurs. Some new fixed connexions are formed, but in the main the normal interaction between the two main psychic spheres is affected and becomes unstable. Stransky called this condition 'intrapsychic ataxia' or 'intrapsychic incoordination'. In his opinion, the striking thing about many dementia praecox patients, especially in the early stages of the illness, was not so much the poverty of affect and affective expression or simple emotional devastation, but dissociation or incoordination between the noöpsychic and thymopsychic contents of the mind.

In 1911 Bleuler made one of the most extensive psychological explanations of schizophrenic symptomatology by means of association psychology. He believed that schizophrenia was due to brain disease, but in some cases there was no pathological brain process, only a mild quantitative deviation of brain function from the normal. He described primary symptoms which he attributed to the direct expression of the disease of the brain and secondary symptoms which could be derived from them. The primary symptoms were:

1. Disturbance of association in so far as it involves a decrease in the number of, or impairment of the quality of, connexions of associations.

2. Clouded states (*Benommenheit*).
3. Affective changes.
4. Possibly hallucinations, although Bleuler considered that everyone had a general predisposition to hallucinations which might be released by schizophrenia.
5. Possibly the tendency to stereotypy.
6. Physical changes such as vasomotor disorders, pupillary changes, and so on.

Bleuler also divided schizophrenic symptoms into fundamental and accessory. A fundamental symptom occurs in schizophrenia and no other disease, while an accessory symptom occurs in other diseases as well. His fundamental symptoms were: (1) Disorder of association. (2) Disorder of affect. (3) Ambivalence.

In this way, Bleuler presented a solution of Schneider's first two tasks for a psychopathological theory. All the symptoms of schizophrenia could be traced back to his primary symptoms which developed understandably into secondary symptoms, or produced secondary symptoms as a result of their interaction with healthy functions. The loosening of associations, for example, leads to the train of thought taking an unusual path and, if it is severe enough, to the fragmentation of thought. Incoherence and illogical thinking occur, since the normal mechanisms of displacement, condensation, and generalization take place readily. The weakness of thinking allows complexes of thoughts to become independent, and the affective loading of these independent complexes leads to their taking over the direction of thinking. This means that psychic activity is now dominated by this complex and now by that, or, in other words, there is a splitting of the personality, which in its turn has an effect on the whole of the symptomatology. The weakening of thinking also allows normal fantasy thinking, or autistic thinking, to dominate psychic activity. This excessive autistic thinking and the disorder of association work together to produce delusions out of the fears and wishes, which are often disguised symbolically and loaded with split-off unconscious affects. In this way Bleuler was able to show psychological connexions between the fundamental and accessory symptoms, but, unfortunately, many important schizophrenic symptoms were left out of consideration, e.g. the apophanous experiences, thought withdrawal, experiences of control, and so on. Nevertheless, his attempt at a psychological interpretation of schizophrenic symptoms is a model of its kind.

Berze (Berze and Gruhle, 1929) attempted to give a complete psychological explanation of schizophrenia and therefore looked for a more general psychological disorder from which all schizophrenic symptoms could be derived. He postulated that this disorder was a primary insufficiency of psychic activity or hypotonia of consciousness. Like Bleuler, he recognized that many other authors had postulated a similar primary schizophrenic disorder. Freusberg had described a diminution of consciousness, Schüle a weakened empty consciousness, Lehmann a decline of the energy of consciousness, Janet a lowering of the mental level, and Masselon an intellectual decline. Whereas Bleuler derived all such disorders from a weakness of logical thinking, Berze considered that such disorders were all attempts to describe a change in the overall state of psychic activity. Many schizophrenics complain of weakness and emptiness in the head, of thought withdrawal, and of disorders of volition. Berze used these common complaints to support his theory of a weakness of psychic activity. Since every voluntary act is associated with a subjective feeling that one is using one's own energy, he assumed that impairment of volition would produce a subjective sense of weakness. Hypotonia of consciousness naturally leads to poor intellectual activity and this in its turn will change affectivity. There is a decrease in the formation of associations and the quality of associations is also affected. Weakness of perception gives rise to incomplete perceptions and hallucinations. The loss of feeling of possession of activity in perception gives rise to a disorder of feeling of recognition and to the feeling of alienation. While Berze succeeds in explaining the negative symptoms, he has to introduce subsidiary theories to explain positive ones. Thus he explains the stiffness and perseveration of affect as a failure of inhibition of the normal tendency of an affect to outlast the event which provokes it. Berze's theory, unfortunately, is too general and vague, and it has not led to any increase in our knowledge of the illness.

Kretschmer (1925), with his concepts of constitution, occupies a special position in the consideration of the theory of schizophrenia. He regards schizophrenia as the extreme end of a continuum, the other end of which is normal. Thus it would appear that the schizoid personality, with the same body type as in the schizophrenic, is virtually a mild variety of schizophrenia. Unfortunately, many schizophrenic syndromes are completely outside any normal pattern of behaviour. If one restricts schizophrenia to quiet hebephrenias and catatonias with a few active symptoms, then it could be considered to be an exaggeration of a schizoid personality, but it is not possible to understand most schizophrenias in this way.

This idea that schizophrenia is grossly exaggerated behaviour of abnormal personalities had been put forward by Adolf Meyer (1910), whose effect on psychiatry in English-speaking countries was very profound. Unfortunately, his writings are opaque and his ideas seem vague and woolly. He adopted a simple general approach which some of his pupils have proudly called the 'common-sense' approach. He looked upon mental illness as a reaction of a patient to stress, or, to quote his own words, a reaction which is a 'faulty response or substitution of an insufficient, or protective, or evasive or mutilated attempt at adjustment'. He distinguished six basic types of reaction and two of these, i.e. 'paranoiac developments' and 'type of defect and deterioration', probably correspond with schizophrenia in the sense used here. Paranoiac development is an anomalous development of a person in which the nature of the reaction depends partly on the individual make-up, but more on the general situation in which he finds himself. The reactions of defect and deterioration are due less to overt and direct over-expression on the part of the patient and more to the faulty substitution of modes of evasion which have been conditioned in various ways.

Meyer regarded dementia praecox as mainly a disorder of the young and this opinion has played a part in discouraging Anglo-American psychiatrists from diagnosing schizophrenia which develops after the age of 40 years. As far as the genesis of dementia praecox is concerned, Meyer looked upon the illness as a breakdown of an abnormal personality under stress, giving rise to a reaction consisting of an excessive use of evasive habits, which had previously been used to deal with the environment. This reaction does not measure up to the situation the patient is facing, and may disrupt his adjustment to the real world far more than the original traumatic situation. Thus the schizophrenic reacts with the inadequate means at his disposal, which are in themselves disorganizing and consequently produce the illness. Meyer compared this with the over-reaction of the body to physical disease processes, such as hyperpyrexia in an infectious illness, which may do more damage to the patient than the direct effect of the bacteria on the tissues. As Meyer himself put it: 'Mind, like any other function, can demoralize and undermine itself and its organ.' Thus it appears that dementia praecox is a direct result of the pre-psychotic personality in that the individual person develops faulty habits of behaviour due to heredity, poor family background, and bad social environment. He is then unable to express his thoughts adequately and acquires faulty habits of thinking and theorizing in an abstract way. The patient becomes excessively self-centred, very sensitive to the opinions of others, develops very poorly integrated social relationships, and usually has undue shyness and over-sensitivity about sexual topics. His faulty thinking and lack of social relationships lead to indulgence in impractical fantasy which cannot be fulfilled. As he matures, he finds difficulty in becoming independent, and cannot stand the normal stresses of maturing and of adult life. Finally, he meets a severe stress and reacts to it with all those faulty habits which he has developed over the years, and which now lead to a disintegration of his personality. The symptoms of dementia praecox can therefore be considered as the faulty habits of a lifetime carried to an extreme. The patient retreats into personal fantasy, which gives rise to delusions and hallucinations. It is difficult to understand the strange acute schizophrenic delusional phenomena and many other symptoms in this simple way. Meyer's insistence on the importance of the individual person and his environment is a useful corrective for the organically minded psychiatrist who cannot lift his eyes from the cerebral cortex. Until our knowledge of schizophrenia is more advanced, we must follow Meyer in his general management and care of any psychiatric patient, i.e. we must take into account all factors which have or may possibly have some bearing on the patient's adjustment to the world.

Jaspers' use of Husserl's and Dilthey's ideas has already been discussed, and there is no doubt that the concept that the true schizophrenic symptoms are non-understandable has allowed our knowledge to be organized and has highlighted the important symptoms. It has also led to the careful descriptions of symptoms by the Heidelberg school, in particular by Gruhle. The symptoms of the first rank of K. Schneider can be regarded as the final product of this school. It is unfortunate that no experimental investigations have been carried out on the non-understandable symptoms isolated by these investigators.

However, Matussek (1952) and Conrad (1958a) have taken the classical symptomatology established by these workers and used *Gestalt* theory to explain it. Conrad regards schizophrenia as due to a disorder of the brain, and uses *Gestalt* theory to explain the psychopathology in the same way as he has used it to explain the psychopathology of other psychological syndromes caused by coarse brain disease. He divides acute schizophrenic shifts into three phases, i.e. the trema, the apophanous phase, and the apocalyptic phase. In the trema the patient experiences a loss of freedom, so that he feels hemmed in, surrounded by barriers, and unable to communicate with others. His environment is changed and has taken on a new foreign aspect which he has never noticed before. He may occasionally behave in a senseless way. Conrad bases his interpretations on the study of a group of 107 schizophrenics in the German Army, and in these cases a senseless breach of military discipline frequently occurred during the trema. In this phase severe anxiety may occur, or marked depression with suicidal ideas, and often with marked ideas of guilt. A general feeling of suspicion may pervade all social contacts and the patient may feel that there is something behind all his experiences and, finally, a delusional mood may occur. The trema may last several months, or may be a very brief prelude to the apophanous phase. Sometimes the illness subsides without passing into the apophanous phase.

Before considering the apophanous phase in detail, it is necessary to consider Matussek's *Gestalt* interpretation of those delusional perceptions in which some aspect of the percept appears to determine the emergence of the new meaning. He follows Metzger (1954) in dividing the properties of *Gestalten* into three groups, i.e. structural properties, total qualities, and essential properties. Structural properties are those properties connected with the arrangement or construction of *Gestalt*, e.g. properties such as straight, round angular, etc. Total qualities are those material properties which concern the total construction of the *Gestalt* and which do not depend on sense qualities which are simple or independent of the structure. Rough, smooth, silky, and transparent are examples of total qualities. Essential properties express the essence of the *Gestalt* and these properties occur in connexion with both animate and inanimate objects. They are expressed in the adjectives when we talk of a 'laughing man', a 'threatening mountain', or a 'sleeping village'. Matussek believes that, in the particular type of delusional perception under discussion, there is a loosening of the coherence of perception which allows the essential properties to acquire an undue prominence and develop a new significance for the patient.

Conrad has accepted Matussek's theory and has developed it to explain the apophanous phase. He recognizes three stages in delusional perception, which are:

1. Pure apophany in which the perceived object indicates something to the patient, but he cannot say what it is.
2. The prefabricated or made experience of Schneider, when the perceived object indicates to the patient that it has been specially put there in order to test him or spy on him.
3. The essential properties have come into undue prominence and the special significance is clearly appreciated by the patient.

The trema can be considered as the phase in which the coherence of the patient's inner and outer world is loosening, while the apophanous phase can be regarded as the phase in which the coherence is so loose that the essential properties stand out in marked relief and become independent. As something is now becoming manifest to the patient, Conrad has suggested the word 'apophany' to designate the delusional and other paranoid experiences of the acute schizophrenic shift. Apophany can affect the patient's outer space (i.e. the objects which he encounters) or his inner space (i.e. the things which he thinks about). Delusional perceptions are the most obvious example of external apophany, but the experiences of false acquaintance and false alienation of people and objects are also of this kind. Here the patient misidentifies persons in his environment and either gives them the identity of someone else or denies their identity, when he has previously known them. These experiences can be explained as being due to the emergence of essential properties, which in the case of previously unknown persons resemble those of acquaintances and in the case of previously known persons give a new foreign quality to the individual.

All these external apophanous experiences give the patient the impression that he is the centre of a changed world. He is surrounded by a set of properties manipulated by some almighty stage manager. On the other hand, many schizophrenics have a feeling of omnipotence which Conrad explains as the reverse side of the experience of being the passive centre of the world. One of Conrad's patients believed that as he urinated he made bombs fall on England. There is a quality of accomplishment in this belief, and urinating and bombing are both activities in which something is caused to fall, so that they both have a common essential property of activity. The effect of the constituents of the world on the patient, which has already been discussed in connexion with delusional perception, is coupled with a reciprocal effect of the patient on the objects of the world. The essential properties of his own actions may become important for the world as he experiences it. This experience of being in the central position of the world leads to anastrophe, or the experience that everything centres around oneself.

In apophany of internal space the represented material becomes manifest. Often external apophany is present for some time before internal apophany, which sometimes does not occur. It seems as if there is a barrier which prevents the process spreading from the sensory aspects to the representational aspects of psychic life. When apophany affects freely rising memory images, some of them come into prominence as delusional inspirations because they are experienced as thoughts inspired from without, so that an ordinary 'brain wave' becomes a delusional inspiration. Thought broadcasting can be explained as the reverse aspect of delusional perception. Instead of a perception becoming manifest to the patient, his thoughts become manifest to his fellows. In general there is a de-differentiation of field structure which explains all apophanous phenomena. In the case of thought, this de-differentiation allows the patient's thoughts to be heard as *Gedankenlautwerden* and, finally, when all personal indication is lost, the thoughts become hallucinatory voices. Thus thought broadcasting, *Gedankenlautwerden*, and voices are connected internal apophanous phenomena of increasing severity, which run parallel with the increasing severity of the *Gestalt* disorder. The bodily hallucinations of schizophrenia can be explained as due to apophany in the sphere of bodily sensations and representations. Taking into account the relative unimportance of formal thought disorder in acute schizophrenia, no attempt will be made to explain this in *Gestalt* terms.

If in delusional perception the perceptional coherence is loosened, then it could be expected that when the schizophrenic process becomes very severe the coherence would break up completely. As Conrad puts it: 'The clouds of essential properties, which every object holds confined within itself, have been set free.' In this case a fragmentation of psychic life takes place which Conrad calls the apocalyptic phase. This is a catatonic illness and the motor disorder can be explained as being due to an apocalyptically changed corporeality or, to put it more intelligibly, the release of representations of bodily sensation and movements. In this apocalyptic or catatonic phase there is a destruction of the sense continuity, so that only fragments of the total experience during such a phase can be subsequently recalled. If this apocalyptic phase progresses it may pass into the terminal phase of acute deadly catatonia.

Conrad has used the concept of energy potential to explain the residual or defect states. Each individual person has his own particular ability to apply and direct his energies; this is his energy potential. In residual states there is a reduction of the energy potential. Conrad has analysed the course of illness in a series of 107 acute schizophrenic soldiers and described 7 types of course, which are illustrated in *Fig*. 8: These are:

Type 1. The process does not pass beyond Phase 1 (trema) and merely touches on Phase 2 before subsiding and returning to its starting point after several weeks. The loss of energy potential is minimal.

Type 2. The process passes through Phase 1 (trema), enters Phase 2, and returns to the starting point after a few weeks without having entered Phase 3. Here again the loss of energy potential is also slight.

Type 3. The process passes through Phases 1 and 2, touches on Phase 3, and then returns to the starting point.

Type 4. Phases 1 and 2 are passed through quickly without the psychosis being recognized. A marked loss of energy potential occurs. In Conrad's patients this residual state made life in the army very difficult.

Type 5. The process does not pass beyond Phase 1, but a severe reduction of energy potential occurs.

Type 6. The process reaches Phase 2 and is arrested in this phase. A severe loss of energy potential occurs.

Type 7. The process reaches Phase 3 and is arrested in this phase. This results in a severe loss of energy potential.

Thus Types 1–3 are acute shifts with almost total recovery, while Types 4–7 correspond to simple, hebephrenic, paranoid, and catatonic defect states respectively.

Other workers, in particular Petrilowitsch (1958a, b) and Pauleikhoff (1957), explained schizophrenic psychopathology in a similar way by means of the concepts of the school of *Ganzheitspsychologie*. This psychology regards psychic events and states (the sphere of

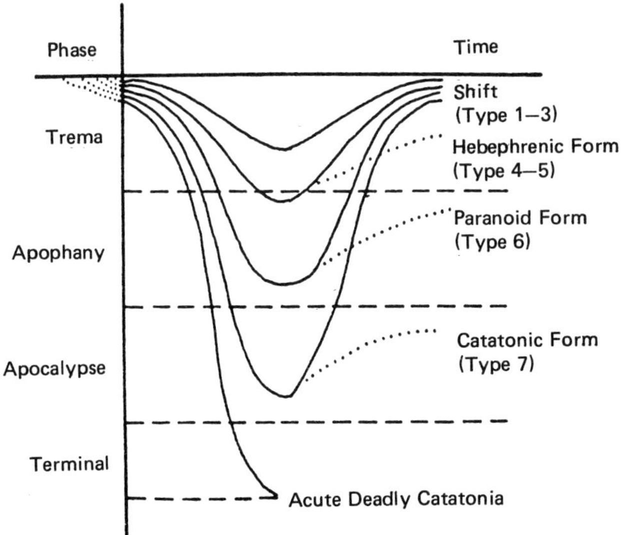

Fig. 8. Varieties of acute schizophrenic shifts. (*After Conrad*.)

experience) in the individual person as figures which occur on a ground or personal structure, usually referred to as the 'structure'. Petrilowitsch regarded manic-depressive insanity as producing an increase or decrease in the sphere of experience, but as having no effect on the personal structure, but in schizophrenia there is a blockade between the 'structure' and the sphere of experience. This leads to the psychic phenomena becoming more independent. At first there is an emotional expectation of a diffuse kind, i.e. delusional mood. In this stage there is an intense personal feeling of concern with few symptoms, new experiences of an 'as if' character, and an insight into illness. As the illness progresses, delusions appear due to the organization and pregnance* of the de-differentiated *Gestalt* qualities which are sharply outlined. In this stage there is usually very little personal concern, the new experiences have the character of reality, there is a wealth of symptoms, and a defective insight into the illness. Petrilowitsch claims that many of the descriptions and explanations of schizophrenic symptomatology by older authors fit in well with his theoretical formulations.

These *Gestalt* theories of schizophrenia are interesting, but their heuristic value is doubtful. The obvious point to be investigated is the

* The German *Gestalt* psychologists used the term '*Pregnänz*' to designate one of the properties which led to a figure being seen as a whole. It roughly means 'good form'. Woodworth, in his standard work (1951), has used the word 'pregnance' as a translation of this German word.

perception of the acute schizophrenic who has external apophany. So far, although changes in perception have been demonstrated in schizophrenics, both acute and chronic, such changes have not been specific.

In order to understand Freudian 'explanations' of psychological illness, it is necessary to understand Freud's ideas about the development and structure of the mind. He believed that adult sexuality is achieved by a process of libidinal development in which the child gets pleasure from different parts of the body and bodily functions. The first stage is the early oral stage in which the infant gets enjoyment from sucking. In this stage the infant has no concept of an object, so that neither love nor ambivalence can exist. The next stage is the late oral sadistic phase which has been rather fancifully called the 'cannibalistic' stage. The infant now has teeth and derives sexual satisfaction from biting and swallowing. No object relations are possible in the early oral stage and, since differentiation between the ego and the world has not yet occurred, the infant is in a state of primary narcissism. In the late oral stage the only way in which an object can be dealt with is by total incorporation. In the next stage, the early anal sadistic stage, the infant gets pleasure from controlling his bowels, more particularly in the elimination and pinching off of the faeces. He is now capable of partial object love with incorporation. This is followed by the late anal sadistic stage, in which the infant gets satisfaction from retaining his faeces. Then the child passes into the early genital phase in which sexual gratification is obtained from the genitals. The child is now capable of love for an object, but this object love is limited by the fear of castration. The final genital stage is achieved when this fear is overcome and sexual gratification is connected with the genitals. The child is then capable of love without ambivalence. Thus as libidinal development progresses, the child becomes more and more able to make reasonable relationships to external objects. Finally, he is able to invest external objects with libido, in other words, to love them without any ambivalence.

Side by side with this libidinal development there is the development of a structure of the mind. The mind when fully developed consists of the ego, the superego, and the id. The ego is the reality-bound part of the mind, and consists roughly of the conscious self, most of the conscious contents of the mind, and those contents which can readily be made available to consciousness. The superego is roughly the conscience, which is partly conscious and partly unconscious. It contains all the punitive and critical thoughts and attitudes which have been taken in or introjected from parental models. The id is entirely unconscious and contains all the instinctive material which has never been allowed to become conscious, and all the material which has been repressed from consciousness. The id tries to gratify the unconscious instinctive drives by means of primary processes which ignore time, reality, and logical connexions.

In the course of libidinal development, a stage may not be properly passed through, so that a fixation point occurs at this level of libidinal development. A fixation point may be due to excessive, or inadequate, or alternating excessive and inadequate gratification at the libidinal stage concerned. Freud also believed that the constitution might determine the fixation point.* The psychological illness occurs when there is some disappointment in life and loss of a loved object. The libido which is attached to the object floods the mind, and a regression occurs which leads back to the fixation point, so that the old childhood conflicts at the fixation point are reactivated by this excess of free libido. The situation is complicated by the activation of conflicts at other weak places in libidinal development apart from the main fixation point, and the fact that the organization of the mind in the illness may correspond to a level of libidinal development which is higher than that of the fixation point.

In schizophrenia regression extends back, at least to some degree, to the early narcissistic level. At this stage the child does not distinguish between self and environment, so that in the schizophrenic there is a loss of object relations. When this occurs, the patient attempts to regain his object relations, so that two kinds of symptoms are found in schizophrenia, those due to regression and those due to an attempt to restore the lost object relations. In the neuroses, symptoms are a compromise formation in which faulty repression is countered by fusing the repressed material and the repressing forces into a single symptom. However, in schizophrenia the regression reaches a level of organization of the mind where the reality sense does not exist. Symptom formation in schizophrenia consists of a re-activation of archaic functions. The conflict is solved by an almost complete total denial of it and of reality. The fantasies of world destruction, the bodily hallucinations, depersonalization, feelings of grandeur, schizophrenic thinking, hebephrenic symptoms, and some catatonic symptoms are all considered to be regressive symptoms. Thus the inner perception of the loss of object relations expresses itself as the classical schizophrenic delusion or fear that the world is coming to an end. In fact, as far as the patient is concerned, the objective world has broken down. Now the infant discovers his self and the objective world by his experiences of his own body as something which is separate from the rest of the world, so that he differentiates between the sensations produced from internal and

* This idea that genetic or chance organic factors might play an important part in the genesis of a psychological illness has never been developed by Freud's followers, most of whom look upon the soma as a dirty word.

external events and organizes his internal sensations into a body image which is, so to speak, the nucleus of the ego. Regression to the narcissistic level allows this nucleus to become prominent in an altered form and the increased libidinization of this bodily nucleus leads to depersonalization and bodily hallucinations. Inflation of the ego and delusions of grandeur are produced by three factors. The weakened and disintegrating ego acquires a hypercathexis of libido, the repressive inhibitory effect of the superego declines, giving rise to a new freedom for the ego, and, finally, an effort is made to compensate for the loss of object relations by exaggerating the ego. Schizophrenic formal thought disorder is archaic thinking which corresponds to the form and content of thinking in the normal id. Thus, apart from the conceptual difficulties, the patient may freely express instinctive material which normally could never have become conscious. Since hebephrenia is characterized by marked devastation of thought and affect in the absence of marked symptoms of restitution, psycho-analysis regards hebephrenia as a pure regressive type of schizophrenia. Some catatonic symptoms such as passivity feelings, negativism, and automatic obedience can be considered to be regressive, since they all demonstrate the loss of ego boundaries which is in keeping with primary narcissism. It also is possible to look upon some of the other catatonic motor activities as revivals of archaic types of motor behaviour.

It is usual to regard world reconstruction fantasies, hallucinations, delusions, and some catatonic symptoms as attempts to restore object relations. It is easy to see that ideas of the salvation and reconstruction of the world can be regarded as an attempt at restitution. Some catatonic symptoms, such as stereotypies, can be seen as efforts to regain object relations. For example, the movements may be magical gestures with which the patient is trying to influence his environment. Hallucinations can be regarded as substitutes for perceptions in that objective reality is partly or entirely lost and some ideas obtain a perceptual quality, giving rise to a substitute reality. Sometimes hallucinations are wish-fulfilling, but since auditory hallucinations are usually unpleasant, this can only apply to a small group of hallucinations. Freud suggested that the anxiety connected with hallucinations was produced by the reappearance of a part of the reality which had been repudiated.

Paranoid delusions can be derived from a formerly repressed form of object relationship, namely, homosexuality. They show that the desire for that relationship is still present and they are therefore a form of object relations. Freud (1924a, b) elaborated his theories of the psychopathology of delusions by analysing the autobiographical writings of Paul Schreber, who was a Saxon Supreme Court judge who developed paranoid schizophrenia. A critique of Freud's views and an English translation of Schreber's writings have now been published (1955). Freud's basic idea is that the patient can deny his desired homosexual relationship in four different ways, thus giving rise to paranoid delusions which have four different contents. The initial homosexual thought of the patient is, 'I love him', but this is denied and the thought becomes, 'I do *not* love him'. This may then develop into 'I hate him', and then into 'He hates me', so that a delusion of persecution occurs. However, 'I do not love him' may develop into 'She loves him and not me', in which case there is a delusion of jealousy. If the thought, 'I do not love him', develops into 'I love her. She loves me', then an amorous delusion or erotomania has developed. Finally, the thought, 'I do not love him', can develop into 'I love no one', which is naturally followed by 'I only love myself', in which case a grandiose delusion has developed. Apart from these explanations, paranoid delusions can also be regarded as projections of elements of the patient's body or personality. Thus the persecutor may be the homosexual object, which is a narcissistically hypercathected organ such as faeces or the buttocks. This object is projected and also represents the projected superego.

The psycho-analytic theories, so far discussed, are the classical theories of schizophrenia. Since then some psycho-analysts have revised Freud's basic ideas, produced new theories of schizophrenia and have developed and modified his theories of the structure of the mind. Federn (1952), who is the outstanding representative of this trend, has put forward a new concept of the ego. For him, ego feeling or the feeling of 'self-ness' permits the individual to distinguish between himself as the subject and the external world as the object, and also to distinguish between himself as an object and the representations of objects. The ego thus experiences itself as both subject and object.* The ego acquires its energy from the libido, the destructive drives, and the life processes. The limits of the penetration of psychic material by the ego-feeling mark the boundary of the ego. This boundary acts as a sensory organ and monitors all events occurring outside the ego. As a result, thought is that which appears to occur inside this boundary while reality is that which occurs outside. In schizophrenia the energy supply of the ego is weakened, so that the ego boundary breaks up, giving rise to an inability to distinguish the self from the environment. The objective cannot be distinguished from the subjective, so that the patient's conception of reality is falsified. This break-up of the ego leads to those ego states which normally occur in infancy. Thus, for Federn, schizophrenia begins with the development of a false reality, while for Freud the false reality is a reconstruction following the initial regression to

* This is very reminiscent of Sartre's earlier views on the ego.

primary narcissism. Freeman et al. (1958a, b), who have studied a group of disturbed chronic schizophrenics, believe that Federn's views are very useful in understanding chronic schizophrenia.

Freud's theories of libidinal development have also been modified. Klein (1952) and Fairbairn (1952) are the most outstanding analysts in Britain who have written on this theme. Klein has pushed back the development of object relations and ego functions into a period of infancy which is so early that her ideas are beyond proof. She considers that the infant can relate to part-objects from birth and that he mainly uses the mechanisms of introjection and projection. The part-object with which the child first relates is the breast, and if he obtains satisfaction from it he acquires the idea of a 'good breast' which he introjects. On the other hand, if the breast does not satisfy him, then he develops the idea of a 'bad breast', which is the object of his oral sadistic drives. The child fears that the hated object may retaliate, so he fears an attack from the outside, but when he introjects the 'bad breast', he fears attack from within. Klein also postulates that the child has innate ideas of a good and a bad penis, which he regards as being inside his mother. The fear of attack from within and without which follows the idea of the bad breast, and the introjection of it is the paranoid position and occurs about the third month of life. This is followed by the depressive position, in which the child has become aware of his mother as a whole object. Klein's view of mental structure is necessarily considerably different from that of Freud. She believes the ego is present from birth and that it has mechanisms of defence, chiefly projection, which have to deal with the fear of destruction produced by the destructive instincts from within. These destructive drives are projected first of all on to the breast which then becomes a bad object which produces fear of destruction. The child not only directs his aggressive and sadistic drives on to his mother, but also his anal and urethral ones, so that the mother's body is penetrated by the anal and urethral products feared by the child. Apart from drives, feared and rejected parts of the ego are projected on to the mother, and this process has been called 'projection and identification'. Despite this defence mechanism of projection, the infantile ego is weak and tends to disintegrate because there are still the destructive drives from within the organism which are directed against it. This stage, where there is a tendency of the ego to fall to pieces, is the paranoid schizoid position. If fixation occurs at this point, then reactivation of the conflicts will lead to schizophrenia, which explains the breaking up of the ego and the paranoid phenomena in schizophrenia.

Many other psycho-analytic theories of schizophrenia have been produced. Unfortunately, it would take another volume to review them critically. The main objection to psycho-analytic theories of schizophrenia is that, like most other psychological theories of schizophrenia, they gloss over many of the outstanding acute symptoms and do not take into account the great diversity of the chronic clinical pictures. There is also the basic objection to all Freudian theory, that aspects of mental functioning, such as unconscious cerebration or self-awareness, are turned into fixed entities with some inner source of perpetual motion. To trace all schizophrenic symptoms to a loss of ego boundaries is to have a startling glimpse of the obvious. Such a formulation is so vague that it can account for everything and nothing at the same time, since all the paranoid phenomena are by definition disturbances of the relation of the self to the environment. Much ink has been spilt in Britain in the controversies about Klein's views, and the heat engendered in orthodox psycho-analytic circles is understandable, since these theories are the *reductio ad absurdum* of psycho-analysis.

It is, of course, impossible to discuss the psychology of schizophrenia without mentioning C. G. Jung (1907), who with Eugen Bleuler used psycho-analytic ideas to interpret the delusions and behaviour of schizophrenics. His use of the 'word association test' in schizophrenia was one of the important milestones in the development of experimental psychopathology. Unfortunately, as Freud once said rather bitterly, Jung gave up psychiatry for mythology. On the whole, his views on the psychology of schizophrenia are less complex than Freud's. He originally considered that this illness was psychogenic, but that toxic factors might play a secondary role. Recently he has argued that the immediate cause is a severe affective disturbance which leads to a weakening or destruction of the ego. The affect-laden complexes break down in chaotic and irregular ways and escape from control because the tendency to arrange psychic material in a hierarchical way is absent in the schizophrenic. Jung suggests a toxin which is produced by the excessive affect as an explanatory hypothesis for this psychic break-up. This toxin has an effect on the sphere in which the pathogenic complex is to be found. There is a marked *abaissement du niveau mental*, which leads to the associations of the complex being taken down into the archaic stage and to their fragmentation into their elementary constituent parts. The concept of the *abaissement du niveau mental* comes from Janet, who considered that this lowering of the mental level was due to a weakness of the will. Jung believes that it is so marked in schizophrenia that a fragmentation of the mind occurs, whereas in neurosis the lowering is only mild and reversible. He explains all Bleuler's primary symptoms as being products of this *abaissement du niveau mental* and regards schizophrenia as an emergence of the unconscious which may be due either to a weak ego or to an unusually strong unconscious.

The existentialist approach to schizophrenia cannot be discussed without a brief account of existentialism. The first modern thinker to lay stress on the existence of the individual and his experience of himself in the world was Kierkegaard (1813–55). He was a strange man who had been brought up as a devout Christian by his father, who himself was a grossly abnormal person. In his student years Kierkegaard led a dissolute life and was well known in Copenhagen as a wit and man about town. Later he developed an intense personal belief in Christ and just before he died he conducted a vigorous attack on the State Church of Denmark, which he considered was no longer Christian. He suffered from manic-depressive insanity, and, in his writings, his moods and personal problems are often discussed in a slightly disguised form. In his book *Fear and Trembling* he writes about faith as follows: 'I can stand everything—even though that horrible demon, more dreadful than death, the king of terrors, even though madness were to hold up before my eyes the motley of the fool, and I understood that it was I who must put it on, I am still able to save my soul, if only it is more to me than my earthly happiness that my love to God shall triumph in me.'

Kierkegaard's writings are full of brilliant insights into the problems of the individual and poignant half-veiled descriptions of his personal sufferings. He was not, however, a philosopher with an organized system of thought, but he was a brilliant religious thinker.

Existentialism as a philosophical movement really began in 1927 with the publication of Heidegger's book *Sein und Zeit* ('Being and Time'). This philosopher developed many of Kierkegaard's ideas, but invented a very complicated jargon in order to express them. The other outstanding contributor to existentialism is Jean-Paul Sartre (1957), the contemporary French author and playwright, who published his classic work *L'être et le néant* ('Being and Nothingness') in 1943 during the German occupation of France. There is a striking contrast between Heidegger and Sartre. One is a typical incomprehensible German professor and the other is an active man of affairs. Although Kierkegaard was a Christian, Sartre denies the existence of God, while Heidegger cannot find a place for God in his scheme of things. However, existentialism is not necessarily antagonistic to religion, so that there are prominent religious existentialists, like Martin Buber who is a Jew, and Gabriel Marcel who is a Catholic.

Heidegger wishes to answer the question, 'What is the Being of things which are?' Whereas traditional philosophy looks beyond the physical in its search for the essence of Being, Heidegger considers that the human existing being, the *Dasein* (the Being who is there), is the true source of being. This word '*Dasein*' comes from the two German words *da*, meaning 'there', and *sein*, meaning 'to be or being', since the gerund in German has the form of the infinitive.

The *Dasein* (the existing human being) stands in the world and this 'standing-in' can be understood as based on the human concern for things. There are three aspects of concern and each is a mode of 'standing-in'. These modes may be authentic or inauthentic. In the authentic mode the *Dasein* has full insight into what he is and relates himself to things with this in view. In the inauthentic mode the *Dasein* is lost in the necessities of everyday life and his relationships to things do not take into account his total possibilities.

The three authentic modes are: (1) The discovery of self as already in the world (*Befindlichkeit*), (2) Understanding (*Verstehen*), and (3) Discourse (Rede).

The corresponding three inauthentic modes are: (1) Ambiguity (*Zweideutigkeit*), (2) Curiosity (*Neugier*), and (3) Prattle (*Gerede*).*

Just as past, present, and future are inseparable modes of time, so none of the modes of 'standing-in' can be separated from the other two.

Inauthentic existence is due to *Dasein* being wrapped up in his concern for everyday life. This everyday state of the *Dasein* is *Verfallensein*, the state of being fallen. In this state, true understanding is impossible and ambiguity occurs. The lack of understanding leads to a concern for trivialities which is the mode of curiosity. *Dasein* expresses this curiosity in prattle, i.e. the results of an inauthentic existence are expressed in prattle.

The three authentic modes of 'standing-in' are based on an ontological structure which can be regarded as the basic attitude of the *Dasein*. This is *Sorge* (care). In order to be authentic, the *Dasein* must understand the structure of his own existence. He must achieve a state of care in which he realizes that he alone is responsible for meaning in the world, and in which he realizes his own nothingness as a finite being.

To achieve this, a special act of self-discovery, which throws the whole of *Dasein*'s being-in-the-world into question, is necessary. The first step in self-discovery is *Angst*, a nameless dread which leads the *Dasein* to ask 'Who am I?' and 'What am I doing here?' *Angst* arises from a psychological shock or from disgust produced by an utterly inauthentic existence, which leads to a realization of the *Dasein*'s *Unheimlichkeit* (Un-home-like-ness) in the world. The *Angst* produced by this leads to self-questioning and the discovery of the whole structure of one's own existence.

In *Sorge* (care) the *Dasein* discovers himself in three ways:

1. As being on the way, i.e. projecting himself into the future. This is understanding (*Verstehen*).

---

* It is interesting to note here the verbal tricks of this philosophy. *Rede* (discourse) is the authentic mode and *Gerede* (prattle) is the inauthentic mode. This verbal contrast is lost in translation.

2. As already being in the world. This is the discovery of self (*Befindlichkeit*).
3. As being with things, i.e. living in a reciprocal relationship with the things that are. This is discourse (*Rede*).

We now have to consider the temporality of *Dasein*. He lives in expectation of the future and the only sure thing in the future is death. When the *Dasein* comprehends absolutely his future death he realizes at the same time the whole of his future existence. *Dasein* is thus being-towards-death (*Sein-zum-Tode*) and when he realizes this he is free to engage himself and decide his attitude towards things.

The *Dasein* begins in a state of thrown-ness (*Geworfenheit*) and ends in death, so that he is always haunted by his own nothingness. The *Dasein* is the only creature who can accept the idea of his own nothingness and is therefore able to accept or reject his own destiny. From out of nothing the *Dasein* inserts a disengaging nothing which allows the things that are to be understood. In other words, *Dasein* opens a space within the horizon of time in which the light of being can reveal itself.

Dasein must accept his guilt due to his previous inauthentic existence by means of resolution which is 'an extraordinary mode of the open-ness of *Dasein* . . .'. This resolution produces an authentic existence and allows the being-with-others (*Mitsein*).

Heidegger does not concern himself very much with *Mitsein* (being-with-others). Sartre rejects *Mitsein* and deduces the existence of the other from the Look. Binswanger (1947) has stressed this mode of being and has modified Heidegger's views. He considers that love is the ontological opposite of care and that being-with-others (*Mitsein*) is the basis of love. Love creates an eternity and vanquishes space, time, and history, since the loved one exists as a thou for the loving one and therefore exists after his death. This is merely a verbal trick. It is difficult to see how the *Dasein* can be eternal as an image in the mind of the *Mitseinde* (co-existent) who loves him. Surely the image disappears when the loving co-existent dies or even dements. Binswanger has, in fact, grossly distorted Heidegger's views by shifting the focal point of the philosophy from the predicament of the isolated individual to the difficulties of the social individual.

Time for Heidegger is dependent on the *Dasein* who projects himself into the future by authentic resolution. Since he anticipates his potentialities, his future is partly a now. This is different from the everyday view of the future which regards it as a state of possession of things, which has not yet arrived. The *Dasein* can possess his past now when he realizes he has been thrown into the world and is being-towards-death. *Dasein* must assume responsibility for what he was and is. The present for the authentic *Dasein* is the full moment (*Augenblick*) when he makes the past present by a future which he possesses as a resolute act of projection into the future. This concept of the full moment or *Augenblick* comes from Kierkegaard who was a manic depressive. One wonders if this was not originally based on Kierkegaard's experiences in mania. However, the morbid origin of a concept does not mean that it is untrue.

The modes of 'standing-in' take place in authentic or inauthentic temporality. Understanding depends on projecting resolution into the future. If this is not done, then the future is merely a now which is not yet. Self-discovery is determined by the past which is acknowledged, and its possibilities are used for future projections. The *Dasein* who exists in authentic temporality lives in the moment (*Augenblick*) in which there is a new light on the things which are. This new being is realized in the form of a discursive unveiling of the new reality. This discourse (*Rede*) is expressed in speech. Words play an important role in Heidegger's philosophy. He and his followers attempt to understand concepts by analysing words. As German is a synthetic language, this artificial philological analysis is easy to carry out. Apart from this analysis of words, they invent new words or use established words in an unusual way.

It is now necessary to consider how this philosophy has arisen and how it stands in relation to other philosophies. There are two basic positions in philosophy, realism and idealism. The realist or materialist believes that mind is a product of matter and the sensations are produced by matter. The idealist regards mind as primary and matter as secondary, so that sensations are not entirely produced by a material world which is independent of mind. An extreme variety of idealism is solipsism in which the individual is sure only of his own existence and considers his sensations to be present in his imagination.

Kant produced an interesting variety of idealism which has had a profound effect on modern European thought, but especially on German philosophy and psychology. He suggested that we perceive things as phenomena, but we do not perceive things as they really are, namely things-in-themselves. To know a thing as it really is, we must make a transcendental leap from the thing for us to the thing in itself. Thus human experience consists of the elaboration of perception, so that the mind orders the perception of objects in time and space.

From this it follows that there are two types of psychology, one which deals with mental phenomena and the other which deals with the transcendental mind. The mind in this latter sense cannot be investigated, but only analysed by means of the *a priori* concepts which are present in the mind. If one follows this kind of philosophy, one is entitled to erect one's own concepts about the mind and to organize them into a system without any need to appeal to empirical facts.

This is what Heidegger does when he tries to derive the way in which the human being exists from pure contemplation of the problems of the existent in terms of philosophical ideas. He imposes an order on things, which is designed to lead to the discovery of the things-in-themselves. He reaches the conclusion that by means of self-discovery one is able to detach onself from the everyday aspect of things, i.e. from the Kantian phenomena. This detachment creates a distance from things which allows of their proper appreciation. This self-detachment is expressed as 'the inserting of a nothing'. Thus the understanding of things-in-themselves is achieved. The weakness of this whole system is the lack of an adequate method of testing the results. How do we know that we really have discovered our true selves, or that our projections into the future are consistent with our potentialities and the situation? Despite Heidegger's protests, one cannot help feeling that his philosophy is really a variety of solipsism.

The most striking feature of this philosophy is its morbid subjectivism. *Dasein* is not 'born of woman', but is thrown into the world. He is not trying to live honestly in harmony with his fellows, but is living towards death. This is the type of thinking which one finds in the shut-in, shy, adolescent who finds it difficult to make interpersonal relationships, and in his utter isolation he asks himself 'Who am I?' and 'Where am I going?' It is not therefore surprising that ideas resembling existentialist thinking are to be found in disturbed adolescents and young intelligent schizophrenics.

So much for a psychiatric criticism of the philosophy; now we must consider its application to the problems of schizophrenia. Binswanger published detailed existential studies of 5 schizophrenic patients during the years 1944 to 1953. In 1958 he republished these studies in book form under the title of *Schizophrenia*, and in his introduction to this book he summarized his findings.

In his investigations he was looking for a *Dasein*-analytic order and structural order of the schizophrenic *Dasein*. He tried to grasp the special structures of the disposition of being. Instead of disease entities, he claims to have discovered a homogeneity of definite structures and developments of the *Dasein*. He claims that the basic concept in the understanding of the schizophrenic development of the *Dasein* is inconsequence of, or the breaking apart of, natural experience which normally proceeds as a natural sequence of connexions. Heidegger expresses this as our abode (*Aufenthalt*) with things and considers that it consists in our allowing the things that are to be as they are. Binswanger's patients wanted to dictate to things and force them to be what they wanted them to be. Since practical experience could not unfold freely, gaps appeared. In most cases this inconsequence could be found in the behaviour in childhood.

This inconsequence of practical experience leads the patient to find out ways which will restore the lost order and fill in the gaps. No satisfactory way out can be found and *Dasein* finally develops a desire for finality, i.e. for an end. The last way out is found in a high-flown or *verstiegene* ideal which gives the patient a base from which he can continue the struggle. However, the high-flown ideal is inadequate for the life situation.

The inconsequence of experience is split into an alternative—a rigid either–or. A new order seems to have emerged in the form of the high-flown ideal, but high-flown-ness offers no way out. In fact, the high-flown ideal is merely one side of the alternative. The opposite side cannot be completely suppressed, but an attempt is made to cover it up. The existential alternative is expressed in some field of activity such as the body or social life. Thus in one patient it was thinness and fatness of the body, while in another it was the choice of being socially superior or inferior.

This insoluble alternative leads to the *Dasein* being in a harassed state. It culminates in a renunciation of the antinomic problem and a withdrawal of the *Dasein* from the accomplishment of his existence. In the case of Ellen West there was a free decision to withdraw from life by ending it. In the case of Jürg Zünd there was a withdrawal from social life and the patient chose life in a mental hospital. In other cases there was a withdrawal from the *Dasein* into the completely involuntary mode of delusion. In this mode, the *Dasein* does not voluntarily renounce actual living or social life, but renounces life as an independent self and surrenders itself to ego foreign powers.

In the case of Ilse, she burnt her hand in order to demonstrate her martyrdom to her co-existents. After this she developed the delusion that she was being put on show. Thus the active behaviour of making a show of herself changed into passive suffering of being put on show. In the mode of martyrdom there was a split in the sequential connexion of practical experience, but not a complete destruction. The martyrdom did not permit of any development of coherent practical experiences which then broke apart, giving rise to an empty place. This was filled by a completely inconsequential mode of experience, namely that of being a sacrifice to others, which had some inner connexion with earlier experiences. The *Dasein* became stuck fast in a model of practical experience which modelled all new experience according to its own model.

Thus the act of sacrifice in this case forms a connecting link between normality and delusional psychosis. In another case the connecting link was an almost delusional superstitious oracle which consisted of the patient extracting meanings from the world by means of a play on words. The resignation of the *Dasein* here took the form of the renouncing of her own decisions in favour of those of her enemies.

Thus delusion is one of the forms of resignation of the *Dasein* in relation to its antinomic tension produced by inconsequence of practical experience. Withdrawal from actual living or from social life are other forms of resignation. In delusion, there is a resignation in the form of a withdrawal from the cohesion of one's own decisions and a complete self-surrender to the power of others. The indications which the delusional patient detects around him are the secondary or tertiary results of the resignation of the *Dasein* in the form of taking oneself out of one's own cohesion of decisions. The content of the delusion depends on the way in which the *Dasein* fills out the gaps created by his withdrawal from the antinomic problem of practical experience. He draws on his fantasies for material to fill these gaps.

In 1956 Binswanger published a book on 'Three Forms of Unsuccessful Existence'—*Verstiegenheit*, *Verschrobenheit*, *Manieriertheit*. Kahn has translated these terms as 'eccentricity', 'queerness', and 'stiltedness', but either they should be left in the German as technical terms or translated into English neologisms. *Verstiegen* comes from the verb *versteigen* which means to climb the wrong way or to go astray on the mountain. This has led to the figurative use of *verstiegen* to mean high flown or eccentric. Since the suffix 'heit' indicates an abstract noun *Verstiegenheit* means 'high-flownness'. *Verschroben* comes from the verb *verschrauben* which means to screw up or screw the wrong way. *Verschrobenheit* is usually translated as 'queerness'. 'eccentricity', or 'crankiness', but could be translated as 'screwiness'. *Manieriertheit* is usually translated as 'mannerism' in the ordinary non-technical sense of the word, but in order to avoid confusion with the symptom of mannerism, I suggest that it be translated as 'manneredness'.

Binswanger considers that high-flownness, screwiness, and manneredness are modes of failure of the *Dasein* in the sense of its historical movement having come to an end, or being stuck fast. Consequently, *Dasein* is not able to be with others in love and friendship. These modes are very close to the modes of schizophrenic *Dasein* such as 'stiffness' and being 'being-at-standstill'. *Verstiegenheit* (high-flownness) is an anthropological disproportion. The normal *Dasein* moves in a horizontal and a vertical plane and his movements in these planes are correlated, but in *Verstiegenheit* the *Dasein* has climbed too high or become stuck in the vertical dimension. In *Verschrobenheit* (screwiness) the *Dasein* is transverse or oblique to the situation and his fellow existents, because he justifies his behaviour, not by relating it to the situation and his co-existents, but by a dominating idea which arises from his fallen state. In *Manieriertheit* (manneredness) the *Dasein* carries on a discussion with himself instead of with others. His existence is split. Binswanger believes that *Verstiegenheit*, *Verschrobenheit*, and *Manieriertheit* are existentially related to schizophrenic inflexibility, stiffness, and splitting.

Stiffness means that the movement of the *Dasein* into the future is cut off. The *verstiegene* (high-flown) ideal and the *Verschrobenheit* are initial stages of schizophrenic stiffness. Thus in *Verschrobenheit* (screwiness) the obliqueness of the patient's world makes authentic self-foundation incomplete. In *Manieriertheit* (manneredness) there is an incessant repeating of the reflection of one's own *Dasein* in the mirror of the pattern or model of Man. The mimicry and gesture of the individual person become a mask and it is as if there were an iron net around all expressive movements. The free play of *Dasein*'s movement is lost.

Binswanger summarizes the relationship of the three unsuccessful forms of existence to schizophrenia as follows:

> The proximity of schizophrenia to the forms of *Dasein* of *Verstiegenheit*, *Verschrobenheit* and *Manieriertheit* and the passing over of these forms into schizophrenia from time to time depends therefore on the fact that these forms represent intermediate existential forms between the authentic historical movement of the *Dasein* and the complete arrest of this movement. These are the forms therefore which somehow make it possible for *Dasein* to hold his own in the world for a variable length of time, although he is not in the homeland of love. This does not occur in the sense of the success of *Dasein* with the development of his freedom, his abundant possibilities and his creative powers, but in the sense of remaining on the edge of the abyss which we call the 'emptiness' or 'stiffness of psychic life', 'schizophrenic thoughtlessness, breakdown or deterioration'.

After all this, have we learned anything new about schizophrenia? Such ideas as a break in the coherence and sequence of experience are not new and do not seem any more profound when expressed in Heideggerian jargon and neologisms. *Verstiegenheit*, *Verschrobenheit*, and *Manieriertheit* are merely long-winded ways of saying that a given person is odd. We know that some people who are odd develop schizophrenia and some do not. It is difficult to see what is to be gained by calling oddness 'an intermediate form of existence between the authentic historical movement of the *Dasein* and the complete arrest of this movement'.

Perhaps Binswanger's criticism of a patient who wrote books can be applied to Binswanger himself. He writes as follows about this patient whom he cites as an example of *Verschrobenheit*:

> Apart from the inconsequent consequence of the mode of communication in the sense of the *Dasein* as *verschroben*, yet another essential characteristic which is connected with *Verschrobenheit* is especially clear in this case. This is the type and manner in which the *Dasein* here handles a precise totality of circumstances. The deficient consideration for the co-existents, even the denial of the basis of communication in general, brings it about that the totality of circumstances, which is in question—i.e. the whole of the historical doctrines and methods of the time—are not preserved in their richness, but are restricted or reduced to a purely formal scheme of thought.

This is precisely what Binswanger himself has done. He has reduced the richness of schizophrenic symptomatology to a simple scheme. The philosophers' stone of schizophrenia, the basic psychological disorder from which all symptoms are derived, is presented to us in a new disguise. Nothing new is said which can help us to understand or explain schizophrenia.

Sartre distinguishes between the being-in-itself, which is non-reflective existence, and the being-for-itself, which is reflective, can ask questions, and can question itself. The being-in-itself is therefore unconscious, while the being-for-itself is conscious. Sartre considers that the ability of the latter to ask questions and question himself is due to the presence of a nothingness within himself. *Angst* occurs where the for-itself becomes aware of the nothingness and he tries to escape from this *Angst* by means of bad faith. Now being-in-itself exists or is present, but being-for-itself is continually developing and is therefore never fixed and definite. In bad faith the being-for-itself is regarded as simply existing as something final and fixed. In other words, a petrification of the being-for-itself occurs in bad faith.

Although Heidegger considers that his philosophy has nothing to do with psychiatry, Sartre is interested in psychology and has developed the idea of existential psycho-analysis. He claims that: 'Existential psycho-analysis seeks to determine the *original* choice.'

This idea of choice or the need for the individual person to choose is a recurrent theme in existentialist writings. Thus Heidegger says that the *Dasein* must choose his heroes. However, he does not tell us whether the *Dasein* should choose Cesare Borgia or St Francis of Assisi. This lack of criteria is typical of the subjective attitude of the existentialists. We are told about various states of being, but we are never told how we know whether we are in one state or another.

An interesting facet of Sartre's work is its morbidity, which is very striking. Thus he discusses the quality of sliminess in great detail and then passes on to discuss the hole as a symbol of a mode of being. Then he says: 'It is only from this standpoint that we can pass on to sexuality. The obscenity of the feminine sex is that of everything which "gapes open". It is an appeal to being as all holes are. In herself woman appeals to a strong flesh which is to transform her into a fullness of being by penetration and dissolution. Conversely, woman senses her condition as an appeal precisely because she is "in the form of a hole". This is the true origin of Adler's complex. Beyond any doubt her sex is a mouth and a voracious mouth which devours the penis—a fact which can easily lead to the idea of castration. The amorous act is the castration of the man; but this is above all, because sex is a hole.'

Zutt and Kuhlenkampf (1958) have analysed the paranoid syndrome using a mixture of concepts derived from Heidegger and

Sartre. They consider that in this syndrome the other appears as an overwhelming one, who penetrates all the patient's boundaries, possesses the patient, and imposes his will upon the patient. Zutt (1952) has introduced the concept of the physiognomic aesthetic sphere of life by which he designates those aspects of experience which are not dependent on emotions or intellect. The living mundane body is experienced as being lived, not as being possessed. Because it is mundane, it signifies that the individual has a specific position in the world, i.e. to be physically manifest. Thus the mundane body becomes fully manifest through the Look and extends as far as the Look. One meets the Look of the other when one encounters the other. The human being can only become manifest in a given position if there is a distance between him and the other which means that boundaries must be maintained. These boundaries not only concern being-there, but also being-on-the-way.

Kuhlenkampf sees the existence of the paranoid patient as a breakdown of these boundaries when he says:

> The breakdown of boundaries leads to an upsetting of the existence orders, described by Zutt as dwelling and status classification. Other's space and own space, inside and outside, lose their separate identities, private and public merge. The familiar gives way to the sinister. In the same manner, friend and foe can no longer be differentiated with certainty. The status classification gives way to an unstable miscellany of persons and forces of indeterminable status. This decisive change of our relationship with other men, with spaces and things in the form of destructive levelling, leads to a loss of any sort of security. Insecure existence can no longer find and establish confidence. In the realm of the originally and basically unfamiliar, in the sphere of suspicion and fear, the human existence is no longer able to cope with the crowding in of the physiognomic; having lost its position, it is physiognomically overpowered.

This description of the changed existence of the paranoid patient appears to be little different from the explanation of schizophrenic symptomatology as due to a breakdown of ego boundaries. It appears that where existentialist formulations are relevant they are merely repeating known facts or Freudian formulations in a more obscure and exotic manner.

POSTSCRIPT

Of many of the theories described in this chapter it can be said that, contrary to the popular expression, the more one sees of them the less one believes in them. It now remains to consider the theories of Laing (1960). He and his colleagues (Laing and Esterson, 1970) have proposed a theory of schizophrenia that is based on a social approach. All societies are founded on accepted rules or norms of conduct, but not all members conform completely; there are always some individuals who deviate more or less. At some point, such deviance becomes unacceptable and social pressures tend to move such individuals into a situation which makes them more socially unacceptable.

The social tensions, exploitation, and 'alienation' of a divided and oppressive society are seen in miniature in the family. The internal strains of society here become perceptible in the contradictory and incoherent communication that exists within the family. The unit of study is therefore not the individual patient but the family. It is the whole family that becomes schizophrenic not merely the patient. Nevertheless, one member is eventually victimized by the others and adopts a special pattern of behaviour in order to cope with an unliveable situation. This pattern may be regarded as a voyage of exploration of 'inner space'. The person returns from this voyage spiritually strengthened and when, or if, he does so, he is specially suited to help other 'schizophrenics', insofar as it can be said that they need help.

There are three distinct features in this theory: the oppressive society, the disorganized family, and the mystical experience. The relative emphasis of them has changed over the years, which makes it difficult to give a non-historical account of them. These theories became very fashionable in the late 1960s among the radical youth and the intelligentsia of the media. It is generally true that an individual's enthusiasm for Laing's ideas is inversely proportional to his contact and experience with schizophrenics.

References

Abe, K. (1969), 'The Morbidity Rate and Environmental Influence in Monozygotic Co-twins of Schizophrenics', *Brit. J. Psychiat.*, **115,** 519–531.

Alanen, Y. O. (1958), 'The Mothers of Schizophrenic Patients', *Acta psychiat. Scand.*, **33,** Suppl. 124.

— — (1966), 'The Family in the Pathogenesis of Schizophrenic and Neurotic Disorders', *Ibid.*, Suppl. 189.

— — (1968), 'From the Mothers of Schizophrenic Patients to the Interactional Family Dynamics', *Transmission of Schizophrenia* (ed. Rosenthal, D., and Kety, S. S.). Oxford: Pergamon.

Allen, G., Harvald, B., and Shields, J. (1967), 'Measures of Twin Concordances', *Acta genet. Statist. med.*, **17,** 475–481.

Andreasen, N. C., Dennert, J. W., Olsen, S. A., and DiMascio, A. R. (1982), 'Hemispheric Asymmetries and Schizophrenia', *Amer. J. Psychiat.*, **139,** 427–430.

Angrist, B., Rotrosen, J., and Gershon, S. (1980), 'Differential Effects of Amphetamine and Neuroleptics on Negative vs. Positive Symptoms in Schizophrenia', *Psychoparmacology*, **72,** 17–19.

Angst, J. (1966), *Zur Atiologie und Nosologie Endogener Depressiver Psychosen.* Berlin: Springer Verlag.

— — (1980), 'Verlauf unipolar depressiver, bipolar manisch-depressiver und schizo-affectiver Erkrankungen und Psychosen. Ergebnisse einer prospectiven Studie' (the course of unipolar depressive, bipolar manic-depressive and schizo-affective disorders and psychoses. Findings of a prospective study), *Fortschr. Neurol. Psychiat.*, **48,** 3–30.

— — Baastrup, P., Grof, P., Hippius, H., Poldinger, W., Varga, E., Weis, P., and Wyss, F. (1973), 'Statistische Aspekte des Beginns und Verlaufs schizophrener Erkrankungen' (statistical aspects of the onset and course of schizophrenic psychoses), in *Verlauf und Ausgang schizophrener Erkrankungen* (course and outcome of schizophrenic disorders) (ed. Huber, G.). Stuttgart: F. K. Schattauer Verlag.

Arnold, O. H. (1955), *Schizophrener Prozess und Schizophrene Symptomgesetze* (schizophrenic process and schizophrenic symptom laws). Vienna: Maudrich.

Astrup, C. (1957a), 'Experimentelle Untersuchungen über die Störungen der höheren Nerventätigkeit bei Defektschizophrenien' (experimental investigations of the disorders of higher nervous activity in defect schizophrenia), *Psychiat. Neurol. u. med. Psychol., Lpz.*, **9,** 9.

— — (1957b), 'Experimentelle Untersuchungen über die Störungen der höheren Nerventätigkeit bei akuten und subchronischen Schizophrenien' (experimental investigations of the disorders of higher nervous activity in acute and sub-chronic schizophrenias), *Ibid.*, **9,** 33.

— — (1975), 'Classification and Prognostic Aspects of Schizophrenia', *Neuropsychobiology*, **1,** 32–40.

Baker, R. (1975), 'Behavioural Techniques in the Treatment of Schizophrenia', in *New Perspectives in Schizophrenia* (ed. Forrest, A., and Afflick, J.). Edinburgh: Churchill Livingstone.

— — Hall, J. W., Hutchinson, K., and Bridge, G. (1977), 'Symptom Changes in Chronic Schizophrenic Patients on a Token Economy: a Controlled Experiment', *Brit. J. Psychiat.*, **131,** 381–393.

BATESON, G., JACKSON, D. D., HALEY, J., and WEAKLAND, J. (1956), 'Toward a Communication Theory of Schizophrenia', *Behav. Sci.*, **1,** 251.

BELMAKER, R., POLLIN, W., WYATT, R. J., and COHEN, S. (1974), 'A Follow-up of Monozygotic Twins Discordant for Schizophrenia', *Arch. gen. Psychiat.*, **30,** 219–222.

BENES, F., SUNDERLAND, P., JONES, B. D., LEMAY, M., COHEN, B. M., and LIPINSKI, J. F. (1982), 'Normal Ventricles in Young Schizophrenics', *Brit. J. Psychiat.*, **141,** 90–93.

BENNETT, D. (1970), 'The Value of Work in Psychiatric Rehabilitation', *Soc. Psychiat.*, **5,** 224–230.

— — and WING, J. K. (1963), 'Sheltered Workshops for the Psychiatrically Handicapped', in *Trends in the Mental Services* (ed. FREEMAN, H., and FARNDALE, J.), Chap. 27. Oxford: Pergamon.

BERZE, J., and GRUHLE, H. W. (1929), *Psychologie der Schizophrenie* (psychology of schizophrenia). Berlin: Springer.

BINSWANGER, L. (1947), *Ausgewählte Vorträge und Aufsätze* (selected lectures and essays). Vol. I. Berne: Francke.

— — (1956), *Drei Formen missglückten Daseins: Verstiegenheit, Verschrobenheit und Manieriertheit* (three forms of unsuccessful existence, highflowness, screwiness and manneredness). Tübingen: Niemeyer.

— — (1958), *Schizophrenie* (schizophrenia). Pfüllingen: Neske.

BLAND, R. C., and ORN, H. (1979), 'Schizophrenia: Diagnostic Criteria and Outcome', *Brit. J. Psychiat.*, **134,** 34–38.

BLEULER, E. P. (1911), *Dementia Praecox or the Group of Schizophrenias* (trans. ZINKIN, J., International Universities Press, New York, 1950). Leipzig: Deuticke.

— — (1924), *Textbook of Psychiatry* (trans. BRILL, A. A.). New York: Macmillan. (Reissued by Dover Publications, London, 1951.)

BLEULER, M. (1943), 'Die spätschizophrenen Krankheitsbilder' (the late schizophrenic clinical pictures), *Fortschr. Neurol. Psychiat.*, **15,** 259.

BOKLAGE, C. E. (1977), 'Schizophrenia, Brain Asymmetry Development, and Twinning: Cellular Relationship with Etiological and Possibly Prognostic Implications', *Biol. Psychiat.*, **12,** 19–35.

BÖÖK, J. A. (1953), 'Schizophrenia as a Gene Mutation', *Acta genet. Statist. med.*, **4,** 133–139.

BROCKINGTON, I., KENDELL, R. E., and LEFF, J. P. (1978), 'Definitions of Schizophrenia: Concordance and Prediction of Outcome', *Psychol. Med.*, **8,** 387–398.

— — — — and WAINWRIGHT, R. S. (1980), 'Depressed Patients with Schizophrenic or Paranoid Symptoms', *Psychol. Med.*, **10,** 665–675.

— — and LEFF, J. P. (1979), 'Schizo-affective Psychosis: Definitions and Incidence', *Psychol. Med.*, **9,** 91–99.

— — PERRIS C., KENDELL R. E., HILLIER V. E., and WAINWRIGHT, S. (1982), 'The Course and Outcome of Cycloid Psychoses', *Psychol. Med.*, **12,** 97–105.

BROWN, G. W., BIRLEY, J. L. T., and WING, J. K. (1972), 'Influence of Family Life on the Course of Schizophrenic Disorders: A Replication', *Brit. J. Psychiat.*, **121,** 241–258.

— — HARRIS, T. D., and PETO, J. (1973), 'Life Events and Psychiatric Disorders. Part 2, Nature of Causal Link', *Psychol. Med.*, **3,** 159–176.

BUCK, C., HOBBS, G. E., SIMPSON, H., and WANKLIN, J. M. (1975), 'Fertility of Sibs of Schizophrenic Patients', *Brit. J. Psychiat.*, **127,** 235–239.

CADORET, R. J. (1973), 'Toward a Definition of the Schizoid State: Evidence from Studies of Twins and their Families', *Ibid.*, **122,** 679–685.

CAMERON, N. (1947), *The Psychology of the Behaviour Disorders.* Boston: Houghton Mifflin.

CARPENTER, W. T., STRAUSS, J. S., and BARTKO, J. J. (1973), 'Flexible System for the Diagnosis of Schizophrenia: Report from the WHO International Pilot Study of Schizophrenia', *Science*, **182,** 1275–1278.

CARPENTER, W. T., STRAUSS, J. S., and BARTKO, J. J. (1974), 'An Approach to the Diagnosis and Understanding of Schizophrenia. Part 1. Use of Signs and Symptoms for the Identification of the Schizophrenic Patients', *Schiz. Bull.*, **11,** 37–49.

CARTER, M., and WATTS, C. A. H. (1971), 'Possible Biological Advantages among Schizophrenics' Relatives', *Brit. J. Psychiat.*, **118,** 453–460.

CHAUGULE, V. B., and MASTER, R. S. (1981), 'Impaired Cerebral Dominance and Schizophrenia', *Ibid.*, **139,** 23–24.

CIOMPI, L. (1980), 'The Natural History of Schizophrenia in the Long Term', *Ibid.*, **136,** 413–420.

— — and MÜLLER, C. (1976), *Lebensweg und Alter der Schizophrenien* (the life and old age of schizophrenics). Berlin: Springer Verlag.

CLANCY, J., CROWE, R., WINOKUR, G., and MORRISON, J. (1973), 'The Iowa 500: Precipitating Factors in Schizophrenia and Primary Affective Disorder', *Compreh. Psychiat.*, **14,** 197–202.

COHEN, S. M., ALLEN, M. G., POLLIN, W., and HRUBEC, Z. (1972), 'Relationship of Schizo-affective Psychosis to Manic-depressive Psychosis and Schizophrenia. Findings in 15,909 Veteran Pairs', *Arch. Gen. Psychiat.*, **26,** 539–545.

CONNELL, P. H. (1958), *Amphetamine Psychosis.* Maudsley Monographs No. 5. London: Oxford University Press.

CONRAD, K. (1958a), *Die beginnende Schizophrenie. Versuch einer Gestaltanalyse des Wahns* (commencing schizophrenia. An attempt at a *Gestalt* analysis of delusion). Stuttgart: Thieme.

— — (1958b), 'Über Begriff und Wesen der Apophanie' (on the concept and essence of apophany), in *Mehrdimensionale Diagnostik und Therapie.* Festschrift zum 70. Geburtstag Ernst Kretschmer. Stuttgart: Thieme.

COOPER, A. F., and CURRY, A. R. (1976), 'The pathology of deafness in the paranoid and affective psychoses of later life', *J. psychosom. Res.*, **20,** 97–105.

COOPER, J. E., KENDELL, R. E., GURLAND, B. J., COPELAND, J. R. M., and SIMON, R. J. (1972), *Psychiatric Diagnosis in New York and London: A Comparative Study of Mental Hospital Admissions.* London: Oxford University Press.

COX, S. M., and LUDWIG, A. M. (1979), 'Neurological Soft Signs and Psychopathology. 1. Findings in Schizophrenia', *J. nerv. ment. Dis.*, **167,** 161–165.

CREER, C., and WING, J. K. (1974), *Schizophrenia at Home.* National Schizophrenia Fellowship, 1974.

CREESE, I., BURT, D. R., and SNYDER, S. (1976), 'Dopamine Receptor Binding Predicts Clinical and Pharmacological Potencies of Anti-schizophrenic Drugs', *Science,* **192,** 481–483.

CRITCHLEY, E. M., DENMARK, J. C., WARREN, F., and WILSON, K. A. (1981), 'Hallucinatory Experiences of Prelingually Profoundly Deaf Schizophrenics', *Brit. J. Psychiat.*, **138,** 30–32.

CROW, T. J. (1980), 'Molecular Pathology of Schizophrenia: More than One Disease Process?, *Brit. med. J.*, **i,** 66–68.

— — (1981), 'Biological Basis of Mental Disorders: The Case for Viral Aetiology', in *Epidemiological Impact of Psychotropic Drugs* (ed. TOGNONI, G., BALLANTUONO, C., and LADER, M.). Amsterdam: Elsevier/North Holland Biomedical Press.

— — DEAKIN, J. F. W., and LONGDEN, A. (1977), 'The nucleus accumbens—possible site of antipsychotic action of neuroleptic drugs?', *Psychol. Med.* **7,** 213–221.

— — and MITCHELL, W. S. (1975), 'Subjective Age in Chronic Schizophrenia: Evidence for a Sub-group of Patients with Defective Learning Capacity', *Brit. J. Psychiat.*, **126,** 360–363.

— — and STEVENS, M. (1978), 'Age Disorientation in Chronic Schizophrenia: The Nature of the Cognitive Defect', *Ibid.*, **133,** 137–142.

CUTTING, J. C., CLARE, A. W., and MANN, A. H. (1978), 'Cycloid Psychosis: An Investigation of the Diagnositic Concept', *Psychol. Med.*, **8,** 637–648.

CUTTING, J. C., and RYAN, K. (1982), 'The Appreciation of Imagery by Schizophrenics: An Interpretation of Goldstein's Impairment of the Abstract Attitude', *Ibid.*, **12,** 585–590.

DAVISON, G. C. (1969), 'Appraisal of Behaviour Modification Techniques with Adults in Institutional Settings', in *Behaviour Therapy: Appraisal and Status* (ed. FRANKS, C. M.). New York: McGraw-Hill.

DAVISON, K., and BAGLEY, C. R. (1969), 'Schizophrenia-like Psychoses associated with Organic Disorders of the Central Nervous System. A Review of the Literature', in *Recent Advances in Neuropsychiatry* (ed. HETHERINGTON, N.). London: Royal Medico-Psychological Association.

DIEM, O. (1903), 'Die einfach demente Form der Dementia Praecox (Dementia Simplex)' (the simple demented form of dementia praecox (dementia simplex)), *Arch. Psychiat. Nervenkr.*, **37,** 111.

DOANE, J. A., WEST, K. L., GOLDSTEIN, M. J., RODNICK, E. H., and JONES, J. E. (1981), 'Parental Communication Deviance and Affective Style. Predictors of Subsequent Schizophrenia Spectrum Disorders in Vulnerable Adolescents', *Arch. gen. Psychiat.*, **38,** 679–685.

DUNHAM, H. W. (1956), 'Current Status of Ecological Research in Mental Disorder', in *Mental Health and Mental Disorder* (ed. ROSE, A. M.). London: Routledge & Kegan Paul.

— — (1965), *Community and Schizophrenia: An Epidemiological Analysis*. Detroit: Wayne University Press.

EKBLAD, M. (1948), *A Psychiatric and Sociologic Study of a Series of Swedish Naval Conscripts*. Copenhagen: Munksgaard.

EKDAWI, M. Y. (1972), 'The Netherne Resettlement Unit: Results of 10 Years', *Brit. J. Psychiat.*, **121,** 417–424.

ELSÄSSER, G., and GRÜNEWALD, H. W. (1953), 'Schizophrene oder schizophrenieähnliche Psychosen bei Hirntraumatikern' (schizophrenic and schizophrenia-like psychoses in patients with brain injury), *Ibid.*, **190,** 134.

FAIRBAIRN, W. R. D. (1952), *Psychoanalytic Studies of the Personality*. Tavistock Publications. London: Routledge & Kegan Paul.

FALCONER, M. A., SERAFETINIDES, E. A., and CORSELLIS, J. A. N. (1964), 'Etiology and Pathogenesis of Temporal Lobe Epilepsy', *Arch. Neurol.*, **10,** 233–248.

FALLOON, I. R., BOYD, J. L., MCGILL, C. W., RAAZANI, J., MOSS, H. B., and GILDERMAN, A. M. (1982), 'Family Management in the Prevention of Exacerbations of Schizophrenia', *N. Engl. J. Med.*, **306,** 1437–1440.

— — WATT, D. C., and SHEPHERD, M. (1978), 'The Social Outcome of Patients in a Trial of Long-term Continuation Therapy', *Psychol. Med.*, **8,** 265–274.

FARIS, R. E. L., and DUNHAM, H. W. (1939), *Mental Disorders in Urban Areas*. Chicago: University Press.

FARLEY, I. J. and HORNYKIEWICZ, O. (1977), 'Noradrenaline Distribution in Subcortical Areas of the Human Brain', *Brain Research* **126,** 52–62.

FEDERN, P. (1952), *Ego Psychology and the Psychoses*. London: Imago.

FEIGHNER, J. P., ROBINS, E., GUZE, S. B., WOODRUFF, R. A., WINOKUR, G., and MUNOZ, R. (1972), 'Diagnostic Criteria for Use in Psychiatric Research', *Arch. gen. Psychiat.*, **26,** 57–63.

FEINSILVER, D. B., and GUNDERSON, J. G. (1972), 'Psychotherapy for Schizophrenics—Is it Indicated? A Review of the Relevant Literature', *Schizophrenia Bulletin No. 6*, 11–23.

FEITEL, B., HAMILTON, M., SCHMADER, L. and SHAH, B. K. (1982), 'Consultation to Line Staff and its Impact on the Care of Chronic Patients', *J. Nerv. Ment. Dis.*, **170,** 561–564.

FEUCHTWANGER, E., and MAYER-GROSS, W. (1938), 'Hirnverletzung und Schizophrenie' (brain injury and schizophrenia), *Schweiz. Arch. Neurol. Psychiat.*, **41,** 17.

Fischer, M. (1971), 'Psychoses in the Offspring of Schizophrenic Monozygotic Twins and their Normal Co-Twins', *Brit. J. Psychiat.* **118,** 43–52.

Fish, F. J. (1958a), 'A Clinical Investigation of Chronic Schizophrenia', *Ibid.*, **104,** 34.

— — (1958b), 'Leonhard's Classification of Schizophrenia', *Ibid.*, **104,** 944.

Flor-Henry, P. (1969), 'Psychoses and Temporal Lobe Epilepsy: A Controlled Investigation', *Epilepsia*, **10,** 363–395.

— — (1972), 'Ictal and Interictal Psychiatric Manifestations in Epilepsy: Specific or Non-specific?', *Ibid.* **13,** 773–783.

Franzén, G., and Ingvar, D. H. (1975), 'Absence of Activation in Frontal Structures during Psychological Testing of Chronic Schizophrenics', *J. Neurol. Neurosurg. Psychiat.*, **38,** 1027–1032.

Freud, S. (1924a), 'Certain Neurotic Mechanisms in Jealousy, Paranoia, and Homosexuality', in *Collected Papers*, Vol. II. London: Hogarth Press.

— — (1924b), 'Psychoanalytic Notes upon an Autobiographical Account of a Case of Paranoia', *Ibid.*, Vol. III. London: Hogarth Press.

Garmezy, N. (1977), 'On some Risks in Risk/Research', *Psychol. Med.*, **7,** 1–6.

Gjessing, R. (1932a), 'Beiträge zur Pathophysiologie des katatonen Stupors. I. Mitteilung. Über periodisch rezidivierend katatonen Stupor mit kritischem Beginn und Abschluss' (contributions to the pathophysiology of catatonic stupor. Communication I, on periodic recurrent catatonic stupor with suddent onset and termination), *Arch. Psychiat. Nervenkr.*, **96,** 319.

— — (1932b), 'Beiträge zur Pathophysiologie des katatonen Stupors. II. Mitteilung. Über aperiodisch rezidivierend verlaufenden katatonen Stupor mit lytischem Beginn und Abschluss' (contributions to the pathophysiology of catatonic stupor. Communication II, on a periodic recurrent catatonic stupor with gradual onset and termination), *Ibid.*, **96,** 393.

Goldberg, E. M., and Morrison, S. L. (1963), 'Schizophrenia and Social Class', *Brit. J. Psychiat.*, **109,** 785–807.

Goldberg, S. C., Schooler, N. R., Hogarty, G. E., and Roper, M. (1977), 'Prediction of Relapse in Schizophrenic Outpatients Treated by Drug and Sociotherapy', *Arch. gen. Psychiat.*, **3,** 171–184.

Goldstein, K. (1944), 'Methodological Approach to the Study of Schizophrenic Thought Disorder', in *Language and Thought in Schizophrenia* (ed. Kasanin, J. S.). Berkeley: University of California Press.

Gomes, U. C. R., Sanney, B. C., Potgieter, L., and Roux, J. T. (1980) 'Noradrenergic Overactivity in Chronic Schizophrenia', *Brit. J. Psychiat.*, **137,** 346–351.

Gottesman, I. I., and Shields, J. (1966), 'Contributions of Twin Studies to Perspectives on Schizophrenia', in *Progress in Experimental Personality Research* (ed. Maher, B. A.). New York: Academic.

— — — — (1973), 'Genetic Theorizing and Schizophrenia', *Brit. J. Psychiat.*, **122,** 15–30.

— — — — (1976), 'A Critical Review of Recent Adoption, Twin and Family Studies of Schizophrenia: Behavioural Genetics Perspectives', *Schiz. Bull.*, **2,** 360–401.

Green, P., and Preston, M. (1981), 'Reinforcement of Vocal Correlates of Auditory Hallucinations Using Auditory Feedback: A Case Study', *Brit. J. Psychiat.*, **139,** 204–208.

Grinspoon, J., Ewalt, J., and Shaker, R. (1968), 'Psychotherapy and Pharmacotherapy in Chronic Schizophrenia', *Amer. J. Psychiat.*, **124,** 1645–1652.

Gruhle, H. W. (1936), 'Über den Wahn bei Epilepsie' (on delusions in epilepsy), *Z. ges. Neurol. Psychiat.*, **154,** 395.

Gruzelier, J. H., and Venables, P. H. (1974), 'Bimodality and Lateral Symmetry of Skin Conductance Orienting Activity in Schizophrenics', *Biol. Psychiat.*, **8,** 55–73.

Hajioff, J., and Wallace, M. (1983), 'Effect of Co-dergocrine Mesylate on Tardive Dyskinesia: A Preliminary Report', *Psychopharmacology*, **79,** 1–3.

HALL, H. A., and LEVIN, S. (1980), 'Affect and Verbal–Non Verbal Discrepancy in Schizophrenic and Non-schizophrenic Family Communication', *Brit. J. Psychiat.*, **137,** 78–92.

HALL, J., and BAKER, R. (1973), 'Token Economy Systems: Breakdown and Control', *Behav. Res. Ther.*, **11,** 253–263.

HAMILTON, M., SMITH, A. L. G., LAPIDUS, H. E., and CADOGAN, E. P. (1960), 'A Controlled Trial of Thiopropazate dehydrochloride (Dartalan), Chlorpromazine and Occupational Therapy in Chronic Schizophrenics', *J. ment. Sci.*, **106,** 40–55.

HANSEN, L. B., LARSEN, N. E., and VESTERGÅRD, P. (1981), 'Plasma Levels of Perphenazine (Trilafon) Related to Development of Extrapyramidal Side Effects', *Psychopharmacology*, **74,** 36–309.

HANSON, D. R., GOTTESMAN, I. I., and HESTON, L. L. (1976), 'Some possible childhood indicators of adult schizophrenia inferred from children of schizophrenics', *Brit. J. Psychiat.*, **129,** 142–154.

HARE, E. H. (1956), 'Family Setting and the Urban Distribution of Schizophrenia', *J. ment. Sci.*, **102,** 753.

HASSOL, L., MAGARET, A., and CAMERON, N. (1952), 'The Production of Language Distortion through Personalized Distraction', *J. Psychol.*, **33,** 289.

HAUG, J. (1962), 'Pneumoencephalographic Studies in Mental Disease', *Acta psychiat. Scand.*, **38,** Suppl. 165, 66–86.

HAWK, A. B., CARPENTER, W. T., and STRAUSS, J. S. (1975), 'Diagnostic Criteria and Five-year Outcome in Schizophrenia', *Arch. gen. Psychiat.*, **32**, 343–347.

HEIDEGGER, M. (1953), *Sein und Zeit* (being and time). Pfullingen: Neske.

HELMCHEN, H., and HIPPIUS, H. (1967), 'Depressive Syndrome im Verlauf neuroleptischer Therapie', (Depressive syndromes in the course of neuroleptic therapy.) *Nervenarzt*, **38,** 455–458.

HESTON, L. L. (1966), 'Psychiatric Disorders in Foster Home-reared Children of Schizophrenic Mothers', *Brit. J. Psychiat.*, **112,** 819–825.

HILLBOM, E. (1960), 'After-effects of Brain Injuries. Research on the Symptoms causing Invalidism of Persons in Finland having sustained Brain-injuries during the Wars of 1939–1940 and 1941–1944', *Acta psychiat. Scand.*, Suppl. **142**.

HIRSCH, S. R., GAIND, R., ROHDE, P. D., STEVENS, B. C., and WING, J. K. (1973), 'Outpatient Maintenance of Chronic Schizophrenic Patients with Long-acting Fluphenazine: Double-blind Placebo Trial', *Brit. med. J.*, **1,** 633–637.

— — and LEEF, J. (1975), 'Abnormalities in the Parents of Schizophrenics'. Maudsley Monograph No. 22. London: Oxford Univ. Press.

HOCH, P. H., and POLATIN, P. (1949), 'Pseudoneurotic Forms of Schizophrenia', *Acta psychiat. Scand.*, **23,** 248.

HOLMBOE, R., and ASTRUP, C. (1957), 'A Follow-up Study of 255 Patients with Acute Schizophrenia and Schizophreniform Psychoses', *Ibid.*, Suppl. **115**.

HORN, A. S., and SNYDER, S. H. (1971), Chlorpromazine and Dopamine: Confirmational Similarities that correlate with the Anti-schizophrenic Activity of Phenothiazine Drugs', *Proc. natn. Acad. Sci. U.S.A.*, **68,** 2325–2328.

HORN, J. M., GREEN, M., CARNEY, R., and ERIKSON, M. T. (1975), 'Bias against Genetic Hypotheses in Adoption Studies', *Arch. gen. Psychiat.*, **32,** 1365–1367.

HORVATH, T., and MEARES, R. (1979), 'The Sensory Filter in Schizophrenia: A Study of Habituation, Arousal, and the Dopamine Hypothesis', *Brit. J. Psychiat.*, **134,** 39–45.

HOUSTON, F. (1954), 'Relationship between Deafness and Psychotic Illness', *J. ment. Sci.*, **100,** 990–993.

HUBER, G., GROSS, G., and SCHÜTTLER, R. (1975a), 'A Long-term Follow-up Study of Schizophrenia: Psychiatric Course and Prognosis', *Acta psychiat. Scand.*, **52,** 49–57.

— — — — — — (1975b), 'Spät Schizophrenie' (late schizophrenia), *Arch. Psychiat. Nervenkr.*, **22,** 53–66.

INGVAR, D. H. (1974), 'Abnormalities of Cerebral Blood Flow Distribution in Patients with Chronic Schizophrenia', *Acta psychiat. Scand.*, **50,** 425–462.

INGVAR, D. H., and FRANZÉN, G. (1974), 'Distribution of Cerebral Activity in Chronic Schizophrenia', *Lancet*, **ii,** 1484–1486.

IVERSON, L. L., HORN, A. S., and MILLER, R. J. (1975) 'Structure Activity Relationships for Agonist and Antagonist Drugs, at Pre- and Post-synaptic Dopamine Receptor Sites in Rat Brain', in *Pre- and Post-Synaptic Receptor Mechanisms* (ed. USDIN, E.). New York: Deckers.

JACOBSEN, B. (1975), *Genetic Research in Psychiatry* (ed. FIEVE, R. R., ROSENTHAL, D., and BRILL, H.). Baltimore: Johns Hopkins University Press.

JASPERS, K. (1910), 'Eifersuchtswahn. Ein Beitrag zur Frage "Entwicklung einer Persönlichkeit oder Prozess"' (delusions of jealousy. A contribution to the question 'development of a personality or process'), *Z. ges. Neurol. Psychiat.*, **1,** 567.

— — (1953), *Allgemeine Psychopathologie* (general psychopathology), 6th ed. Berlin: Springer. (1st ed. 1913.)

JOHANSON, E. (1958), 'A study of Schizophrenia in the Male', *Acta psychiat. Scand.*, Suppl. **125**.

JOHNSON, D. A. W. (1979), 'Further Observations on the Duration of Depot Neuroleptic Maintenance Therapy in Schizophrenia', *Brit. J. Psychiat.*, **135,** 524–530.

JOHNSTONE, E. C., CROW, T. J., FRITH, C. D., HUSBAND. J., and KREEL, L. (1976), 'Cerebral Ventricular Size and Cognitive Impairment in Chronic Schizophrenia', *Lancet*, **iv,** 924–926.

— — — — — — CARNEY, M. W. P., and PRICE, J. S. (1978) 'Mechanism of the Antipsychotic Effect in the Treatment of Acute Schizophrenia', *Ibid.*, **i,** 848–851.

— — FRITH, C. D., GOLD, A., and STEVENS, M. (1979), 'The Outcome of Severe Acute Schizophrenic Illness after One Year', *Brit. J. Psychiat.*, **134,** 28–33.

JUNG, C. G. (1907), *The Psychology of Dementia Praecox* (trans. BRILL, A. A.). Nervous Mental Disease Monograph, Series No. 3. New York: Nervous and Mental Disease Publishing Co.

KANNER, L. (1948), *Child Psychiatry* (2nd ed.). Springfield, Ill.: Thomas.

KARLSSON, J. L. (1966), *The Biologic Basis of Schizophrenia.* Springfield, Ill.: Thomas.

— — (1970), 'Genetic Association of Giftedness and Creativity with Schizophrenia', *Hereditas*, **66,** 177–182.

— — (1973), 'An Icelandic Family Study of Schizophrenia', *Brit. J. Psychiat.*, **123,** 549–554.

— — (1982), 'Family Transmission of Schizophrenia: A Review and Synthesis', *Ibid.*, **140,** 600–606.

KAY, D. W. K., and ROTH, M. (1961), 'Environmental and Hereditary Factors in the Schizophrenias of Old Age', *J. ment. Sci.*, **107,** 649–686.

KETY, S. S., ROSENTHAL, D., WENDER, P. H., and SCHULSINGER, F. (1968), 'The Types and Prevalence of Mental Illness in the Biological and Adaptive Families of Adopted Schizophrenics', *Int. J. Psychiat.*, **1,** 345–362.

— — — — — — — — and JACOBSEN, B. (1975), *Genetic Research in Psychiatry* (ed. FIEVE, R. R., ROSENTHAL, D., and BRILL, H.) Baltimore: Johns Hopkins University Press.

KLEIN, M. (1952), *Developments in Psycho-Analysis* (RIVIERE, JOAN). London: Hogarth.

KLEIST, K. (1914), 'Aphasie und Geisteskrankheit' (aphasia and mental illness), *Münch. med. Wschr.*, **61,** 8.

— — (1921), 'Autochthonone Degenerationspsychosen' (autochthonous degeneration psychoses), *Z. ges. Neurol. Psychiat.*, **69,** 1.

— — (1923), 'Die Auffasung der Schizophrenien als Systemkrankheiten (Heredodegenerationen)' (the concept of the schizophrenias as system diseases (heredodegenerations), *Klin. Wschr.*, **1,** 962.

— — (1927), 'Gegenhalten (motorischer negativismus), Zwangsgreifen und Thalamus Opticus' (opposition (motor negativism), forced grasping and the optic thalamus), *Mschr. Psychiat. Neurol.*, **65,** 317.

KLEIST, K. (1960), 'Schizophrenic Symptoms and Cerebral Pathology', *J. ment. Sci.*, **106,** 246.

KLETT, C. J., and CAFFEY, E. M., jun. (1972), 'Evaluating the Long-term Need for Anti-Parkinson Drugs by Chronic Schizophrenics', *Arch. gen. Psychiat.*, **26,** 374.

KNIGHTS, A., and HIRSCH, S. R. (1981), '"Revealed" Depression and Drug Treatment of Schizophrenia', *Ibid.*, **38,** 806–811.

KOLLE, K. (1931), *Die Primäre Verrücktheit* (primary madness (paranoia)). Leipzig: Thieme.

—— (1957), *Der Wahnkranke in Lichte alter und neurer Psychopathologie* (the delusional patient in the light of the old and the new psychopathology). Stuttgart: Thieme.

KORNETSKY, G. (1976), 'Hyporesponsivity of Chronic Schizophrenic Patients to Dextroamphetamine', *Arch. gen. Psychiat.*, **33,** 1425–1428.

KRAEPELIN, E. (1913), *Psychiatrie, ein Lehrbuch für Studierende und Ärtzte* (psychiatry, a text-book for students and practitioners) (8th ed.), Vol. 3. Leipzig: Barth.

—— (1919), *Dementia Praecox and Paraphrenia* (trans. BARCLAY, R. M.). Edinburgh: Livingstone.

—— (1921), *Manic Depressive Insanity and Paranoia* (trans. BARCLAY, R. M.). Edinburgh: Livingstone.

KRETSCHMER, E. (1925), *Physique and Character* (trans. SPROTT, W. J. H.). London: Kegan Paul, Trench & Trubner.

—— (1950), *Die Sensitive Beziehungswahn* (sensitive delusions of reference) (3rd ed.) Berlin: Springer. (1st ed. 1918.)

LAING, R. D. (1960), *The Divided Self. An Existential Study in Sanity and Madness.* London: Tavistock Publications.

—— and ESTERSON, A. (1970), *Sanity, Madness and the Family.* Harmondsworth: Penguin.

LANGFELDT, G. (1939), *The Schizophreniform States.* Copenhagen: Munksgaard.

LAUTIN, A., ANGRIST, B., STANLEY, M., GERSHON, S., HECKL, K., and KAROBATH, M. (1980), 'Sodium Valproate in Schizophrenia: Some Biochemical Correlates', *Brit. J. Psychiat.*, **137,** 240–244.

LEFF, J. P., KUIPERS, L., BERKOWITZ, R., EBERLEIN-VRIES, R., and STURGEON, D. (1982), 'A Controlled Trial of Social Intervention in the Families of Schizophrenic Patients'. *Ibid.*, **141,** 121–134.

—— and VAUGHN, C. (1981), 'The Role of Maintenance Therapy and Relatives' Expressed Emotion in Relapse of Schizophrenia: A Two-year Follow-up', *Ibid.*, **139,** 102–104.

——, and WING, J. K. (1971), 'Trial of Maintenance Therapy in Schizophrenia', *Brit. med. J.*, **3,** 599–604.

LEONHARD, K. (1934), 'Atypische endogene Psychosen im Lichte der Familienforschung' (atypical endogenous psychose in the light of familial studies), *Z. ges. Neurol. Psychiat.*, **149,** 520.

—— (1936), *Die Defektschizophrenen Krankheitsbilder* (the clinical pictures in schizophrenic defect states). Leipzig: Thieme.

—— (1959), *Aufteilung der endogenen Psychosen* (classification of the endogenous psychoses) (2nd ed.). Berlin: Akademie Verlag.

—— (1979), *The Classification of Endogenous Psychoses* (5th ed.). Chichester: Wiley.

LETEMENDIA, F. J., HARRIS, A. D., and WILLIAMS, P. J. (1967), 'The Clinical Effects on a Population of Chronic Schizophrenic Patients of Administrative Changes in Hospital', *Brit. J. Psychiat.*, **113,** 959–971.

LEVY, L., and ROWITZ, L. (1973), *The Ecology of Mental Disorder.* New York: Behavioral Publications.

LEWINE, R., RENDERS, R., KIRCHOFER, M., MONSOUR, A., and WATT, N. (1982), 'The Empirical Heterogeneity of First Rank Symptoms in Schizophrenia', *Brit. J. Psychiat.*, **140,** 498–502.

LEWIS, A. (1934), 'Melancholia. A Clinical Survey of Depressive States', *Ibid*, **80,** 277.

LIDZ, T. (1968), 'The Family Language and the Transmission of Schizophrenia', in *The Transmission of Schizophrenia* (ed. ROSENTHAL, D., and KETY, S.) Oxford: Pergamon.

— — CORNELISON, A. T., FLECK, S., and TERRY, D. (1957a) 'The Intrafamilial Environment of the Schizophrenic Patient. I. The Father', *Psychiatry*, **20,** 329.

— — — — — — — — — (1957b), 'The Intrafamilial Environment of Schizophrenic Patients. II. Marital Schism and Marital Skew', *Amer. J. Psychiat.*, **114,** 241.

LORR, M. (ed.) (1966), *Explorations in Typing Psychotics.* New York: Pergamon.

MADEW, L., SINGER, G., and MACINDOE, I. (1966), 'Treatment and Rehabilitation in the Therapeutic Community: A Progress Report', *Med. J. Aust.*, **1,** 1112–1114.

MALAMUD, N. (1967), 'Psychiatric Disorder with Intracranial Tumors of Limbic System', *Arch. Neurol. Chicago*, **17,** 113–123.

MARICQ, H. R. (1975), 'A Two-gene Model for Schizophrenia with the Possibility to Detect Carriers of the Modifier Gene', *Acta psychiat. Scand.*, **52,** 264–282.

MARKOWE, M., STEINERT, J., and HEYWORTH-DAVIES, F. (1967), 'Insulin and Chlorpromazine in Schizophrenia: A Ten-year Comparative Study', *Brit. J. Psychiat.*, **113,** 1101–1106.

MATUSSEK, P. (1952), 'Untersuchungen über die Wahnwahrnehmung. I. Mitteilung. Veränderungen der Wahrnehmungswelt bei beginnenden schizophrenen Wahn' (investigations into delusional perception. Communication I, changes in the perceptual world in commencing schizophrenic delusion), *Arch. Psychiat. Nervenkr.*, **189,** 279.

MAY, P. R. A. (1969), *Treatment of Schizophrenia: A Comparative Study of Five Treatment Methods*, New York: Science House.

— — TUMA, A. H., DIXON, W. J., with YALE, C., THIELE, D. A., and KRAUDE, W. H. (1981), 'Schizophrenia. A Follow-up Study of the Results of Five Forms of Treatment', *Arch. gen. Psychiat.*, **38,** 776–784.

MAYER, W. (1921), 'Über paraphrene Psychosen', *Z. ges. Neurol. Psychiat.*, **71,** 187.

MAYER-GROSS, W. (1924), *Selbstschilderung der Verwirrtheit. Das oneiroide Erlebnis.* (Self descriptions in confusional states. The oneroid experience). Berlin: Springer.

MEDNICK, S. A. (1970), 'Breakdown in Individuals at High Risk for Schizophrenia: Possible Predispositional Perinatal Factors', *Mental Hyg.*, **54,** 50–63.

— — and MCNEIL, T. F. (1968), 'Current Methodology in Research on the Etiology of Schizophrenia', *Psychol. Bull.*, **70,** No. 6, 681–693.

— — SCHULSINGER, F., TEASDALE, T. W., SCHULSINGER, H., VENABLES, P. H., and ROC, D. R. (1978), 'Schizophrenia in High-risk Children: Sex Differences in Predisposing Factors', in *Cognitive Defects in the Development of Mental Illness* (ed. SERBAN, G. S.). New York: Brunner/Mazel.

MEDUNA, L. J., and MCCULLOCH, W. S. (1945), 'The Modern Concept of Schizophrenia', *Med. Clin. N. Amer.*, **29,** 147.

MELLOR, C. S., SIMS, A. C. P., and COPE, R. V. (1981), 'Change of Diagnosis in Schizophrenia and First-rank Symptoms: An Eight-year Follow-up', *Compreh. Psychiat.* **22,** 184–188.

METZGER, W. (1954), *Psychologie* (2nd ed.). Darmstadt: Steinkopf.

MEYER, A. (1906), 'Fundamental Conceptions of Dementia Praecox', *J. nerv. ment. Dis.*, **34,** 331.

— — (1910), 'The Nature and Conception of Dementia Praecox', *J. abnorm. (soc.). Psychol.*, **5,** 274.

MITSUDA, H. (ed.) (1967), *Clinical Genetics in Psychiatry. Problems in Nosological Classification.* Tokyo: Igaku-Shoin.

MORGAN, R. (1974), 'Industrial Therapy', *Brit. J. Hosp. Med.*, **11,** 231.

MORRISON, J., WINOKUR, G., CROWE, R., and CLANCY, J. (1973), 'The Iowa 500: The First Follow-up', *Arch. gen. Psychiat.*, **29,** 678–682.

MOSHER, L., POLLIN, W., and STABENAU, J. R. (1971), 'Identical Twins Discordant for Schizophrenia: Neurological Findings', *Ibid.*, **24,** 422–430.

MUNRO, A. (1982), 'Paranoia revisited', *Brit. J. Psychiat.*, **141,** 344–349.

NAMYSLOWSKA, I. (1975), 'Thought Disorders in Schizophrenia Before and After Pharmacological Treatment', *Compreh. Psychiat.*, **16,** 37–42.

NASRALLAH, H. A., JACOBY, C. G., McCALLEY-WHITTERS, M., and KUPERMAN, S. (1982), 'Cerebral Ventricular Enlargement in Subtypes of Chronic Schizophrenia', *Arch. gen. Psychiat.*, **39,** 774–777.

NATIONAL INSTITUTE OF MENTAL HEALTH, 1964 Collaborative Study Group (1964), 'Phenothiazine Treatment in Acute Schizophrenia: Effectiveness', *Ibid.*, **10,** 246–261.

NITSON, M., STAPLETON, J. H., and BENDER, M. P. (1974), 'Movement and Drama Therapy with Long-standing Schizophrenics', *Brit. J. med. Psychol.*, **47,** 101–119.

O'BRIEN, C. P., HAMM, K. B., RAY, B. A., PIERCE, J. F., LUBORSKY, L., and MINTY, J. (1972), 'Group vs. Individual Psychotherapy with Schizophrenics', *Arch. gen. Psychiat.*, **27,** 474–478.

O'CONNOR, N., HERON, A., and CARSTAIRS, G. M. (1956), 'Work Performance of Chronic Schizophrenics', *Occup. Psychol.*, **30,** 153–164.

ØDEGAARD, Ø. (1970), 'The Multifactorial Theory of Inheritance in Predisposition for Schizophrenia', in *Genetic Factors in Schizophrenia* (ed. KAPLAN, A. R.). Springfield, Ill.: Thomas.

OWEN, F., CROSS, A. J., CROW, T. J., LONGDEN, A., POULTER, M., and RILEY, G. J. (1978), 'Increased Dopamine-receptor Sensitivity in Schizophrenia', *Lancet*, **ii,** 223–226.

PARNAS, J., SCHULSINGER, F., TEASDALE, T. W., SCHULSINGER, H., FELDMAN, P. M., and MEDNICK, S. A. (1982), 'Perinatal Complications and Clinical Outcome within the Schizophrenic Spectrum', *Brit. J. Psychiat.*, **140,** 416–420.

PAULEIKHOFF, B. (1957), *Atypische Psychosen* (atypical psychoses). Basle: Karger.

PAYNE, R. W., and HIRST, H. (1957), 'Over inclusive Thinking in a Depressive and a Control Group', *J. Consul. Psychol.*, **21,** 186–188.

PERRIS, C. (1973), 'Cycloid Psychoses: Historical Background and Nosology', *Nord. psychiat. Tidsskr.*, **27,** 369–378.

— — (1974), 'A Study of Cycloid Psychoses', *Acta psychiat. Scand.*, Suppl. **253.**

— — (1978), 'Morbidity Suppressive Effect of Lithium Carbonate in Cycloid Psychoses', *Arch. gen. Psychiat.*, **35,** 328–331.

PETRILOWITSCH, N. (1958a), *Beiträge zu einer Struktur-Psychopathologie* (contributions to a structure psychopathology). Basle: Karger.

— — (1958b), 'Zur Strukturtheorie der endogenen Psychosen' (a contribution to the structure theory of the endogenous psychoses), *Schweiz. Arch. Neurol. Psychiat.*, **81,** 312.

PINARD, G., PRENOVEAU, Y., FLIESEN, W., ELIE, E., et al. (1972), 'Le Pimozide et la Réintégration Sociale des Schizophrènes Chroniques', *Encèphale*, **61,** 53–66.

POLLIN, W., ALLEN, M., HEFFER, A., STABENAU, J., and HRUBEC, Z. (1969), 'Psychopathology in 15,909 Pairs of Veteran Twins: Evidence for a Genetic Factor in the Pathogenesis of Schizophrenia and its Relative Absence in Psycho-neuroses', *Amer. J. Psychiat.*, **126,** 597–609.

PRIEN, R. F., and KLETT, C. J. (1972), 'An Appraisal of the Long-Term Use of Tranquillizing Medication with Hospitalized Chronic Schizophrenics: A Review of the Drug Discontinuation Literature', *Schizophrenia Bull.*, **5,** 64–73.

PRITCHARD, M. (1967a), 'Prognosis of schizophrenia before and after pharmacotherapy. I. Short-term Outcome', *Brit. J. Psychiat.*, **113,** 1345–1352.

— — (1967b), 'II. Three-year Follow-up', *Ibid.*, **113,** 1353–1359.

PROCCI, W. R. (1976), 'Schizo-affective Psychosis: Fact or Fiction?', *Arch. gen. Psychiat.*, **33,** 1167–1178.

QUITKIN, F., RIFKIN, A., and KLEIN, D. F. (1976), 'Neurologic Soft Signs in Schizophrenia and Character Disorders', *Ibid.*, **33,** 845–853.

REICH, L., WEISS, B. L., COBLE, P., McPARTLAND, R., and KUPFER, D. J. (1975), 'Sleep Disturbance in Schizophrenia. A Revisit', *Ibid.*, **32,** 51–55.

RIFKIN, A., QUITKIN, F., and KLEIN, D. F. (1975), 'Akinesia. A Poorly Recognized Drug-induced Extra-pyramidal Disorder', *Ibid.*, **32,** 672–674.

RIMMER, J., COLE, S., JACOBSON, B., KETY, S. S., ROSENTHAL, D., and SCHULSINGER, F. (1979), Personal and social characteristics differentiating adoptive relatives of schizophrenics and non-schizophrenics: a preliminary report based on interviews. *Compr. Pyschiatry*, **20,** 151–158.

ROCHFORD, J. M., DETRE, T., TUCKER, G. J., and HARRAOW, M. (1970), 'Neuropsychological Impairments in Functional Psychiatric Diseases', *Arch. gen. Psychiat.*, **22,** 114–119.

ROGERS, C. R., GENDLIN, E. G., KIESLER, D. J., and TRUAX, C. B. (1967), *The Therapeutic Relationship and its Impact: A Study of Psychotherapy with Schizophrenics*. Wisconsin: University of Wisconsin Press.

ROSENTHAL, D. (1962), 'Familial Concordance by Sex with Respect to Schizophrenia', *Psychol. Bull.*, **59,** 401–421.

— — WENDER, P. H., KETY, S. S., SCHULSINGER, F., WELNER, J., and ØSTERGAARD, L. (1968) 'Schizophrenics' offspring reared in adoptive homes'. In *The Transmission of Schizophrenia* (ed. ROSANTHAL, D., and KETY, S. S.). Oxford: Pergamon.

— — — — — — WELNER, J., and SCHULSINGER, F. S. (1971), 'The Adopted-away Offspring of Schizophrenics', *Amer. J. Psychiat.*, **128,** 307–311.

ROTH, M. (1955), 'The Natural History of Mental Disorder in Old Age', *J. ment. Sci.*, **101,** 281.

— — (1957), 'Interaction of Genetic and Environmental Factors in the Causation of Schizophrenia', in *Schizophrenia—Somatic Aspects* (ed. RICHTER, D.). London: Pergamon Press.

ROTROSEN, J., ANGRIST, B. M., GERSHON, S., SACHAR, E. J., and HALPERN, F. S. (1976), 'Dopamine Receptor Alteration in Schizophrenia: Neuroendocrine Evidence', *Psychopharmacology*, **51,** 1–7.

ROWNTREE, D. W., and KAY, W. W. (1952), 'Clinical Biochemical and Physiological Studies in Cases of Recurrent Schizophrenia', *J. ment. Sci.*, **98,** 100.

RÜMKE, H. C. (1957), 'The Clinical Differentiation within the Group of Schizophrenias', *Second International Congress for Psychiatry* (*Zürich*, 1957) *Report*, **1,** 302. Orell Füssli.

SALETU, B., SALETU, M., MARASA, J., MEDNICK, S., and SCHULSINGER, F. (1975), 'Acoustic Evoked Potentials in Offspring of Schizophrenic Mothers ("High Risk" Children for Schizophrenia)', *Clin. Electroencephalog.*, **6,** 92–102.

SARTORIUS, N., JABLENSKY, A., and SHAPIRO, R. (1977), Two-year follow-up of the patients included in the WHO International Pilot Study of Schizophrenia. *Psychol. Med.*, **7,** 529–541.

SARTRE, J. P. (1957), *Being and Nothingness* (trans. BARNES, H. E.). London: Methuen.

SCHARFETTER, C. (1981), 'Subdividing the Functional Psychoses: A Family Heredity Approach', *Psychol. Med.*, **11,** 637–640.

SCHELDRICK, C., JABLENSKY, A., SARTORIUS, N., and SHEPHERD, M. (1977), 'Schizophrenia Succeeded by Affective Illness: Catamnestic Study', *Ibid.*, **7,** 619–624.

SCHMIDT, L. J., REINHARDT, A. M., KANE, R. L., and OLSEN, D. M. (1977), 'The Mentally Ill in Nursing Homes, New Back Wards in the Community', *Arch. gen Psychiat.*, **34,** 687–691.

SCHNEIDER, C. (1930), *Die Psychologie der Schizophrenen* (the psychology of schizophrenics). Leipzig: Thieme.

— — (1942), *Die schizophrenen Symptomverbände* (the schizophrenic symptom complexes). Berlin: Springer.

SCHNEIDER, K. (1957), 'Primäre und sekundäre Symptomen bei Schizophrenie' (primary and secondary symptoms in schizophrenia), *Fortschr. Neurol. Psychiat.*, **25,** 487.

— — (1958), *Psychopathic Personalities* (trans. HAMILTON, M. W.). London: Cassel.

SCHNEIDER, K. (1959), *Clinical Psychopathology* (trans. HAMILTON, M. W.). New York: Grune & Stratton.

SCHREBER, D. P. (1955), *Memoirs of my Nervous Illness* (trans. MACALPINE, I., and HUNTER, R. A.). London: Dawson.

SCHRÖDER, P. (1920a), 'Degeneratives Irresein und Degenerationspsychosen' (degenerative insanity and degeneration psychoses), *Z. ges. Neurol. Psychiat.*, **60,** 119.

— — (1920b), *Die Spielbreite der Symptome bei Manisch-Depressiven Irresein und den Degenerationspsychosen* (the range of symptoms in manic depressive insanity and the degeneration psychoses). Berlin: Karger.

— — (1926a), 'Das Halluzinieren' (hallucinating), *Z. ges. Neurol. Psychiat.*, **101,** 599.

— — (1926b), 'Über Degenerationspsychosen (Metabolische Erkrankungen)' (on degeneration psychoses (metabolic illnesses)), *Ibid.*, **101,** 539.

SCHULSINGER, H. (1976), 'A Ten-year Follow-up of Children of Schizophrenic Mothers (1976)', *Acta psychiat. Scand.*, **53,** 371–386.

SEEMAN, P., LEE, T., CHAU-WONG, M., and WONG, K. (1976), 'Antipsychotic Drug Doses and Neuroleptic/Dopamine Receptors', *Nature*, **21,** 717–718.

SERAFETINIDES, E. A., COGER, R. W., MARTIN, J., and DYMOND, M. A. (1981), 'Schizophrenic Symptomatology and Cerebral Dominance Patterns: A Comparison of EEG, AER and BPRS Measures', *Compreh. Psychiat.*, **22,** 218.

SHIELDS, J. (1977), 'High Risk for Schizophrenia', *Psychol. Med.*, **7,** 7–10.

SINGER, M. T. (1967), 'Family Transactions and Schizophrenia: I, Recent Research Findings', in *The Origins of Schizophrenia*, pp. 147–164. Amsterdam: Excerpta Medica International Series No. 151.

— — and WYNNE, L. C. (1963), 'Differentiating Characteristics of Parents of Childhood Schizophrenics, Childhood Neurotics, and Young Adult Schizophrenics', *Amer. J. Psychiat.*, **120,** 234–243.

— — — — (1965), 'Thought Disorder and Family Relations of Schizophrenics: IV, Results and Implications', *Arch. gen. Psychiat.*, **12,** 201–212.

SLATER, E. (1953), *Psychotic and Neurotic Illnesses in Twins*. Special Report of the Medical Research Council, 278. London: H.M.S.O.

— — (1958), 'The Monogenic Theory of Schizophrenia', *Acta genet., Basel*, **8,** 50.

— — (1968), 'A Review of Earlier Evidence on Genetic Factors in Schizophrenia', in *The Transmission of Schizophrenia* (ed. ROSENTHAL, D., and KETY, S.). Oxford: Pergamon.

— — (1969), 'The Schizophrenia-like Illnesses of Epilepsy', in *Current Problems in Neuropsychiatry* (ed. HERRINGTON, R. N.). London: RMPA.

— — BEARD, A. W., and GLITHERO, E. (1963), 'The Schizophrenia-like Psychoses of Epilepsy', *Brit. J. Psychiat.*, **109,** 95–150.

— — and COWIE, V. (1971), *The Genetics of Mental Disorders*. London: Oxford University Press.

SPECHT, G. (1905), 'Chronische Manie und Paronoia' (chronic mania and paranoia), *Zbl. Nervenheilk.*, **28,** 590.

SPITZER, R. L., ENDICOTT, J., and ROBINS, E. (1975), 'Research Diagnostic Criteria (RDC)', *Psychopharmacol. Bull.*, **11,** 22–24.

STABENAU, J., and POLLIN, W. (1967), 'Early Characteristics of Monozygotic Twins Discordant for Schizophrenia', *Arch. gen. Psychiat.*, **17,** 723–734.

STEPHENS, J. H., ASTRUP, C., and MANGRUM, J. C. (1966), 'Prognostic Factors in Recovered and Deteriorated Schizophrenics', *Amer. J. Psychiat.*, **122,** 1116–1121.

STEVENS, B. (1969), *Marriage and Fertility of Women suffering from Schizophrenia or Affective Disorders*. London: Oxford University Press.

STRANSKY, K. (1904), 'Zur Lehre von der Dementia Praecox' (a contribution to the theory of dementia praecox), *Zbl. Nervenheilk.*, **27,** 1.

STRAUSS, J. S., and CARPENTER, W. T. (1974), 'Characteristic symptoms and outcome in schizophrenia', *Arch. gen. Psychiat.*, **30,** 429–434.

SUNDBY, P. (1955), 'Occupation and Insanity. The Frequency Distribution of Psychoses within Different Occupational Groups, with Special Reference to Psychosis among Ordinary Seamen', *Acta psychiat. Scand.,* Suppl. **106**.

TANAKA, Y., HAZAMA, H., KAWAHARA, R., and KOBAYASHI, K. (1981), 'Computerized Tomography of the Brain in Schizophrenic Patients: A Controlled Study', *Ibid.*, **63,** 191–197.

TAYLOR, D. C. (1975), 'Factors Influencing the Occurrence of Schizophrenia-like Psychosis in Patients with Temporal Lobe Epilepsy', *Psychol. Med.*, **5,** 249–254.

TAYLOR, F. KRAUPL (1981), 'On Pseudo-hallucinations', *Ibid.*, **11,** 265–271.

TORREY, E. F. (1980), 'Neurological Abnormalities in Schizophrenic Patients', *Biol. Psychiat.*, **15,** 381–388.

TSUANG, M. T. (1979), 'Schizo-affective Disorder—dead or alive', *Arch. gen. Psychiat.*, **36,** 633–634.

— — DEMPSEY, G. M., DVOREDSKY, A., and STRUSS, A. (1977), 'A Family History Study of Schizo-affective Disorder', *Biol. Psychiat.*, **12,** 331–338.

— — — — —and RAUSCHER, F. (1976), 'A study of "atypical schizophrenia",' *Arch. gen. Psychiat.*, **33,** 1157–1160.

VAILLANT, G. E. (1963), 'Manic-depressive Heredity and Remission in Schizophrenia', *Brit. J. Psychiat.*, **109,** 746–749.

VAUGHN, C. E., and LEFF, J. P. (1976), 'The Influence of Family and Social Factors on the Course of Psychiatric Illness', *Ibid.*, **129,** 125–137.

VENABLES, P. H., MEDNICK, S. A., SCHULSINGER, F., RAMAN, A. C., BELL, B., DALAIS, J. C., and FLETCHER, R. P. (1978), 'Screening for Risk of Mental Illness', in *Cognitive Defects in the Development of Mental Illness* (ed. SERBAN, G.). New York: Brunner/Mazel.

— — and WING, J. K. (1962), 'Level of Arousal and the Sub-classification of Schizophrenia', *Arch. gen. Psychiat.*, **7,** 114–119.

WADSWORTH, M. V., WELLS, B. W. P. and SCOTT, R. F. (1962), 'Quantity and Quality of Industrial Therapy', *Lancet*, **2,** 1375–1376.

WALLIS, G. G. (1972), 'Stress as a predictor in schizophrenia'. *Brit. J. Psychiat.*, **120,** 375–384.

WEINBERGER, D. R., BIGELOW, L. B., KLEINMAN, J. E., KLEIN, S. T., ROSENBLATT, J. R., and WYATT, R. J. (1980a), 'Cerebral Ventricular Enlargement in Chronic Schizophrenia: An Association with Poor Response to Treatment', *Arch. gen. Psychiat.*, **37,** 11–13.

— — CANNON-SPOOR, E., POKIN, S. G., and WYATT, R. J. (1980b), 'Premorbid Adjustment and CT Scan Abnormalities in Chronic Schizophrenia', *Amer. J. Psychiat.*, **137,** 1410–1413.

— — TORREY, F. E., NEOPHYTIDES, A. N., and WYATT, R. J. (1979a), 'Lateral Cerebral Ventricular Enlargement in Chronic Schizophrenia', *Arch. gen. Psychiat.*, **36,** 735–739.

— — — — — — — — (1979b), 'Structural Abnormalities in the Cerebral Cortex of Chronic Schizophrenic Patients', *Ibid.*, **36,** 935–939.

WELNER, A., CROUGHAN, J., FISHMAN, R., and ROBINS, E. (1977), 'The Group of Schizo-affective and Related Psychoses: A Follow-up Study', *Compreh. Psychiat.*, **18,** 413–422.

WELZER, Z., and FISHMAN, R. (1979), 'The Group of Schizoaffective and Related Psychoses: IV. A Family Study', *Ibid.*, **20,** 21–25.

WENDER, P. H., ROSENTHAL, D., and KETY, S. S. (1968), 'A Psychiatric Assessment of the Adoptive Parents of Schizophrenics', in *The Transmission of Schizophrenia* (ed. ROSENTHAL, D., and KETY, S. S.), p. 235. Harmondsworth: Penguin.

— — — — — — SCHULSINGER, F., and WELNER, J. (1974), 'Cross Fostering. A Research Strategy for Clarifying the Role of Genetic and Experiential Factors in the Etiology of Schizophrenia', *Arch. gen. Psychiat.*, **30,** 121–128.

WENDER, P. H., ROSENTHAL, D., ZAHU, T. P., and KETY, S. S. (1971), 'The Psychiatric Adjustment of the Adopting Parents of Schizophrenics', *Amer. J. Psychiat.*, **127,** 1013–1018.

WEYGANDT, W. (1907), 'Kritische Bemerkungen zur Psychologie der Dementia Praecox' (critical observations on the psychology of dementia praecox), *Mschr. Psychiat. Neurol.*, **22,** 289.

WILD, C., SINGER, M., ROSMAN, B., RICCI, J., and LIDZ, T. (1965), 'Measured Disordered Styles of Thinking', *Arch. gen. Psychiat.*, **13,** 471.

WING, J. K. (1966), 'Five-year Outcome in Early Schizophrenia', *Proc. R. Soc. Med.*, **59,** 17–18.

WING, J. K., COOPER, J. E., and SARTORIUS, N. (1974), *The Measurement and Classification of Psychiatric Symptoms*. London: Cambridge University Press.

— — and NIXON, J. (1975), 'Discriminating Symptoms in Schizophrenia', *Arch. gen. Psychiat.*, **32,** 853–859.

WINOKUR, G., and TSUANG, M. T. (1975), 'A Clinical and Family History Comparison of Good Outcome and Poor Outcome Schizophrenia', *Neuropsychobiology*, **1,** 59–64.

WORLD HEALTH ORGANIZATION (1973), *Report of the International Pilot Study of Schizophrenia*, Vol. 1. Geneva: WHO Press.

— — (1979), *Schizophrenia. An International Follow-up Study*. Chichester: Wiley.

WYNNE, L. C. (1967), 'Family Transactions and Schizophrenia: Conceptual Considerations for a Research Strategy', in *The Origins of Schizophrenia*, pp. 165–178. Amsterdam: Excerpta Medica International Series No. 151.

YORKSTON, N. J., GRUZELIER, J. H., ZAKI, S. A., HOLLANDER, D., PITCHER, D. R., and SERGEANT, H. G. S. (1977), Propanolol as an adjunct to the treatment of schizophrenia', *Lancet*, **ii,** 575–578.

ZAHN, T. P. (1964), 'Autonomic Reactivity and Behaviour in Schizophrenia', *Psychiat. Res. Rep.*, **19,** 156–173.

ZERBIN-RÜDIN, E. (1967), 'Endogene Psychosen', In: *Handbuch der Humangenetik* (ed. BECKER, P. E.), Vol. 2, p. 446. Stuttgart: Thieme.

ZUTT, J. (1952), 'Der ästhetische Erlebnisbereich und seine krankhafte Abwandlungen. Ein Beitrag zum Wahnproblem' (the aesthetic zone of experience and its morbid modifications), *Nervenarzt*, **23,** 163.

— — and KUHLENKAMPF, C. (1958), *Das paranoide Syndrom in anthropologischer Sicht* (the paranoid syndrome from the anthropological point of view). Berlin: Springer.

Further Reading

ACKNER, B. (1954), 'Depersonalisation I', *J. ment. Sci.*, **100,** 838.

— — (1954), 'Depersonalisation II', *Ibid.*, **100,** 854.

ASTRUP, C. (1958), 'Klinisch-experimentelle Untersuchungen bei verschiedenen Formen von Schizophrenien' (clinical-experimental investigations in different forms of schizophrenia), *Psychiat. Neurol. u. med. Psychol., Lpz.*, **10,** 355.

— — (1979), *The Chronic Schizophrenias*. Oslo: Universitetforlaget.

BLEULER, M. (1951), 'The Psychiatry of Cerebral Diseases', *Brit. med. J.*, **2,** 1233.

— — (1955), 'Research and Changes in Concepts in the Study of Schizophrenia 1941–1950', *Bull. Isaac Ray Med. Lib.*, **3,** 1.

— — (1978), *The Schizophrenic Disorders: Long-term Patient and Family Studies* (trans. CLEMENS, S. M.). New Haven: Yale University Press.

BUMKE, O. (1932), *Handbuch der Geisteskrankheiten* (handbook of mental disorders): Vol. 9, *Schizophrenie*. Berlin: Springer.

CONRAD, K. (1959), 'Bemerkungen zum psychopathologischen Problem des Beziehungswahns' (observations on the psychopathological problem of delusions of reference), *Dtsch. med. Wschr.*, **84,** 1.

CORNU, F. (1958). 'Katamnestische Erhebungen über den Verlauf einfacher Schizophrenien' (the course of simple schizophrenia as revealed by follow-up studies), *Psychiat. et neurol. Basel*, **135,** 129.

FEINBERG, I., and GARMAN, E. M. (1961), 'Studies of Thought Disorder in Schizophrenia II. Plausible and Implausible Errors on a Modification of the Progressive Matrices Test', *Arch. gen. Psychiat.*, **4,** 191.

— — and MERCER, M. (1960), 'Studies of Thought Disorder in Schizophrenia, I. Chapman's Test of Distractability and Associative Intrusion in Schizophrenia and Organic Brain Disease'', *Ibid.*, **2,** 504.

FISH, F. J. (1957), 'The Classification of Schizophrenia—The Views of Kleist and his Co-Workers', *J. ment. Sci.*, **103,** 443.

— — (1959), 'Senile Paranoid States', *Geront. clin.*, **1,** 127.

— — (1960), 'Senile Schizophrenia', *J. ment. Sci.*, **106,** 938.

— — (1961), 'Existentialism and Psychiatry', *Ibid.*, **107,** 978.

FREEMAN, T., CAMERON, J. L., and MCGHIE, A. (1958a), *Chronic Schizophrenia*. London: Tavistock Publications.

— — — — — — (1958b), *Chronic Schizophrenics*. London: Tavistock Publications.

FREYHAN, F. A. (1958), 'Eugene Bleuler's Concept of the Group of Schizophrenias at Mid Century', *Amer. J. Psychiat.*, **114,** 769.

GJESSING, R. (1935), 'Beiträge zur Pathophysiologie der katatonen Erregung. III. Mitteilung. Über periodisch rezidivierende katatone Erregung, mit kritischen Beginn und Abschluss' (contributions to the pathophysiology of catatonic excitement. Communication III, on periodic recurrent catatonic stupor with sudden onset and termination), *Arch. Psychiat.*, **104,** 355.

— — (1939), 'Beiträge zur Kenntnis der Pathophysiologie periodisch katatoner Zustände. IV. Mitteilung. Versuch einer Ausgleichung der Funktions-störungen' (contributions to the knowledge of the pathophysiology of periodic catatonic states. Communication IV, an attempt at an adjustment of the disorders of function), *Ibid.*, **109,** 525.

GJESSING, R. (1953a), 'Beiträge zur Somatologie der periodischen Katatonie. Mitteilung V. Verlaufstypen B' (contributions to the pathophysiology of periodic catatonia. Communication V, the B type course of illness), *ibid.*, **191,** 191–219.

— — (1953b), 'Beiträge zur Somatologie der periodischen Katatonie: Mitteilung VI. Umweltfactoren die sich nicht beiseitigen lassen' (contributions to the pathophysiology of periodic catatonia. Communication VI, environmental factors which cannot be ignored), *Ibid.*, **191,** 220.

— — (1953c), 'Beiträge zur Somatologie der periodischen Katatonie. Mitteilung VII. Wertung der Befunde, I' (contributions to the pathophysiology of periodic catatonia. Communication VII, evaluation of the findings, I), *Ibid.*, **191,** 247.

— — (1953d), 'Beiträge zur Somatologie der periodischen Katatonie. Mitteilung VIII. Wertung der Befunde, II' (contributions to pathophysiology of periodic catatonia. Communication VIII, evaluation of the findings, II), *Ibid.*, **191,** 297.

GOLDSTEIN, K., and SCHEERER, M. (1941), 'Abstract and Concrete Behaviour. An Experimental Study with Special Tests', *Psychol. Monogr.*, **53,** No. 239.

GORNAL, A. G., EGLETIS, B., MILLER, A., STOKES, A. B., and DEWAN, J. G. (1953), 'Longterm Clinical and Metabolic Observations in Periodic Catatonia', *Amer. J. Psychiat.*, **109,** 584.

HANFMANN, E., and KASANIN, J. S. (1942), *Conceptual Thinking in Schizophrenia.* Nervous and Mental Diseases Monograph, No. 67. New York: Nervous and Mental Disease Publishing Co.

HEDENSTRÖM, V., and SCHORSCH, G. (1959), 'E.E.G.—Befunde bei epileptischen Dämmer- und Verstimmungszuständen' (E.E.G. findings in epileptic twilight states and dysthymic states), *Arch.-Psychiat. Nervenkr.*, **199,** 311.

HOHLENBERG, J. (1954), *Sören Kierkegaard* (trans. CROXALL, T. H.). London: Routledge & Kegan Paul.

HUBER, G. (1955), 'Das Wahnproblem (1939–1954)' (the problem of delusions), *Fortschr. Neurol. Psychiat.*, **23,** 6.

— — (1957), 'Die coenästhetische Schizophrenie' (coenaesthetic schizophrenia), *Ibid.*, **25,** 491.

JANZARIK, W. (1950), 'Die Paranoia (Gaupp)', *Arch. Psychiat. Nervenkr.*, **183,** 328.

— — (1955), 'Der Wahn schizophrener Prägung in den psychotischen Episoden der Epileptiker und die schizophrene Wahnwahrnehmung' (delusions with a schizophrenic character in epileptic psychotic episodes and schizophrenic delusional perception), *Fortschr. Neurol. Psychiat.*, **23,** 533.

JOST, F., and GIBITZ, H. J. (1957), 'Über grundsätzliche Unterschiede zwischen hypochondrischen Zustände und Körper-Organ Halluzinationen' (on the basic differences between hypochondriacal conditions and body-organ hallucinations), *Wien. Z. Nervenheilk.*, **14,** 249.

JUNG, C. G. (1939), 'On the Psychogenesis of Schizophrenia', *J. ment Sci.*, **85,** 999.

— — (1958), 'Die Schizophrenie', *Schweiz. Arch. Neurol. Psychiat.*, **81,** 163.

KAHN, E. (1959), 'An Appraisal of Existential Analysis I and II', *Psychiat. Quart.*, **31,** 203, 417.

KASANIN, J. S. (ed.) (1944), *Language and Thought in Schizophrenia.* Berkeley: California University Press.

KISKER, K. P. (1960), *Der Erlebniswandel des Schizophrenen* (the change in experience of the schizophrenic). Berlin: Springer.

— — MEYER, J.-E., MÜLLER, M., and STRÖMGREN, E. (1972), *Klinische Psychiatrie I.* Berlin: Springer.

— — and STRÖTZEL, L. (1960), 'Zur vergleichenden Situationsanalyse beginnender Schizophrenien und erlebnisreaktiver Fehlentwicklungen bei Jugendlichen' (a contribution to a comparative analysis of the situation in commencing schizophrenias and faulty developments in adolescents occurring as a reaction to experience), *Arch. Psychiat. Nervenkr.*, **202,** 1.

KLEIST, K. (1928), 'Über zykloide, paranoide und epileptoide Psychosen und über die Frage der Degenerationspsychosen' (on cycloid, paranoid and epileptoid psychoses and the question of degeneration psychoses). *Schweiz. Arch. Neurol. Psychiat.*, **23**, 1.

— — (1930), 'Zur hirnpathologischen Auffassung der schizophrenen Grundstörungen: Die alogische Denkstörung' (a contribution to the interpretation of the fundamental disorders in schizophrenia on the basis of brain pathology: the alogical thought disorder), *Ibid.*, **26**, 99.

— — (1935), 'Leitvortrag über Gehirnpathologie und Klinik der Persönlichkeit und Körperlichkeit' (opening lecture on brain pathology and clinical disorders of the personality and bodily awareness), *Arch. Psychiat. Nervenkr.*, **103**, 301.

— — (1939), 'Störungen des Denkens und ihre hirnpathologische Grundlagen' (thought disorder and its basis in brain pathology), in *Gegenwartsprobleme der psychiatrisch-neurologisch Forschung* (ed. ROGGENBAU, C. H.). Stuttgart: Enke.

— — (1943), 'Die Katatonien', *Nervenarzt*, **16**, 1.

— — (1947), 'Die paranoiden Schizophrenien', *Ibid.*, **18**, 481, 544.

— — (1954a), 'Beitrag zur gerichtlichen Bedeutung der Angstpsychose (contribution to the legal significance of the anxiety psychosis), in *Richter und Arzt* (ed. KLEIST, K.). Munich: Reinhardt.

— — (1954b), 'Die gerichtliche und praktische Bedeutung von atypischen seelischen Störungen (ängstliche-ekstatische und ratlose Psychosen)' (the legal and practical significance of atypical psychological disorders (anxious-ecstatic and perplexed psychoses), *Ibid.* Munich: Reinhardt.

— — and DRIEST, W. (1937), 'Die Katatonien auf Grund katamnestischer Untersuchungen. I. Teil. Die als Katatonien verkannten Degenerationspsychosen' (catatonias as revealed by follow-up studies. Part I, degeneration psychoses which were mistaken for catatonias), *Z. ges. Neurol. Psychiat.*, **157**, 479.

— — FAUST, E., and SCHÜRMANN, C. (1960a), 'Weitere klinisch-katamnestische Untersuchungen an Hebephrenien. I. Mitteilung Die Hebephrenien' (further clinical follow-up studies in hebephrenias. Communication I, the hebephrenias), *Arch. Psychiat. Nervenkr.*, **200**, 541.

— — — — — — (1960b), 'Weitere klinisch-katamnestische Untersuchungen an Hebephrenien. II. Mitteilung. Als Hebephrenien verkannte andere Arten von Schizophrenien' (further clinical follow-up studies in hebephrenias. Communication II, other kinds of schizophrenia mistaken for hebephrenia), *Ibid.*, **200**, 653.

— — LEONHARD, K., and FAUST, E. (1950), 'Die Hebephrenien auf Grund von katamnestischen Untersuchungen. I. Teil' (follow-up studies of the hebephrenias, Part I), *Ibid.*, **185**, 773.

— — — — — — (1951), 'Die Hebephrenien auf Grund von katamnestischen Untersuchungen. II. Teil' (follow-up studies of the hebephrenias, Part II), *Ibid.*, **186**, 1.

— — — — and SCHWAB, H. (1940), 'Die Katatonien auf Grund katamnestischer Untersuchungen. III. Teil. Formen und Verläufe der eigentlich Katatonie' (follow-up studies of catatonia, Part III, forms and courses of illness of true catatonia), *Z. ges. Neurol. Psychiat.*, **168**, 535.

— — and SCHWAB, H. (1950), 'Die verworrenen Schizophrenien auf Grund katamnestischer Untersuchungen. II. Teil. Die denkverwirrten Schizophrenien' (follow-up studies on confused schizophrenics, Part II, the thought confused schizophrenics), *Arch. Psychiat. Nervenkr.*, **184**, 28.

KOEHLER, K. (1979), 'First-rank Symptoms of Schizophrenia: Questions Concerning Clinical Boundaries', *Brit. J. Psychiat.*, **134**, 236–248.

KOLLE, K. (1955), *Die endogenen Psychosen—das delphische Orakel der Psychiatrie* (the endogenous psychoses—the delphic oracle of psychiatry). Munich: Lehrmanns.

KRAPF, E. (1928), 'Differential diagnostische Schwierigkeiten in Grenzgebiet von Epilepsie und Schizophrenie' (differential diagnostic difficulties in the boundary area between epilepsy and schizophrenia), *Zbl. ges. Neurol. Psychiat.*, **48**, 12.

KRETSCHMER, E. (1952), *A Textbook of Medical Psychology* (trans. STRAUSS, E. B.). London: Hogarth Press.

KUROSAWA, R. (1960), 'Untersuchung der atypischen endogenen Psychosen (periodischen Psychosen)' (investigation of atypical endogenous psychoses), *Mie med. J.*, **10,** 303.

LANDOLT, H. (1955), 'Über Verstimmungen Dämmerzustände und schizophrene Zustandbilder bei Epilepsie' (dysthymic states, twilight states and schizophrenic clinical pictures in epilepsy), *Schweiz. Arch. Neurol. Psychiat.*, **76,** 313.

—— (1958), 'Serial Electroencephalographic Investigations during Psychotic Episodes in Epileptic Patients and during Schizophrenic Attacks: in Lectures on Epilepsy', *Folia psychiat. neerl.*, Suppl. **4**.

—— (1960), *Die Temporallappenepilepsie und ihre Psychopathologie* (temporal lobe epilepsy and its psychopathology). Basle: Karger.

LANGAN, T. (1959), *The Meaning of Heidegger*. London: Routledge & Kegan Paul.

LANGFELDT, G. (1952), 'Some Points regarding the Symptomatology and Diagnosis of Schizophrenia', *Acta psychiat. Scand.*, Suppl. **80**.

—— (1956), 'The Prognosis in Schizophrenia', *Ibid.*, Suppl. **110**.

LEONHARD, K. (1948), *Grundlagen der Psychiatrie* (the fundamentals of psychiatry). Stuttgart: Enke.

—— (1950), 'Eine Sippe affektvoller Paraphrenie mit gehäuften Erkrankungen aus Verwandte-Ehen. Zugleich ein Beitrag zur Frage der Paranoia' (a sibship with affect-laden paraphrenia and an excess of illness in consanguineous marriages (also a contribution to the question of paranoia)), *Arch. Psychiat. Nervenkr.*, **184,** 291.

—— (1960), 'Die Atypische Psychosen und Kleist's Lehre von Endogenen Psychosen' (the atypical psychoses and Kleist's views on endogenous psychoses), in *Psychiatrie der Gegenwart*, Vol. II (ed. GRUHLE, H. W., JUNG, R., MAYER-GROSS, W., and MÜLLER, M.). Berlin: Springer.

—— (1961), 'Cycloid Psychoses—Endogenous Psychoses which are neither Schizophrenic nor Manic Depressive', *J. ment. Sci.*, **107,** 633.

LIDZ, T., CORNELISON, A. R., TERRY, D., and FLECK, S. (1958), 'The Intra-familial Environment of the Schizophrenic Patient VI. The Transmission of Irrationality', *Arch. Neurol. Psychiat., Chicago*, **79,** 305.

—— FLECK, S., CORNELISON, A., and TERRY, D. (1958), 'Schizophrenia and the Family', *Psychiatry*, **21,** 21.

——PARKER, B., and CORNELISON, A. R. (1956), 'Role of the Father in the Family Environment of the Schizophrenic Patient', *Amer. J. Psychiat.*, **113,** 126–132.

MATUSSEK, P. (1953), 'Untersuchungen über die Wahnwahrnehmung. II. Mitteilung. Die auf einem abnormen Vorrang von Wesenseigenschaften beruhrenden Eigentümlichkeiten von Wahnwahrnehmung' (investigations into delusional perception. Communication II, the characteristics of delusional perception which depend on an abnormal precedence of essential properties), *Schweiz. Arch. Neurol. Psychiat.*, **71,** 189.

MAYER-GROSS, W., SLATER, E., and ROTH, M. (1972), *Clinical Psychiatry*. London: Baillière, Tindall and Cassell.

MEDUNA, L. J. (1950), *Oneirophrenia*. Urbana: Illinois University Press.

MEYER, A. (1951), *The Collected Papers of Adolf Meyer*, Vol. II: *Psychiatry*. Baltimore: Johns Hopkins Press.

MEYER, G., LEONHARD, K., and KLEIST, K. (1944), 'Die paranoiden Schizophrenien auf Grund katamnestischer Untersuchungen, IV. Teil. Die paranoide Demenz (Progressive Auto-und Somatopsychose)' (follow-up studies of paranoid schizophrenia. Part IV, paranoid dementia (progressive auto and somatopsychosis)), *Z. ges. Neurol. Psychiat.*, **177,** 114.

MILGRAM, N. A. (1959), 'Preference for Abstract versus Concrete Word Meanings in Schizophrenic and Brain-damaged Patients', *J. clin. Psychol.*, **15,** 201.

MORAN, L. J. (1953), 'Vocabulary Knowledge and Usage among Normal and Schizophrenic Subjects', *Psychol. Monogr.*, **67,** No. 20.

MÜLLER-SUUR, H. (1961), 'Das sogennante Praecoxgefühl' (the so-called praecox-feeling), *Ibid.*, **29,** 145.

ØDEGARD, Ø. (1957), 'The Epidemiology of Schizophrenia in Norway'. *Second International Congress for Psychiatry (Zürich, 1957) Report*, **3,** 49. Zürich: Orell Füssli.

PASSMORE, J. (1957), *A Hundred Years of Philosophy* London: Duckworth.

PAULEIKHOFF, B. (1957), 'Über die seelischer Struktur Wahnkranker' (the psychic structure of delusional patients), *Arch. Psychiat. Nervenkr.*, **196,** 356.

PAYNE, R. W., MATUSSEK, P., and GEORGE, E. I. (1959), 'An Experimental Study of Thought Disorder', *J. ment. Sci.*, **105,** 627.

PENFIELD, W., and JASPER, H. (1954), *Epilepsy and the Functional Anatomy of the Human Brain*. London: Churchill.

RITTER, M. R., and KLEIST, K. (1956), 'Psychosen der Ratlosigkeit' (perplexity psychoses), *Arch. Psychiat. Nervenkr.*, **195,** 163.

SAHLI, H. R. (1959), 'Übergänge manisch-depressiver und schizophrener Verläufe' (change-over to the other functional psychosis occurring in the course of manic depressive and schizophrenic illnesses), *Psychiat. et Neurol. Basel*, **138,** 98.

SCHRÖDER, P. (1922), 'Degenerationspsychosen und Dementia Praecox' (degeneration psychoses and dementia praecox), *Arch. Psychiat. Nervenkr.*, **66,** 1.

— — (1928), 'Fremddenken und Fremdhandeln' (alienation of thinking and acting), *Mschr. Psychiat. Neurol.*, **68,** 515.

SEDGEWICK, P. (1982), *Psychopolitics*. London: Pluto Press.

SHAKOW, D. (1946), *The Nature of Deterioration in Schizophrenic Conditions*. Nervous and Mental Disorders Monograph Series, No. 40. New York: Nervous and Mental Disease Publishing Co.

SHEPHERD, M. (1959), 'The Social Outcome of Early Schizophrenia', *Psychiat. et Neurol., Basel*, **137,** 224.

SPIEL, W. S. (1961), *Die endogenen Psychosen des Kindes und Jugendalters* (the endogenous psychoses of childhood and adolescence). Basle: Karger.

STENGEL, E. (1945), 'A Study of Some Clinical Aspects of the Relationship between Obsessional Neurosis and Psychotic Reaction Types', *J. ment. Sci.*, **91,** 166.

STRAUS, E. W., and GRIFFITH, R. M. (1955), 'Pseudoreversibility of Catatonic Stupor', *Amer. J. Psychiat.*, **111,** 680.

SULLIVAN, H. S. (1953), *The Interpersonal Theory of Psychiatry*. New York: Norton.

ULMER, R. A. (1976), *On the Development of a Token Economy Mental Hospital Treatment Program*. New York: Wiley.

VERBEEK, E. (1959a), 'De la Paranoia', *Psychiat. et Neurol., Basel*, **137,** 257.

— — (1959b), 'Le délire dermatozoaire et le problème de l'hallucinoze tactile chronique' (the delusion of infestation and the problem of chronic tactile hallucinosis), *Ibid.*, **138,** 217.

VIGOTSKY, L. S. (1934), 'Thought in Schizophrenia', *Arch. Neurol. Psychiat., Chicago*, **31,** 1063.

WAKOH, T., TAKEKOSHI, A., YOSHIMOTO, S., HIRAMOTO, K., and KUROSAWA, R. (1960), 'Pathophysiological Study of the Periodic Psychosis (Atypical Endogenous Psychosis) with Special Reference to the Comparison with the Chronic Schizophrenia', *Mie med. J.*, **10,** 317.

WALTHER-BÜEL, H. (1951), *Die Psychiatrie der Hirngeschwülste* (the psychiatry of brain tumours). Vienna: Springer.

WOGGON, B. (1979), 'Neuroleptika-Absetzversucherei chronisch schizophrenen Patienten I. Literaturzusammenfassung' (investigations on discontinuation of neuroleptic drugs for chronic schizophrenic patients. I. Summary of the literature), *Int. Pharmacopsychiat.*, **14,** 34–56.

WYRSCH, J. (1960), 'Klinik der Schizophrenie' (clinical aspects of schizophrenia), in *Psychiatrie der Gegenwart* (present-day psychiatry), Vol. II (ed. GRUHLE, H. W., JUNG, R., MAYER-GROSS, W., and MÜLLER, M.). Berlin: Springer.

ZANETTI, G. (1957), 'Le schizophrenie 'post-traumatiche'. Rivista sinteticocritica. Considerazione su di un caso personale' (the 'post-traumatic' schizophrenias. A synthetic critical review. Consideration of one personal case), *G. med. Marca. trevig.*, **14,** 1.

ZUTT, J. (1957), 'Blick und Stimme. Beitrag zur Grundlegung einer verstehenden Anthropologie' (look and voice. A contribution to the foundation of understanding anthropology), *Nervenarzt*, **28,** 350.

INDEX

abstract attitudes, Goldstein's, 40, 41
abstract thinking, disorders of, 78, 94
accessory symptoms, 90, 177
acetylcholine, 28
acute schizophrenia
  anxiety in, 62, 90
  depression in, 53, 54, 62
  diagnostic problems in, 90
  oneiroid states in, 74, 119–20
  outcome after, 135
  relation to chronic states 12, (*Table* 7) 95–7
  suicide attempts, 74
  treatment, 140–2, 149–51
acute schizophrenic shifts
  Conrad's theories on, 128, 180, (*Fig.* 8) 181–5
  levels of awareness in, 74
  misidentifications in, 76
  and phases in course of illness, (*Figs.* 3 and 4) 128–32
adience, 79
adolescent crises, 32, 63, 164–5
adoption studies, 10–13
advertence, attitude of, 69–70, 79
affect, blunting of, 64
  in hebephrenia, 87–8, 89, 95
  in paraphrenia, 92, 95
  violent crime with, 74, 167
affect, disorders of, 63–5
  in catatonia, 71, 78, 86
  as fundamental symptoms, 177
  in hebephrenia, 78, 87–8, 89
  in paraphrenia, 82–3, 90, 92, 93, 95
  prognosis and, 135–6
affect, dissociation of, in violent criminals, 63, 167
affect, flattening of, 63
  in desultory syndrome, 80
  in hebephrenia, 88
  prognosis and, 135
  in proskinetic catatonia, 86
affect, incongruity of, 63, 135
affect, stiffening of, 63
affect-laden paraphrenia, 82–3, 164
affective ambivalence, 64
affective disorders (*see also* depression, mania and schizo-affective psychoses)
  differential diagnosis, 103, 163–4
  paranoid schizophrenia and, 90, 103–5
  precipitating factors in, 37
affective loading of delusions, 64, 82–3
age disorientation, 23, 25
age of onset
  concept of dementia praecox and, 1, 98–9
  prognosis and, 101–2, 134–5
  of schizo-affective psychoses, 113
  of schizophrenia, (*Table* 8) 99–100, 123, 127
aggressive behaviour, 82, 89
aggressive schizophrenia, 79
agrammatism, 43, 44, 85
agranulocytosis after neuroleptics, 154
akathisia after neuroleptics, 147, 153
akinesia, 72
  after neuroleptics, 152, 153
  in motility psychosis, 116–7
  in periodic catatonia, 83–4
alcoholism, 30, 168
alogia, Kleist's 43–4, 45
ambitendency, 64, 66, 86
ambivalence, 64, 120, 177
amphetamine
  experimental administration of, 26, 28–9
  psychosis, 25–6, 30–1, 170–1
amylobarbitone, sodium, in stupor, 70, 72
anastrophe, 182
anoxia, hippocampal damage after, 16
anti-cholinergic drug effects, 28, 153
anti-parkinsonian drugs, 28, 150, 153
anti-social behaviour, 73–4, 88
  in psychopaths, 167
anxiety
  in affect-laden paraphrenia, 82
  at onset of illness, 58, 62

anxiety (*cont.*)
in 'paranoid depression' 104–5
in pseudoneurotic schizophrenia, 120
psychoses, 115
reducing level of awareness, 74
anxiety-elation psychosis, 82, 115–6
aphasic symptoms in schizophrenia, 42–3
apocalyptic phase, Conrad's 183, (*Fig.* 8) 184
apomorphine, growth hormone responses to, 28
apophany, Conrad's 50, 180–2, (*Fig.* 8) 184
apperception, Wundt's concept of, 176
'approximate answers', syndrome of, 167
Argwöhnische depression, 104
arousal, high state of, 16
asphyxia, neonatal, 22
association psychology, Bleuler's 39, 48, 176–7
Astrup's classification of schizophrenia, (*Table* 7) 95–7
asyndetic thinking, 39
attention, disorders of, 75
atypical schizophrenia, 81
auditory hallucinations, 56–60
aversion induced by, 57, 69, 70, 92
in catatonia, 87
continuous, 56, 57, 92
neologisms and, 44
in paranoid states, 52
in paraphrenia, 90, 91, 92, 93
prognosis and, 135
relation to formal thought disorder, 46, 57
autism, infantile, 124, 125
autistic hebephrenia, 89, 97
autistic thinking, 39
autochthonous delusions (*see also* delusional ideas), 51
automatic obedience, 67, 86
aversion
attitude of, 69
hallucinatory, 57, 69, 70, 92
awareness, levels of *see* consciousness

baclofen, 29
behaviour disorder(s) (*see also* motor activity and individual disorders)
childhood, 125, 166
in schizophrenia, 65–74
behavioural therapy, 157–9
benzamides, 147
benzhexol, 153
benztropine, 153
Berze's theory of schizophrenia, 177–8
beta-adrenergic blockers, 29
Binswanger's theory of schizophrenia, 193, 195–9
biochemical changes in schizophrenia, 25–30, 122–3
bipolar psychoses (*see also* cycloid psychoses), 115
birth complicatins, 15–16, 22
Bleuler('s),
on ambivalence, 64, 177
concepts of schizophrenia, 1–2, 99, 176–7
on disorders of association, 39, 45, 48, 176–7
on 'double book keeping', 75
latent schizophrenia, 120
simple schizophrenia, 78, 79
blood flow, regional cerebral, 24
bodily hallucinations, 60–1
in fantastic paraphrenia, 93
in hypochondriacal paraphrenia, 54, 90
in paranoid states, 52
prognosis and, 135
in Schneider's desultory syndrome, 80
symptom of first rank, 102
body build, 33, 134
bouffée délirante, 111
brain development, symmetry of (*see also* left/right...), 10
brain disease, coarse (*see also* epilepsy)
in aetiology of schizophrenia, 21, 176
clouding of consciousness in, 74–5
hallucinations in, 30, 56, 163, 168
schizophrenic-like psychoses in, 21, 168–9
thought disorder in, 38, 41
brain function in schizophrenia (*see also* neuro-transmitters), 23–5
brain injury, association with schizophrenia, 16, 21–3, 169–70
bromide psychosis, 163, 170
butaclamol, 27
butyrophenones, 26, 29, 147, (*Table* 11) 148

Cameron
on childhood schizophrenia, 124–6
classification by, 79

Cameron (*cont.*)
on formal thought disorder, 39–40, 46
Capgras syndrome, 76
Carpenter's diagnostic criteria, 161, 162
catatonia, 78
age of onset, (*Table* 8) 100, 127
behaviour disorders, 64, 65–74
classification, 81, 83–4, 85–7
course of illness, (*Figs.* 3 and 4) 130–1
epileptic twilight states resembling, 169
manneristic, 86
negativistic, 86
parakinetic, 85
periodic, 83–4, 122–3
pernicious, 123, 132
prognosis and outcome, 132, 135
in schizo-affective psychoses, 112
speech-inactive, 87
speech-prompt, 87
theories of, 183, (*Fig.* 8) 184, 187
thought disorders, 42, 43, 44, 45
catatonic psychoses, Astrup's, (*Table* 7) 95–7
'Catcher in the Rye' syndrome, 164
CATEGO diagnostic criteria, 161, 162
caudate nucleus, 26, 27, 28
cerebral organic pseudoschizophrenia, 118, 119
characterogenic pseudoschizophrenia, 118, 119
childbirth precipitating schizophrenia, 15–16, 22
childhood
behaviour disorder, 125, 166
development
family relationships and, 33–5
Freud's theory of, 185–6
schizophrenia, 121, 124–5
children of schizophrenics (*see also* parents)
adoption studies on, 10–13, 19
electrodermal studies on, 15–17
risks to, (*Table* 3) 7, 13–14, 17–19
chlorpromazine
in acute schizophrenia, 149, 150
mode of action, 27, 29
outcome after, 132
side-effects, 153–4
structure, 27, (*Table* 11, *Fig.* 6) 148, (*Fig.* 7), 149
chlorprothixene, (*Table* 11) 148, 150
choreiform movements
in parakinetic catatonia, 85
choreiform movements (*cont.*)
in tardive dyskinesia, 154
chronic schizophrenia
amphetamine response in, 28–9
brain changes, 24–5
course, (*Fig.* 2) 128–9
delusions in, 52, 53, 54
depressive symptoms in, 62
drug therapy, 151–2
hallucinations in, 57, 58, 60
memory falsification, 76
rehabilitation, 138, 155–9
relation to acute states, 12, (*Table* 7) 95–7
cingulate gyrus, 26
clozapine, anti-cholinergic effect of, 28
coarsening of thinking, 95
collecting and hoarding, 72–3, 74, 88
command automatism, 67
community psychiatry, 143–4
computer-assisted tomography (CAT scans), 24–5
conceptual thinking, disorder of, 38, 47, 71
concrete attitudes, Goldstein's, 40–41, 45
concrete thinking in confabulatory paraphrenia, 94
condensation in thought disorder, 39, 45
confabulations, 76
in anxiety-elation psychosis, 116
in speech-inactive catatonia, 87
confabulatory paraphrenia, 93–4, 97
confused schizophrenia, Kleist's, 81, 90
confusion
in cycloid psychoses, 114
in epilepsy, 169
in oneiroid states, 119
as a prognostic sign, 135, (*Table* 10) 136
psychoses, 112, 116
in puerperal affective psychoses, 112
of speech in schizophasia, 83
confusional hallucinosis, 55
Conrad's theory of schizophrenia, 128, 180, (*Fig.* 8) 181–4
consciousness, clouding of, 55, 74–5, 120
consciousness, disorders of, 38, 74–5
in epileptics, 168
in oneiroid states, 119–20
in theories of schizophrenia, 177–8
consciousness, restriction of, 74

constitutional (predisposing) factors (*see also* brain disease, brain injury, genetic factors, personality and physique), 6–33
control, loss of
of thought, 48–9
of voluntary acts, 65–6, 80
co-operation (*Mitmachen*), 67, 68
and advertance, 69
in proskinetic catatonia, 86
in stupor, 72
corpus striatum, 28
criminal(s)
behaviour in schizophrenics, 74, 87–8
hysterical pseudodementia in, 167
lack of emotion in, 63, 167
crisis intervention, 144
critical flicker fusion theshold, 16
cycloid psychoses (*see also* anxiety-elation psychosis, confusion psychoses and motility psychosis), 3, 81, 111
classification, 114–8
prognosis, 135
schizophreniform psychoses and, 118
treatment, 152

Dasein
Binswanger's schizophrenic, 193–8
Heidegger's concept of, 191–4, 195, 199
day hospital in rehabilitation, 143, 155
deafness
in aetiology of schizophrenia, 36–7
auditory hallucinations in, 56
degeneration psychoses *see* schizo-affective psychoses
déjà vécu and *déjà vu* experiences, 75–6
delusional beliefs, 70, 74
delusional experiences in oneiroid states, 119–20
delusional ideas, 51, 75
becoming memories, 76
in paraphrenia, 90
in thought withdrawal syndrome, 80
delusional memories, 76–7
delusional misinterpretations, 50, 52
delusional mood, 50
delusional perceptions, 50–2
Conrad on, 181, 182
first rank symptom, 103
Matussek's interpretation of, 180–1
misidentifications, 76–7
delusions, 49–55, 78
in affect-laden paraphrenia, 82–3
affective loading, 64, 82–3
in amphetamine psychosis, 170
autochthonous (*see also* delusional ideas), 51
back-dating of, 76
in cycloid psychoses, 114
in depression, 62, 104–5
in epilepsy, 168
in expansive paraphrenia, 94–5
in fantastic paraphrenia, 93
Freudian theory on, 187
of grandeur, 53–4, 93, 94–5
hypochondriacal, 54
of jealousy, 171
in organic hallucinosis, 168
in paranoia, 98, 99, 101
paranoid *see* paranoid delusions
persecutory *see* persecutory delusions
primary, 49, 51, 52, 80, 168
secondary, 52
of self-reference, 50, 53, 106
démence précoce, 1
dementia, silly 79
dementia infantilis 124–5
dementia praecox 1–2, 98, 175
dementia precocissima, 124
depersonalization, 64–5, 116
depot neuroleptics, 62, 151–2
depression
Argwöhnische, 104
differential diagnosis, 163–4
paranoid symptoms in, 104–5
in schizo-affective psychoses, 111–7
in schizophrenia, 61–2, 105
hallucinations causing, 58, 62
prognosis and, 135, (*Table* 10) 136
treatment, 154
stupor in, 72
derailment of speech, 42, 45
in hypnagogic and hypnopompic states, 46
in paraphrenia, 91, 93
in thought withdrawal syndrome, 80
derealization, 65, 116
dereistic thinking, 39
desultory syndrome, Schneider's, 80, 95
desultory thinking, 80
detached schizophrenia, 79
developmental pseudoschizophrenia, 118, 119
diagnosis
differential, 163–71
and rapport with patient, 63–4

diagnosis (*cont.*)
of schizo-affective psychoses, 111–5
of schizophrenia, 101–3, 160–3
'diathesis-stress' model, 16
dibenzothiazepines, 147
diethylpropion abuse, 26
diphenyl-butyl-piperidines, 147
dipropylacetic sodium (sodium valproate), 29
Disablement Resettlement Officer, 143
disease, definition of, 174–5
displacement in thought disorder, 39
dopamine hypothesis of schizophrenia, 25–9
'double-bind' relationship, 35
'double book keeping' (orientation), 75, 119
dream-like changes of consciousness, 74, 119–20
drivelling speech, 42
drivelling syndrome, Schneider's, 80, 97
drug action and the dopamine hypothesis, 25–9
drug 'holiday', 151
drug intoxications simulating schizophrenia, 25–6, 30–1, 112, 163, 170–1
drug therapy (*see also* anti-parkinsonian drugs and neuroleptic drugs), 146–54
and outcome, 136–7
versus psychotherapy, 145
dyskinesia, tardive, 154
dystonia, acute, 153

eccentric hebephrenia, 88, 97
écho de pensée, 59
echolalia, 69
echopraxia, 67, 69
ecstasy, mood of, 61
in affect-laden paraphrenia, 82
in anxiety-elation psychosis, 115–6
in oneiroid states, 119
ego in theories of schizophrenia, 185, 187, 188, 189
electrical hallucinations, 60
electroconvulsive therapy (ECT)
compared with other therapies, 145
in cycloid psychoses, 152
for depressive symptoms, 105, 154
in stupor, 72, 154
electrodermal responses, 14–17
electroencephalographic (EEG) changes
in epileptics, 168, 169
in high-risk children, 15
in periodic catatonia, 123
in schizo-affectives, 113
in schizophrenia, 23–4
elevated mood, 61, 94
emotion
disorders of (*see also* affect and mood), 61–5
expressed (EE), and rehabilitation, 137–8
endocrine disorders and schizophrenia, 30
endogenous pseudoschizophrenia, 118–9
energy potential, Conrad's, 183
environment, family *see* family environment
environmental (precipitating) factors (*see also* physical illness, psychogenic reactions, social isolation and stress, psychological), 33–7
in periodic catatonia, 122
and prognosis, 113, 135
and reactions in schizophrenia, 175
epilepsy
association with schizophrenia, 20–1, 22
schizophrenic-like psychoses in, 4, 20, 30, 168–9
Epstein Test of Over-inclusion, 45
ethical deterioration, 73, 74, 87, 88
exacerbation, definition of, 128
excitements
catatonic, 71, 86, 87
hallucinatory, 57
in hebephrenia, 88, 89
in negativism, 72
in periodic catatonia, 83, 84, 122
in pernicious catatonia, 123
existentialism, 196–5
existentialist theories of schizophrenia, 195–200
exogenous pseudoschizophrenia, 118, 119
expansive autopsychoses, 115
expansive paraphrenia, 94–5, 97
extra-pyramidal side-effects
and dopamine activity, 26, 27, 28
and molecular structure of neuroleptics, 147
treatment, 149, 150, 152–3

facial expression
  in catatonia, 68–9, 83, 85, 87
  in hebephrenia, 88, 89
  in stupor, 71–2
family (*see also* children)
  advice to, before discharge of patient, 143
  schizophrenic, Laing's theory of, 201
family environment (*see also* twin studies)
  in aetiology of schizophrenia, 10–13, 33–5, 125
  and hospital admission, 141
  in success of rehabilitation, 137–9, 157
family history and prognosis, 134
family incidence
  of paranoia, 101
  of schizo-affective psychoses, 113–4
  of schizophrenia, (*Table* 3) 6–7, 17–19, 81, 83
fantasiophrenia, 164
fantastic confabulations, 76, 87, 93
fantastic hallucinosis, 55, 56
fantastic paraphrenia, 82, 93, 97
fantastic symptoms in affect-laden paraphrenia, 82–3
fantasy thinking, 39
Federn's theory of schizophrenia, 188–9
Feighner's St Louis criteria, 162
fertility in schizophrenics, 19
figure-ground relationships, 41
fixation point, Freudian, 186
flexibilities cerea (waxy flexibility), 68, 72
flight of ideas, 70
flupenthixol, 27, 28, (*Table* 11) 148, 152
fluphenazine, 27, (*Table* 11) 148–9, 152
fluspirilene, 147, 152
forced grasping, 67–8, 69
forced responsiveness (*see also* individual symptoms), 67–8, 69–70
formal thought disorder, 38–47
  Bleuler on, 39, 48, 176–7
  causing confusion, 119
  Freud on, 45, 46, 187
  in letter writing, 71
  in paraphrenia, 93, 94
  positive and negative, 45
  in simple schizophrenia, 79
Frankfurt school, 81
Fregoli syndrome, 76
Freudian theories on schizophrenia, 185–90
functional hallucinations, 59
functional pseudoschizophrenia, 119
functional psychosis, 118
fundamental symptoms, Bleuler's, 177
fusion of speech and thought, 42, 45, 46

galvanic skin responses (GSR), 15, 16
gamma-aminobutyric acid (GABA), 29
ganser states, 167
Ganzheitspsychologie, school of, 183–4
Gedankenlautwerden (thoughts spoken aloud), 59, 91
  Conrad's theory of, 182
  in desultory syndrome, 80
  diagnostic significance of, 102, 161, 163
  in paranoid epileptic psychosis, 168
Gegenhalten (opposition), 67, 68, 86
genes, advantages of schizophrenic, 19
genetic factors (*see also* family incidence and twin studies)
  in schizo-affective psychoses, 113–4
  in schizophrenia, 6–20
genetic models of schizophrenia, 17–20
Gestalt theories of schizophrenia, 40, 51, 180–5
Gjessing, on periodic catatonia, (*Fig.* 1) 122–3
Goldstein on thought disorder, 40–1, 45
Goldstein-Sheerer Object Sorting Test, 45
grafted schizophrenia, 121–2
grandiose delusions, 53–4, 93, 94–5
grimacing, 69, 83, 85
group psychotherapy, 145–6
growth hormone responses
  after neuroleptics, 30
  to apomorphine, 28
guilt
  paranoid delusions related to, 104
  prognosis and, 135, (*Table* 10) 136

hallucinations, 55–61
  anxiety caused by, 58, 62
  auditory *see* auditory hallucinations
  bodily *see* bodily hallucinations
  Conrad's theory of, 182
  in cycloid psychoses, 116
  definition, 55
  and depression, 62, 163
  in diagnosis, 78–9, 102, 161, 162

hallucinations (*cont.*)
in epileptic paranoid psychosis, 168
Freudian theory on, 187
functional, 59
in hebephrenia, 89
in oneiroid states, 119–20
in paraphrenia, 82, 90–1, 92, 93, 124
prognosis and, 135
pseudo-, 55, 89, 116
reflex, 60–1
sexual, 60, 135
of smell and taste, 61, 90
visual *see* visual hallucinations
hallucinatory aversion, 57, 69, 70, 92
hallucinatory excitements, 57
hallucinatory instructions, 58
hallucinatory voices (*see also* auditory hallucinations), 56–9
hallucinogens, 30
hallucinosis
confusional, 55
drug-induced, 30–1, 170–1
fantastic, 55, 56
organic, 30, 112, 168
Schröder's syndromes of, 55–6
self-reference, 55–6, 62
verbal, 55, 56
haloperidol, 26, 28, 147, (*Table* 11) 148, 150
Haltungsverharren, 68, 86
handling, catatonic, 66–7
hebephrenia, 1, 78–9, 81
age of onset, (*Table* 8) 100, 127
autistic, 89, 97
classification, 87–9
Conrad's theory of, 183, (*Fig.* 8) 184
depressive mood in, 62
eccentric, 88, 97
ethical deterioration, 73, 74, 87, 88
Freudian theory of, 187
prognosis, 135
ranking of severity in, 97
shallow, 88–9, 97
silly, 87–8, 97
hebephrenic psychoses in Astrup's classification, (*Table* 7) 95–7
Heidegger and existentialism, 191–3, 195, 199
Heidelberg school, 180
Heller's dementia infantilis, 124–5
heredity *see* genetic factors and family incidence
high-risk children, studies on, 13–14, 15–17
hippocampus, damage to, 16
hoarding and collecting, 72–3, 74, 88
homosexuality, Freudian theory on, 187–8
hospital
admission, 140–2
discharge, preparation for, 142–3, 155–7
hyperkinesia, 83–4, 116–7
hypnagogic states, 46
hypnopompic states, 46
hypochondriacal delusions, 54
hypochondriacal paraphrenia, 85, 90–1, 97
hypomanic mood, 61
hypotension after neuroleptics, 149, 153
hypotonia of consciousness, 177–8
hypoxia and development of epilepsy, 22
hysteria, diagnosis of, 166–7
hysterical pseudodementia, 47, 167

id, in Freudian theory of schizophrenia, 185–6, 187
idealism, 194
ideas of self-reference (*see also* delusional ideas), 53
in affect-laden paraphrenia, 82
in cycloid psychoses, 115–6
in hebephrenia, 89
in paranoid states, 90, 106
illness, definition of, 174–5
illusions, 55, 116
impulsive behaviour, catatonic, 72, 84
incoherence
caused by hallucinatory voices, 57, 92
in cycloid psychoses, 116, 117
of thought, 43–4, 45
incoherent paraphrenia, 90, 92, 97
incontinence, double, 72, 73, 92
industrial therapy units, 156–7
infantile autism, 124, 125
inhibition of thought, 47–8
insight
lack of, in mania, 164
in pseudo-hallucinations, 55
institutionalization, 155–6, 158
intellectual ambivalence, 64
intelligence (*see also* mental defect)
and abstract attitude, 40
in late paraphrenia, 124
and prognosis, 134

International Pilot Study of Schizophrenia (IPSS), 103, 160–2
interpenetration of themes, 39–40, 46
interpretative psychology, 173–4
intertwining movements, 66–7, 86
intoxications *see* drug intoxications
isolation
  Goldstein's concept of, 41
  social *see* social isolation
isomeric forms of neuroleptics, 27

Jasper('s)
  concept of understandability, 2–3, 49, 102, 105, 180
  on psychic process, 107, (*Table* 9) 108
  'understanding' psychology, 49, 102, 172–4
jaundice, obstructive, 154
jealousy, morbid, 171
Jung's theory of schizophrenia, 190

Kanner's infantile autism, 124, 125
Kant's idealism, 194–5
Kierkegaard and existentialism, 191, 194
Klein's theory of schizophrenia, 189
Kleist
  on classification, 2, 81
  on cycloid marginal psychoses, 3, 115, 117
  on speech disorders, 42–3
  on thought disorders, 43–4, 45
Kraepelin's
  classification of schizophrenia, 78
  concept of paranoia and paraphrenia, 99, 101, 105
  definition of dementia praecox, 1, 98–9
  paranoid depression, 104
  schizophasia, 83
Kretschmer's
  sensitive Beziehungswahn, 106
  theory of schizophrenia, 178
Kuhlenkamf's concept of paranoia, 200

L-dopa
  growth hormone response to, 28
  schizophrenic symptoms after, 26
Laing's theory of schizophrenia, 200–1
Langfeldt's schizophreniform psychoses, 118
late paraphrenia, 36–7, 100, 123–4
latent schizophrenia, 120
left/right handedness, 10, 23
left/right hemisphere symptoms, 23–4
Leonhard
  classification of schizophrenia by, 81–97
  on cycloid psychoses, 115, 117
letter writing, 70–1
leucotomy, prefrontal, 154
libidinal development, Freudian, 185–6, 189
life-stresses *see* stress, psychological
limbic system, 16, 22, 26
literal paraphasia, 42, 44
lithium carbonate, 152
lysergic acid diethylamide (LSD), 30

magnet reaction, 67–8
mania
  differential diagnosis, 163, 164
  excitement in, 71
  in mixed affective states, 61
  paranoid attitudes in, 104, 164
manic-depressive symptoms in schizo-affective psychoses, 111–2, 114–5, 116, 117
mannerisms
  in eccentric hebephrenia, 88
  in letter writing, 70
  of movement, 66
  of posture, 68
  of speech, 45, 70, 88
manneristic behaviour patterns, 72–3
manneristic catatonia, 86
marginal psychoses *see* schizo-affective psychoses
Matussek on delusional perception, 51–2, 180–1
Mayer-Gross on oneiroid states, 119–20
memory, delusional, 76–7
memory disorders (*see also* confabulations and misidentifications), 38, 75–7
memory distortion, 76
memory falsifications, 76, 82
  in confabulatory paraphrenia, 93–4
  in morbid jealousy, 171
mental defect (*see also* intelligence), childhood schizophrenia with, 121–2, 125, 126

mental deterioration as a diagnostic criterion, 101
mental set, perseveration of, 67
mental slowness of schizophrenics, 45
mescaline, 30
metabolic changes in periodic catatonia, 30, (*Fig.* 1) 122–3
methotrimeprazine, (*Table* 11) 148
methylphenidate, 26
metonyms, 39
Meyer's theory of schizophrenia, 6, 178–80
milieu treatment, 145
mimic expression, 68–9, 84, 117
mind, development of, Freudian, 185
misidentifications, delusional, 76–7
  Conrad's theory on, 181–2
  in fantastic paraphrenia, 93
  transient, in confusion psychosis, 116
Mitgehen, 67, 69, 86
Mitmachen see co-operation
mixed psychoses (*see also* schizo-affective psychoses), 111
mood, disorders of (*see also* anxiety, delusional mood, depression, ecstasy and perplexity), 61–2
  in anxiety-elation psychosis, 115–6
  in hebephrenia, 87, 88, 89
morbid jealousy, 171
motility psychosis, 84, 111–2, 116–7
motor activity, disorders of (*see also* movement disorders and speech disorders), 65–72
  in catatonia, 78, 83, 86, 87
  in childhood schizophrenia, 124, 125
  in motility psychosis, 116–7
  in paranoid schizophrenia, 78
movement blocking, 66
movement disorders (*see also* individual symptoms), 66–8
  after neuroleptics, 152–3, 154
  in catatonia, 83–4, 85, 86
  in motility psychosis, 116–7
muteness, 70, 116

negative formal thought disorder, 45
negativism, 69, 72, 86, 135
negativistic catatonia, 86
neologisms, 44–5
  in dementia infantilis, 125
  in schizophasia, 83
  technical, 44, 90
neostratum, neuroleptic action on, 27
nervous system disorders (*see also* brain disease and brain injury)
  in aetiology of schizophrenia, 21–5
  Kleist's theory of, 81
neuro-transmitters in aetiology of schizophrenia, 25–9
neuroleptic drugs (*see also* individual agents), 146–52
  in acute schizophrenia, 141, 149–51
  anti-dopaminergic effect, 26–8
  chemical structure, 27, (*Figs.* 5–7, *Table* 11) 146–9
  depot, 62, 151–2
  differences in response to, 28
  and gamma-aminobutyric acid, 29
  and noradrenaline, 29
  and outcome, 132–3
  side-effects (*see also* extrapyramidal side-effects), 152–4
  thought disorders after, 39
neurological 'soft sign' deficits, 23
neurosis in psuedoneurotic schizophrenia, 120
nitrogen balance in periodic catatonia, (*Fig.* 1) 122
non-organic psychoses, 103
non-systematic schizophrenia, 81, 82–4
non-understandable symptoms *see* Jasper's concept of understandability
noöpsyche, Stransky's, 176
noradrenaline, 29
nucleus accumbens, 27

obedience, automatic, 67, 86
obsessional states, 165–6
obsessional symptoms in schizophrenia, 48–9, 51, 88
obstruction of movement, 66
occupational therapy, 142, 143
odour, hallucinations of, 61
omission in speech, 42, 45
oneiroid states (oneirophrenia), 74, 111, 119–20
opposition (*Gegenhalten*), 67, 68, 86
organic hallucinosis, 30, 112, 168
organic psychiatric syndromes, 41
orientation (*see also* age disorientation)
  double, 75, 119
  false, 23, 75
orphenadrine, 153
out-patient treatment, 141, 142–3, 151, 154

over-activity, catatonic, 71
over-inclusion (*see also* derailment and fusion), 39, 40, 45, 47

paragrammatism, 42–3
parakinesia, 66–7, 69, 83, 135
parakinetic catatonia, 85
paralogia, 43–4, 45, 47
paranoia
  concepts of, 98–9, 101
  definition, 108
  morbid jealousy resembling, 171
paranoid delusions (*see also* persecutory delusions), 52–3, 54–5
  affective loading, 64, 82, 83
  Freudian theory on, 187–8
  in late paraphrenia, 123–4
paranoid depression, 98, 104–5
  prognosis, 105, 109
paranoid personality, 98
  abnormal, development of psychosis in, (*Table* 9) 105–9, 128
  querulous, 105, 106–7
paranoid psychoses
  after bromide, 170
  in amphetamine addicts, 25–6, 30–1, 170–1
  Astrup's classification, (*Table* 7) 95–7
  epileptic, 30, 168
paranoid schizophrenia (*see also* paraphrenia), 78
  affective loading, 64, 82
  age of onset, (*Table* 8) 99–100, 127
  classification, 81, 82–3, 89–95
  Conrad's theory on, 183, (*Fig.* 8) 184
  course of illness, (*Figs.* 3 and 4) 130–1
  delusions of jealousy, 171
  illusions, 55
  letter writing, 70–1
  memory falsifications, 76–7
  perseveration of theme, 47
  prognosis, 109, 135
  speech disorders, 70
paranoid states, 98–110
paranoid symptoms (*see also* delusions and hallucinations), 78
  in affective disorders, 103–5, 163, 164
  and limbic dysfunction, 22
  in senile schizophrenia, 124
paraphasia, literal, 42, 44
paraphasia, verbal, 42–3, 44
paraphrenia (*see also* paranoid schizophrenia)
  affect-laden, 82–3, 97, 164
  concepts of, 1, 99
  confabulatory, 93–4, 97
  definition, 107–8
  depression in, 62
  expansive, 94–5, 97
  fantastic, 70, 93, 97
  hypochondriacal, 85, 90–1, 97
  incoherent 90, 92, 97
  late, 36–7, 100, 123–4
  'phonemic', 85, 91–2, 97
  ranking of severity in, 97
parent-child relationships, 33–4, 35
parents of schizophrenics (*see also* children)
  behaviour of, 33–5, 125
  risk to, (*Table* 3) 7
Parkinsonism, symptoms of *see* extra-pyramidal side-effects
Parkinson's disease, dopamine deficiency in, 26
passivity, feelings of, 52, 65–6, 163
perception, disorders of (*see also* delusional perception, hallucinations and illusions), 55–61, 94
pericyazine, (*Table* 11) 148
periodic catatonia, 83–4, 122–3
pernicious catatonia, 123, 132
perphenazine, (*Table* 11) 148
perplexity, 62, 116
  reducing level of awareness, 74
  in thought withdrawal syndrome, 80
persecutory delusions (*see also* paranoid delusions), 52–3, 54
  in amphetamine psychosis, 170
  in organic hallucinosis, 112, 168
  with anxiety and depression, 62, 104–5
perseveration, 67
  of theme of thought, 47, 67
  of words or phrases, 67, 70
personality
  abnormal, in morbid jealousy, 171
  deterioration and age of onset, 78, 101–2, 109
  development in theories of schizophrenia, 6, 32, 178–9
  paranoid *see* paranoid personality
  in paranoid depressions, 105
  pre-morbid, (*Table* 6) 31–3, 36, 134
  psychopathic *see* psychopathic personality

personality (*cont.*)
  schizoid *see* schizoid personality
Petrilowitsch's theory of schizophrenia, 183–4
Pfropf schizophrenia, 121–2
phase, definition of, 128
phenmetrazine, 26
phenothiazines (*see also* individual agents)
  in acute schizophrenia, 149–50
  in hysteria, 167
  side-effects, 153–4
  structure, 27, (*Figs.* 5 and 6, *Table* 11) 146–9
'phonemic' paraphrenia, 85, 91–2, 97
physical illness
  precipitating schizophrenia, 37
  transient paranoid states after, 109
physique in schizophrenia, 33, 134
pimozide, 26, 29, 147, 151
positive formal thought disorder, 45
posture, disorders of (*see also* *Haltungsverharren*, psychological pillow and waxy flexibility), 68
  in motility psychosis, 117
  in periodic catatonia, 84
posture, perseveration of, 67
precipitating factors *see* environmental factors
predisposing factors *see* constitutional factors
prefrontal leucotomy, 154
pregnancy complications, 15–16
Present State Examination, 160–1
process
  definition of, 128
  psychic, Jaspers on, 107, (*Table* 9) 108
prochlorperazine, (*Table* 11) 148, (*Fig.* 7) 149
procyclidine, 153
prodromal symptoms of schizophrenia, 127–8
prognosis, 133–9
  of paranoid states, 109, 135
  precipitating stresses and, 37, 133, 135
  in schizo-affective psychoses, 112–3, 133
prolactin, 30
promazine (*Table* 11), 148
promethazine, 27
prompt speech, 69, 87
propranolol in schizophrenia, 29
prosectic speech, 69, 86
proskinetic catatonia, 86
pseudo-hallucinations, 55, 89, 116
pseudodementia, hysterical, 47, 167
pseudoneurotic schizophrenia, 120–1
pseudoschizophrenia, 118–9
  post-analytic, 121
psychiatric social worker, 143
psychiatrist in out-patient management, 143, 144
psychic activity, primary insufficiency of, 177–8
psychic process, Jaspers on 107, (*Table* 9) 108
psycho-analysis
  in pseudoneurotic schizophrenia, 121
  in pseudoschizophrenia, 119
psycho-analytical theories of schizophrenia, 185–90
psycho-physiological research, 14–17, 97
psychodrama, treatment by, 146
psychogenic psychosis, 111
psychogenic reactions (*see also* environmental factors)
  in obsessional states, 166
  paranoid, 106, 109
  in pseudoschizophrenia, 119
  in schizophreniform psychoses, 118
psychological pillow, 68, 72, 86
psychological stress *see* stress, psychological
psychological theories of schizophrenia, 172–99
psychopathic personality
  hysterical pseudodementia in, 167
  latent schizophrenia, 120
  psychogenic reactions, 118, 166
  sensitive, 106
  transient psychoses in, 167
psychopathic traits, pre-morbid, 36
psychopathology, search for causal connexions in, 172–4
psychopathy
  inadequate, 79
  incidence of, 32
psychotherapy, 145–6
  in hysteria, 167
puerperal affective psychoses, 37, 112
putamen, dopamine receptors in, 27

querulous attitudes, 88, 91
querulous paranoid personality, 105, 106–7

rage, senseless outbursts of, 63
rapport between patient and interviewer, 63–4, 165, 166
reaction, ambiguity of word (*see also* psychogenic reactions), 175
reactive inhibition, 45
reactive psychosis, 111
realism in philosophy, 194
reference *see* self-reference
reflex hallucinations, 60–1
regression in Freudian theory, 186–7
rehabilitation methods, 155–9
relatives *see* family
reserpine, 146
reticular system, activity of, 16
retinitis pigmentosa, 154
right handedness *see* left/right handedness
Rümke on pseudoschizophrenia, 118–9

saliva, dribbling of, 72
de Sanctis's dementia precocissima, 124–5
Sartre and existentialism, 193, 199
schizo-affective (marginal) psychoses (*see also* cycloid psychoses, oneiroid states and schizophreniform psychoses)
  age of onset, 127
  course of illness, (*Figs.* 3 and 4) 130–1
  definitions, 103, 111–5, 117–8
  outcome, 112–3, 132, 133
schizoid personality
  depersonalization in, 65
  pre-morbid, 31, 134
  in relation to schizophrenia, 178
schizophasia, 81, 83, 97
schizophrenia
  acute *see* acute schizophrenia
  aetiology (*see also* constitutional factors and environmental factors), 5–37
  age of onset *see* age of onset
  atypical, 81
  catatonic *see* catatonia
  childhood, 121, 124–6
  chronic *see* chronic schizophrenia
  classification, 78–97
  course, (*Figs.* 2–4) 128–32
  development of concepts of, (*Table* 1) 1–4, 98–101
  diagnosis *see* diagnosis
  grafted, 121–2
schizophrenia (*cont.*)
  hebephrenic *see* hebephrenia
  latent, 120
  non-systematic, 81, 82–4
  onset, mode of, 127–8, (*Fig.* 2) 129, 135, (*Table* 10) 136
  outcome, 132–3, 162
  paranoid *see* paranoid schizophrenia and paraphrenia
  Pfropf, 121–2
  prognosis *see* prognosis
  pseudo-, 118–9, 121
  pseudoneurotic, 120–1
  senile (*see also* late paraphrenia), 123–4
  simple, 78, 79, 101
  symptomatology (*see also* symptoms), 38–77
  systematic, 81, 84–97
  theories of, 172–99
  treatment (*see also* electroconvulsive therapy and neuroleptic drugs), 140–59
  typical, 81
schizophrenic-like psychoses, differential diagnosis of (*see also* brain disease, brain injury, drug intoxications, epilepsy and organic hallucinosis), 163–71
schizophreniform psychoses, 111, 118–9
Schnauzkrampf (snout spasm), 69, 72
Schneider('s)
  on aims of psychopathology, 175
  classification, 79–80
  on delusional perception, 50–1, 77
  first rank symptoms, 102–3, 161, 162–3, 180
  on schizophrenic speech, 41–2
  on thought disorders, 48, 80
Schröder's hallucinatory syndromes, 55–6
sedative neuroleptics, 147, 149, 150
self-mutilation, 123, 166
self-reference
  delusions of *see under* delusions
  hallucinosis, 55–6, 62
  ideas of *see under* ideas
  of thinking, 47
senile schizophrenia (*see also* late paraphrenia), 123–4
sensitive Beziehungswahn, 106
sexual behaviour in obsessional states, 166
sexual hallucinations, 60, 135
shallow hebephrenia, 88–9, 97

shift, definition of (*see also* acute schizophrenic shifts), 128
siblings of schizophrenics, risk to (*see also* twin studies), (*Table* 3) 7, 17–19
silly dementia, 79
silly hebephrenia, 87–8, 97
simplex syndrome, 1
skin conductance studies, 14–17
sleep disturbance in affective disorders, 113, 163
smell, hallucinations of, 61, 90
snout spasm (*Schnauzkrampf*), 69, 72
social decline in schizophrenia (*see also* anti-social behaviour), 36, 79
social factors
  in Laing's theory of schizophrenia, 200–1
  in prognosis, 135, 136
  in re-adjustment, 137–9, 155, 157
social isolation in causation, 36–7, 124
social therapy, 137, 143–4
sodium valproate (dipropylacetic sodium), 29
'soft signs', neurological, 23
speech, confusion of, in schizophasia, 83
speech, poverty of (*see also* muteness), 116
speech, pressure of, 70, 83, 116
speech, prompt, 69, 87
speech, prosectic, 69, 86
speech, retardation of, 70
speech abnormalities in parents of schizophrenics, 34
speech disorders (*see also* individual disorders)
  in childhood schizophrenia, 125, 126
  in cycloid psychoses, 116, 117
  in parakinesia, 67, 85
  in schizophrenia, 42–5, 69–70
speech-inactive catatonia, 87
speech-prompt catatonia, 87
spiroperidol, 27, 28
Spitzer's diagnostic criteria, 162
stereo-isomerism of neuroleptics, 27
stereotypies
  Freudian theory on, 187
  of movement, 66, 84, 86
  of posture, 68, 84
  prognosis and, 135
  in speech, 45, 70
  in writing, 70
stimulating neuroleptics, 147
stock words, 42–3, 44
Stransky's theory of schizophrenia, 176
stream of thought, disorders of, 47–8
stress, psychological (precipitating) (*see also* psychogenic reactions)
  in Meyer's theory of schizophrenia, 178–9
  in periodic catatonia, 122
  and prognosis, 113, 133, 135
  in schizo-affective disorders, 111, 113, 133
  in schizophrenia, 32–3, 37
stupor (*see also* akinesia), 71–2
  in epileptic twilight states, 169
  muteness during, 70
  in periodic catatonia, 122
submissive schizophrenia, 79
substantia nigra, 26
suicide
  in hysteria, 166–7
  in schizophrenia, 58, 62, 74, 154
superego, Freudian, 185
symbolism in thought disorder, 39, 45
symptoms
  accessory 90, 177
  Bleuler's primary and secondary, 176–7
  diagnostic, 102–3, 161–3
  fundamental, Bleuler's, 177
  'negative' in chronic schizophrenics, 25, 28–9
  non-understandable *see* Jasper's concept of understandability
  prodromal, 127–8
syntonic synchronous catatonia, (*Fig.* 1) 122
systematic schizophrenia, 81, 84–97

talking past the point (*Vorbeireden*), 45, 47, 69–70, 87
tardive dyskinesia, 154
taste, hallucinations of, 61, 90
technical neologisms, 44, 90
temporal lobe
  epilepsy and schizophrenia, 20–1, 22
  lesions and schizophrenia, 21–2, 169
tension insanity, 1
therapeutic community, 144
thiopropazate, (*Table* 11) 148, 154
thioridazine
  in acute schizophrenia, 150
  mode of action, 27, 28
  retinitis pigmentosa after, 154
  structure, (*Table* 11, *Fig.* 6) 148, (*Fig.* 7) 149

thioridazine (*cont.*)
  therapy versus psychotherapy, 145
thiothixene, (*Table* 11) 148
thioxanthenes (*see also* individual agents), 27, (*Fig.* 5) 146–7, (*Table* 11, *Fig.* 6) 148
thought, alienation of, 48
thought, fragmentation of, 80
thought, loss of control of, 48–9
thought, 'my-ness' of, 48, 49
thought, perseveration of theme of, 47, 67
thought, stream of, disorders of, 47–8
thought blocking, 47–8, 80
thought broadcasting, 48, 103, 182
thought content, disorders of *see* delusions
thought deprivation, 48
thought disorders, 38–55
  in diagnosis 78, 103, 162
  formal *see* formal thought disorder
  hallucinatory voices causing, 46, 57, 92
  interference causing, 46, 56–7
  in paranoid schizophrenia, 47, 89–90
  in paraphrenia, 91, 92, 93, 94, 95
  Schneider on, 48, 80
thought insertion, 48, 103
thought withdrawal, 80, 103
  syndrome, 80, (*Table* 7) 95–7
thymopsyche, Stransky's, 176
thyroid treatment in periodic catatonia, 123
time disorientation, 23, 75
token economies in rehabilitation, 158
toxic pseudoschizophrenia, 118, 119
toxic psychoses *see* drug intoxications
trema, Conrad's, 128, 180, 181, 183, (*Fig.* 8) 184
trifluoperazine 28, (*Table* 11) 148
trifluperidol, 147, (*Table* 11) 148
twin studies, (*Tables* 4 and 5) 7–10, 22, 32, 33
  in schizo-affective psychoses, 113
typical schizophrenia, 81

unconcentrated thinking, 91
understandability of symptoms *see* Jasper's concept of understandability
'understanding' (*verstehende*) psychology, 49, 102, 172–4

vagueness of thought, 39
ventricular enlargement, 23, 24–5
verbal derailment *see* derailment of speech
verbal hallucinations *see* hallucinatory voices
verbal hallucinosis, 55, 56
verbal paraphasia, 42–3, 44
verbigeration, 69, 70
verstehende (understanding) psychology, 49, 102, 172–4
violence, senseless, in catatonia, 71, 123
violent criminals, dissociation of affect in, 63, 167
Virchow's definition of disease, 174–5
visual hallucinations, 60
  in fantastic paraphrenia, 93
  in hypochondriacal paraphrenia, 90–1
  in Schröder's hallucinatory syndromes, 55, 56
voices, hallucinatory *see* hallucinatory voices
Vorbeireden (talking past the point) 45, 47, 69–70, 87

waxy flexibility, 68, 72
Weygandt's theory of schizophrenia, 176
white noise improving intellectual test scores, 46
will, ambivalence of, 64
woolliness of thought, 39
woolly thinking, 92
word monstrosity, 44
word storage, disorders of 42–3
word usage in schizophrenia (*see also* speech disorders), 42–5
work, return to, 138, 143
workshop in industrial therapy units, 156–7
writing, letter, 70–1

Zutt's concept of paranoid syndrome, 199–200